atlas of

sexually transmitted diseases

A Slide Atlas of Sexually Transmitted Diseases, based on the material in this book, is also available. The Slide Atlas is organized into 12 topic-based units, each consisting of superbly illustrated text, with 35mm color slides corresponding to the photographs in the text. In this unique format, all of the slides are labeled and numbered for easy reference. In addition, each unit is presented in a durable vinyl binder, and the complete collection comes in an attractive and sturdy presentation slip case.

Unit 1 *Syphilis*
Unit 2 *Genital Herpes*
Unit 3 *Chancroid*
Unit 4 *Granuloma Inguinale*
Unit 5 *Gonorrhea*
Unit 6 *Infections Caused by Chlamydia trachomatis*
Unit 7 *Genital Mycoplasmas*
Unit 8 *The Acquired Immunodeficiency Syndrome*
Unit 9 *Vaginitis*
Unit 10 *Genital Human Papillomavirus Infections*
Unit 11 *Infestations*
Unit 12 *Nonvenereal Genital Dermatoses*

For further information, please contact:
Gower Medical Publishing
101 Fifth Avenue
New York, NY 10003

atlas of

sexually transmitted diseases

Editors

Stephen A. Morse, MSPH, PhD

Director of Sexually Transmitted Diseases, Laboratory Program
Center for Infectious Diseases, Centers for Disease Control
Adjunct Professor of Microbiology and Immunology
Emory University School of Medicine
Atlanta, Georgia

Adele A. Moreland, MD

Assistant Professor of Medicine (Dermatology)
University of Saskatchewan College of Medicine
Saskatoon, Saskatchewan
Canada

Sumner E. Thompson, MD

Associate Professor of Medicine (Infectious Diseases)
Emory University School of Medicine
Director, Infectious Diseases Clinic
Grady Memorial Hospital
Atlanta, Georgia

Foreword by

King K. Holmes, MD, PhD

J.B. Lippincott Company, Philadelphia
Gower Medical Publishing, New York, London

Distributed in USA and Canada by:
J.B. Lippincott Company
East Washington Square
Philadelphia, PA 19105
USA

Distributed in UK and Continental Europe by:
Harper & Row Ltd.
Middlesex House
34-42 Cleveland Street
London W1P 5FB
UK

Distributed in Australia and New Zealand by:
Harper & Row (Australasia) Pty. Ltd.
P.O. Box 226
Artarmon, N.S.W. 2064
Australia

Distributed in Southeast Asia, Hong Kong, India and Pakistan by:
Harper & Row Publishers (Asia) Pty. Ltd.
37 Jalan Pemimpin 02-01
Singapore 2057

Distributed in Japan by:
Igaku-Shoin Ltd.
Tokyo International
P.O. Box 5063
Tokyo
Japan

Library of Congress Cataloging-in-Publication Data
Atlas of sexually transmitted diseases.
A slide atlas of sexually transmitted diseases, based on material in this book, is also available.
Includes bibliographies and index.
1. Sexually transmitted diseases–Atlases. I. Morse, Stephen A. II. Moreland, Adele A. III. Thompson, Sumner E, 1941- . [DNLM: 1. Sexually Transmitted Diseases–atlases. WC 17 A8815]
RC200.A85 1990   616.95'10754   88-81419
ISBN 0-397-44663-2

British Library Cataloguing-in-Publication Data
Atlas of sexually transmitted diseases.
1. Man. Sexually transmitted diseases
I. Morse, Stephen A. II. Moreland, Adele A.
III. Thompson, Sumner E.
616.95'1

ISBN 0-397-44663-2

Editors: **Meryl R.G. Muskin, Joy Noel Travalino**
Art Director: **Jill Feltham**
Illustrators: **Sue Ann Fung, Alan Landau**
Interior Design: **Romi Dorsey**
Layout and Cover Design: **Thomas Tedesco**

Printed in Singapore by: **Imago Productions (FE) PTE, Ltd.**

10 9 8 7 6 5 4 3 2 1

FOREWORD

It was a pleasure to review *Atlas of Sexually Transmitted Diseases* by Stephen Morse, Adele Moreland, and Sumner Thompson. Like the previous books produced by Gower Medical Publishing, this Atlas is beautifully illustrated. There are over 750 useful photographs and figures of high quality. The book is so clearly laid out, and the text so succinct, one can literally go through the book from cover to cover at a single sitting, and view the entire spectrum of characteristic and unusual manifestations of sexually transmitted diseases, including AIDS. I found pictures of a few things I had lectured about, but had not really seen well-photographed previously. The drawings and histopathological photographs that accompany many of the photographs of lesions quickly convey the pathophysiology and laboratory diagnosis of each disease. This book is a must for the dermatologist and the specialist in sexually transmitted diseases, and will be useful to other clinicians as well. Both the Atlas and the accompanying slides, which are also available, should be provided in all medical libraries. The editors and authors, most from the Centers for Disease Control and Emory University, as well as the publishers, should be congratulated for producing a very useful teaching aid for students and clinicians alike.

King K. Holmes, MD, PhD
Professor and Vice-Chairman
Department of Medicine
University of Washington
Chief of Medicine
Harborview Medicine Center
Seattle, Washington

PREFACE

Our concepts of sexually transmitted diseases have changed considerably over the past two decades. Gonorrhea and syphilis have been overshadowed by other sexually transmitted diseases that are actually more common. These diseases, such as chlamydial, papillomavirus, and herpetic infections, have been underdiagnosed because the laboratory methods required are often not routinely available to clinicians. The purpose of this book is to provide a comprehensive pictorial account of sexually transmitted diseases. It is intended to provide a source of visual material for those teaching the subject as well as up-to-date information on the epidemiology, clinical manifestations, laboratory tests, and treatment of these infections.

We have concentrated on the needs of clinicians but there is also much in this book which will be of interest to clinical microbiologists. Almost all broad-based medical specialists are seeing more patients with sexually transmitted diseases as public concern and medical information increase. We have tried to illustrate those diseases of global importance. What may seem an obscure infection to a reader in one part of the world may be of greater significance in another country or continent.

Sexually transmitted diseases now represent the largest proportion of ambulatory patient visits and a growing proportion of hospitalized patients seen by many infectious disease specialists. In addition, these diseases are also implicated in a wide spectrum of acute inflammatory conditions and in a variety of preneoplastic, neoplastic, and postinflammatory complications now seen by many dermatologists, urologists, obstetricians, and gynecologists. Pediatricians are more frequently seeing sexually transmitted infections in the neonate and infant, the abused older child, and the adolescent. Internists already familiar with the varied manifestations of sexually transmitted diseases must now cope with the impact of AIDS.

The rapid application of new technology to the diagnosis of sexually transmitted diseases has led to an increasing number of laboratory tests that require critical evaluation by clinicians, public health specialists, and clinical microbiologists. The global perspective and expertise of the contributors in both clinical and laboratory diagnosis has allowed us to provide a more comprehensive coverage of this subject than other atlases available today. Finally, the Slide Atlas collection offers an extensive library of both the clinical and laboratory aspects of the most common sexually transmitted diseases in the world. We hope that you will enjoy using this Atlas as much as we have enjoyed creating it.

Stephen A. Morse
Adele A. Moreland
Sumner E. Thompson

ACKNOWLEDGMENTS

We wish to thank the clinical, laboratory, and secretarial staff in each of our institutions and clinics, and the patients who have allowed themselves to be photographed.

CONTENTS

CONTRIBUTORS

Robert J. Arko, DVM
Assistant Chief, Bacteriology Research Branch
Sexually Transmitted Diseases Laboratory Program
Center for Infectious Diseases
Centers for Disease Control
Atlanta, Georgia

Robert C. Barnes, MD
Chief, Chlamydia Laboratory
Sexually Transmitted Diseases Laboratory Program
Center for Infectious Diseases
Centers for Disease Control
Atlanta, Georgia

Henry M. Blumberg, MD
Fellow in Infectious Diseases
Emory University School of Medicine
Atlanta, Georgia

John Bryan, MD
Associate Professor
Department of Pathology and Laboratory Medicine
Emory University School of Medicine
Director, Division of Laboratory Medicine
Emory University Hospital
Atlanta, Georgia

Gail H. Cassell, MS, PhD
Professor and Chairman
Department of Microbiology
University of Alabama at Birmingham
Birmingham, Alabama

Wallis E. DeWitt, MSPH, MS
Division of Bacterial Diseases
Center for Infectious Diseases
Centers for Disease Control
Atlanta, Georgia

Mark H. DuPuis, MD
Department of Pathology
Crawford Long Hospital of Emory University
Atlanta, Georgia

Douglas Kellogg, PhD
Sexually Transmitted Diseases Laboratory Program
Center for Infectious Diseases
Centers for Disease Control
Atlanta, Georgia
(retired)

Joan S. Knapp, PhD
Chief, Bacteriology Research Branch
Sexually Transmitted Diseases Laboratory Program
Center for Infectious Diseases
Centers for Disease Control
Atlanta, Georgia

Phyllis E. Kozarsky, MD
Assistant Professor of Medicine (Infectious Diseases)
Emory Unversity School of Medicine
Atlanta, Georgia

Sandra A. Larsen, PhD
Chief, Treponema Research Branch
Sexually Transmitted Diseases Laboratory Program
Center for Infectious Diseases
Centers for Disease Control
Atlanta, Georgia

Joel S. Lewis
Research Microbiologist
Sexually Transmitted Disease Laboratory Program
Center for Infectious Diseases
Centers for Disease Control
Atlanta, Georgia

John G. Long, MD
Medical Director, STD Clinic
DeKalb County Board of Health
Decatur, Georgia

Bhagirath Majmudar, MD
Professor of Pathology and Associate Professor of
Gynecology and Obstetrics
Emory University School of Medicine
Atlanta, Georgia

Marilynne McKay, MD
Associate Professor of Dermatology and Gynecology
Emory University School of Medicine
Chief, Dermatology Section
Grady Memorial Hospital
Atlanta, Georgia

Adele A. Moreland, MD
Assistant Professor of Medicine (Dermatology)
University of Saskatchewan College of Medicine
Saskatoon, Saskatchewan
Canada

Stephen A. Morse, MSPH, PhD
Director of Sexually Transmitted Diseases Laboratory
Program
Center for Infectious Diseases
Centers for Disease Control
Adjunct Professor of Microbiology and Immunology
Emory University School of Medicine
Atlanta, Georgia

Samuel K. Sarafian, PhD
Research Microbiologist
Sexually Transmitted Diseases Laboratory Program
Center for Infectious Diseases
Centers for Disease Control
Atlanta, Georgia

William O. Schalla, MS
Research Microbiologist
Sexually Transmitted Diseases Laboratory Program
Center for Infectious Diseases
Centers for Disease Control
Atlanta, Georgia

George P. Schmid, MD
Division of Sexually Transmitted Diseases
Center for Prevention Services
Centers for Disease Control
Clinical Associate Professor of Medicine and
Microbiology
Morehouse School of Medicine
Atlanta, Georgia

Steve D. Shafran, MD
Assistant Professor
Division of Infectious Diseases
Department of Medicine
University of Alberta
Edmonton, Alberta
Canada

Kay Stone, MD
Clinical Research Investigator
Division of Sexually Transmitted Diseases
Center for Prevention Services
Centers for Disease Control
Atlanta, Georgia

David Taylor-Robinson, MD
Director of Sexually Transmitted Diseases Unit
Medical Research Council
Harrow, Middlesex
England

Sumner E. Thompson, MD
Associate Professor of Medicine (Infectious Diseases)
Emory University School of Medicine
Director, Infectious Diseases Clinic
Grady Memorial Hospital
Atlanta, Georgia

Ken B. Waites, MD
Department of Microbiology and Pathology
University of Alabama at Birmingham
Birmingham, Alabama

Jonathan M. Zenilman, MD
Medical Epidemiologist
Division of Sexually Transmitted Diseases
Center for Prevention Services
Centers for Disease Control
Atlanta, Georgia

Syphilis 1

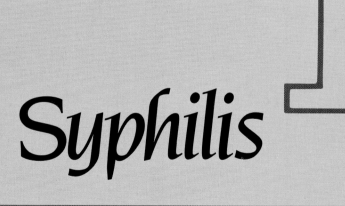

S.E. THOMPSON, S.A. LARSEN, A.A. MORELAND

Introduction

Syphilis is a chronic systemic infectious disease that is transmitted during sexual intercourse or other intimate contact; it also can be transmitted from a pregnant woman to her fetus in utero or by contact of the infant with a maternal lesion during birth. The causative agent of syphilis is *Treponema pallidum* subspecies *pallidum*, a spirochete (Fig. 1.1). This agent has never been cultured successfully on artificial media, and does not take up the Gram stain. Three other treponemes (subspecies *pertenue*, subspecies *endemicum*, and *T. carateum*) are also pathogenic for humans (Fig. 1.2). Infection with these organisms will cause the serologic tests for syphilis to be positive, although the infections are not sexually transmitted.

Epidemiology

In the United States, primary and secondary (infectious) syphilis rates were at a high in 1947, declined sharply over the following 10 years, and have gradually increased again over each suc-ceeding decade to the present (Fig. 1.3). Many factors have undoubtedly contributed to this increase, including earlier age of first intercourse and larger numbers of lifetime partners, high prevalence in homosexual men (although there is evidence that rates among homosexual men are declining since the AIDS epidemic), decreasing federal dollars for control programs, and diversion of control efforts to other STD problems.

Individuals are infectious for their sex partners during the primary and secondary stages, when skin lesions are present. Women are most likely to transmit the infection to their infants during secondary disease when they are spirochetemic, but infection of the fetus during early latency is not impossible.

Clinical Manifestations

Untreated, syphilis is a chronic disease that is spread throughout the body hematogenously and which can produce manifestations in virtually every organ system (Fig. 1.4). The infec-

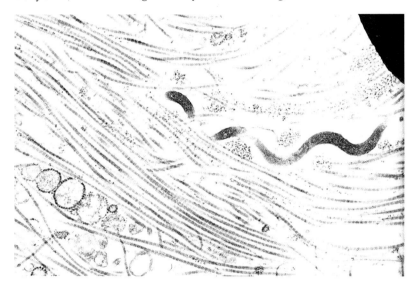

Figure 1.1 Transmission electron micrograph of *Treponema pallidum* subspecies *pallidum* in tissue.

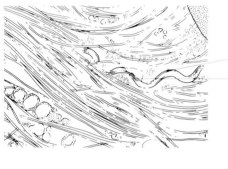

Outer "membrane"

Axial filaments (endoflagella)

Figure 1.2 Pathogenic treponemes of humans.

PATHOGENIC TREPONEMES OF HUMANS				
	SYPHILIS	**YAWS**	**BEJEL**	**PINTA**
ORGANISM	*T. pallidum* subspecies *pallidum*	*T. pallidum* subspecies *pertenue*	*T. pallidum* subspecies *endemicum*	*T. carateum*
TRANSMISSION	Sexual contact	Skin contact	Skin contact, oral?	Skin contact
LESION TYPE				
PRIMARY	Chancre	Crusted papules	Oral mucosal lesions	Crusted papules and plaques
SECONDARY	Macular or papulosquamous	Papillomatous and scarring	Mucous patches and condylomata lata	Scaly plaques
LATE	Gummata and endarteritis	Gummata of bone and skin	Gummata of cartilage, bone, and skin	Dyschromia

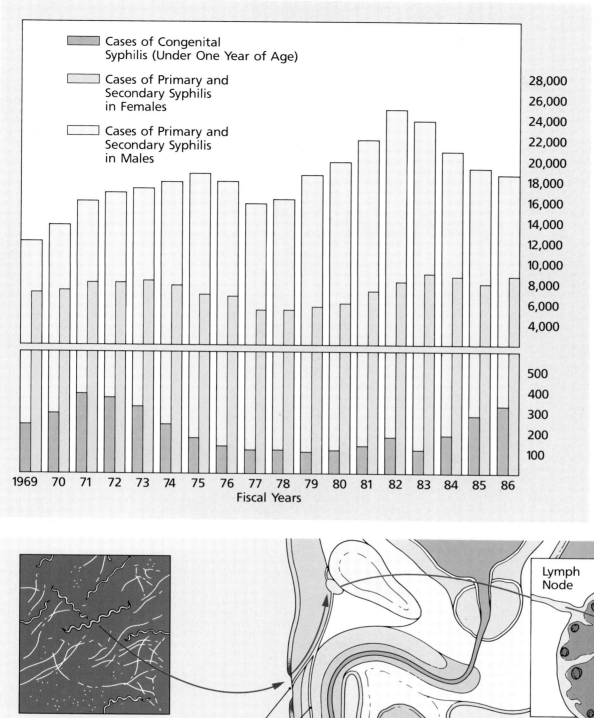

Figure 1.3 Rates of primary and secondary syphilis in men and women compared with the rates of congenital syphilis. Numbers of cases of congenital syphilis are a highly sensitive indicator of the amount of infectious syphilis in a population and the need for control activities.

Legend:
- Cases of Congenital Syphilis (Under One Year of Age)
- Cases of Primary and Secondary Syphilis in Females
- Cases of Primary and Secondary Syphilis in Males

Fiscal Years

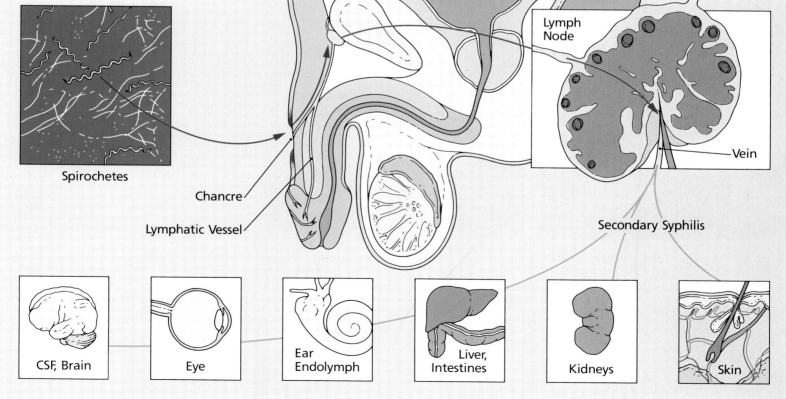

Figure 1.4 Schematic diagram to show how spirochetes enter regional lymph nodes from a skin chancre, and then enter the bloodstream. Organ systems that are involved are shown: CSF, brain, eye, ear endolymph, liver, intestines, kidneys, skin.

tious, clinically manifest stages of the disease—primary and secondary syphilis—are transient events. During latency, by definition, there are no clinical signs or symptoms of infection, despite the fact that T. *pallidum* can be demonstrated in some tissues. Serology is the only available method for accurate diagnosis during this stage of the disease. The clinical course and serologic changes of untreated syphilis are summarized in Figures 1.5 and 1.6.

PRIMARY SYPHILIS

The first clinical manifestation of syphilis, the chancre, develops an average of 3 weeks after infection (10 to 30 days). The chancre appears at the site where treponemal invasion of the dermis first occurred, usually on or near the genitals. However, it may occur on any skin or mucous membrane. Chancres are usually single lesions and are painless (Fig. 1.7) unless superinfected; hence, they may be missed by the patient if they occur on an

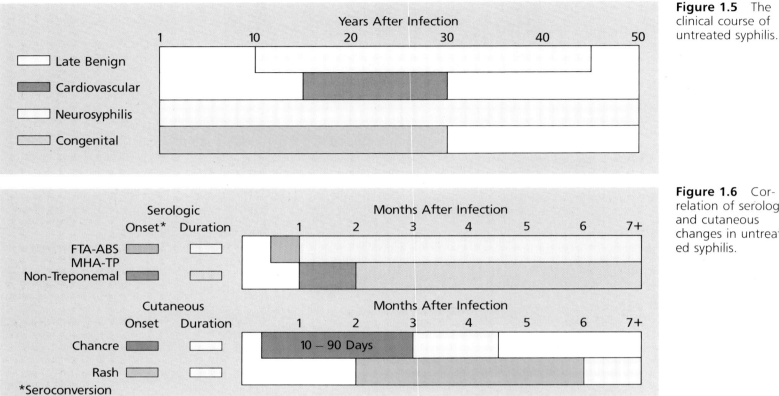

Figure 1.5 The clinical course of untreated syphilis.

Figure 1.6 Correlation of serologic and cutaneous changes in untreated syphilis.

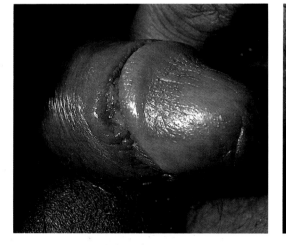

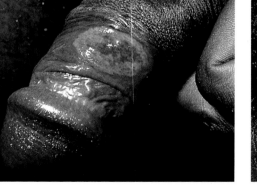

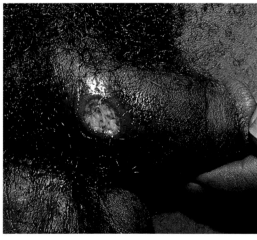

Figure 1.7 Typical syphilitic chancre of the coronal sulcus. This early asymptomatic chancre in the coronal sulcus shows characteristic induration and a "clean" base. Dark-field examination will almost always be positive if no medication has been given or applied topically.

Figure 1.8 Large, indurated primary chancre of the penile shaft. This penile chancre has been present for several weeks, but it is still painless and large. The induration produces a cartilaginous quality.

Figure 1.9 Atypical penile chancre. This chancre appears atypical because it has become secondarily infected with bacteria. Dark-field examination may be difficult because of the presence of nonpathogenic treponemes.

inaccessible region such as the cervix, pharynx, or rectum. Nontender regional adenopathy also is common. If untreated, the chancre will persist for 2 to 6 weeks and heal without scarring. Occasionally a relapsing chancre will occur at the same site. Motile spirochetes should be demonstrable in untreated chancres during most stages of their evolution. They may be difficult to demonstrate in late, healing lesions, and usually are absent if the patient has applied local medications or taken antibiotics.

The typical chancre is indurated, has a clean base, and rolled edges (Fig. 1.8). Secondary infection with bacteria or even herpesviruses occasionally occurs, and may cause the ulcer to appear somewhat atypical (Fig. 1.9). The major confusion would be with chancroid, granuloma inguinale, or occasionally, herpes. The labia and fourchette are the most typical areas for chancres to occur in women (Fig. 1.10). Perianal, anal or rectal chancres occur primarily in homosexual men, and in women who have a history of rectal intercourse (Fig. 1.11). While single lesions are seen most commonly, multiple primary chancres are not uncommon (Fig. 1.12). Healing lesions may present problems in diagnosis, particularly in their later stages when they are dark-field negative, and adenopathy may not be prominent (Fig. 1.13). Acquired syphilis can occur in infants and children (Fig. 1.14). Syphilitic chancres occasionally may occur in extragenital sites, such as the fingers (Fig. 1.15) or oral cavity (Fig.

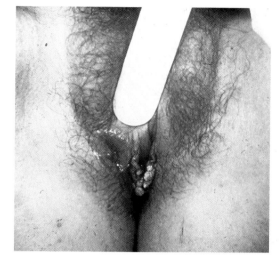

Figure 1.10 Syphilitic chancre of the labia majora. The lower labia and fourchette are the most common locations of primary chancres in women. This lesion was completely asymptomatic.

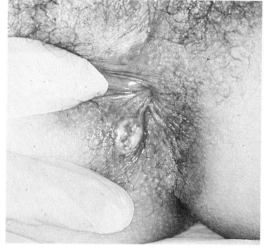

Figure 1.11 Perianal syphilitic chancre. A well-developed anal chancre demonstrating the buttonlike morphology typical of syphilis; however, this same appearance can be seen in granuloma inguinale and in chancroid.

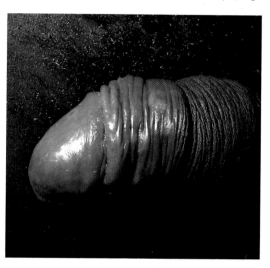

Figure 1.12 Multiple chancres of primary syphilis. Multiple primary chancres are not uncommon in primary syphilis. They occur most frequently on the penis and vulva.

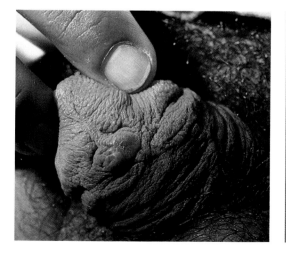

Figure 1.13 Healing chancre. Primary chancres heal spontaneously, as seen here in this almost resolved penile chancre.

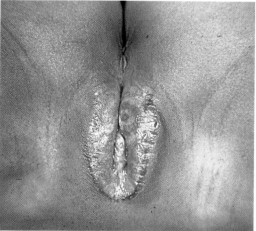

Figure 1.14 Vulvar chancre in a child. A painless ulcer found on the genitals of a child should always raise the possibility of syphilis, but also may be acquired through nonsexual means.

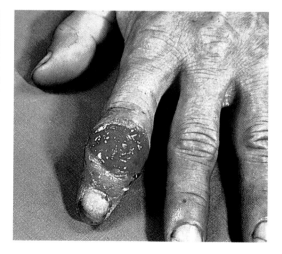

Figure 1.15 Digital syphilitic chancre. Occupational exposure of health care workers may be the cause of chancres on the hands.

1.16). Clinical findings of primary syphilis are summarized in Figure 1.17.

SECONDARY SYPHILIS

Onset of the secondary stage of disease ranges from 6 weeks to 6 months after infection in the untreated patient. The primary chancre may still be present when clinically apparent secondary lesions occur. In this phase of the disease, spirochetes enter the bloodstream from their dermal and lymph node foci and are distributed to most tissues and organs (see Fig. 1.4). After a suitable multiplication period, generalized but nonspecific symptoms occur: fever, malaise, headache, sore throat, arthral-gias and anorexia. Generalized adenopathy occurs in more than half of patients. Hepatomegaly and occasionally splenomegaly also may occur. There may be leukocytosis, anemia, and elevation of the erythrocyte sedimentation rate. Syphilitic hepatitis is characterized by mild derangement of liver enzymes and a markedly elevated alkaline phosphatase. An acute, "viral type" of meningitis may complicate the picture.

A rash, which is sometimes called a syphilid, occurs in about 75% of patients and is extremely variable in appearance. It may be localized or generalized. Symmetrical discrete erythematous, brown or hyperpigmented macules are the earliest generalized syphilid (Fig. 1.18). This eruption commonly begins on the trunk.

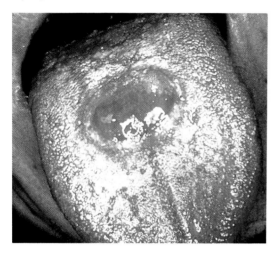

Figure 1.16 Chancre of the tongue. Dark-field examination of mouth lesions may not be reliable due to the presence of saprophytic spirochetes. However, the direct FA test is useful in this situation.

SYNOPSIS OF CLINICAL FINDINGS OF PRIMARY SYPHILIS

I. **ULCER**

   Single genital ulcer most commonly

   Diameter of lesion usually > ½ cm

   Nonpainful

   Indurated, rolled edges

   Clean lesion base

   Dark-field (+) for motile spirochetes

II. **ADENOPATHY**

   Inguinal, ipsilateral to ulcer

   Nontender

   Nonfluctuant

III. **CONSTITUTIONAL SYMPTOMS**

   None

Figure 1.17 Synopsis of clinical findings of primary syphilis.

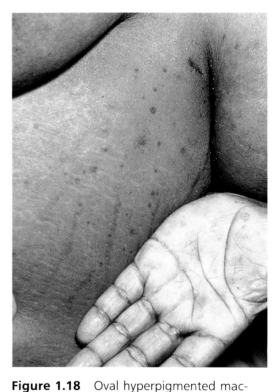

Figure 1.18 Oval hyperpigmented macules of the trunk and extremities in early secondary syphilis. The eruption was generalized, but not readily visible, and therefore unnoticed by the patient.

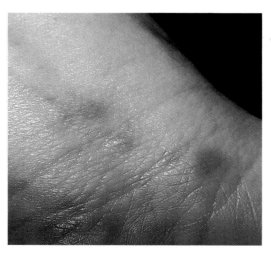

Figure 1.19 Early papular syphilis. The lack of scale suggests that this is an early form of papular syphilis. Erythema and firmness of the papules on palpation are characteristic.

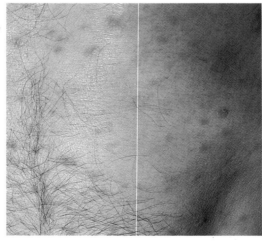

Figure 1.20 Macular and papulosquamous forms of syphilis coexisting in syphilis of 1 month's duration. This eruption was completely asymptomatic.

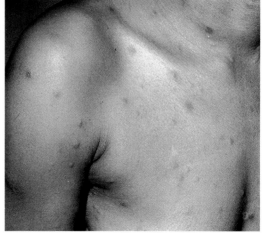

Figure 1.21 Papular secondary syphilis. The generalized erythematous papules are quite obvious to both patient and physician.

The macules may enlarge or become annular; scaling and pruritus are absent. As the eruption progresses, some of the macules may become thickened and papular (Fig. 1.19), and thus macular syphilids may coexist with the papular forms (Fig. 1.20). Papular syphilids (Fig. 1.21) appear to be more common than macular eruptions, perhaps because they are easier to see. If the disease remains untreated for several weeks, the papules may develop a dry, thin collarette of scale, which peels off easily (Fig. 1.22).

Frequent involvement of the palms and soles in macular and papular syphilids may help to distinguish them from other dermatoses (see Fig. 1.23A and the following section on Differential Diagnosis). Many varieties of papular syphilids have been described, and include, among others, the papulosquamous (Fig. 1.23B), annular (Fig. 1.23C), lenticular (Fig. 1.23D), syphilis cornee, in which the lesions resemble clavi (see Figs. 1.22B and 1.23A), psoriasiform (Fig. 1.23E), and framboesiform (Fig. 1.23F) types.

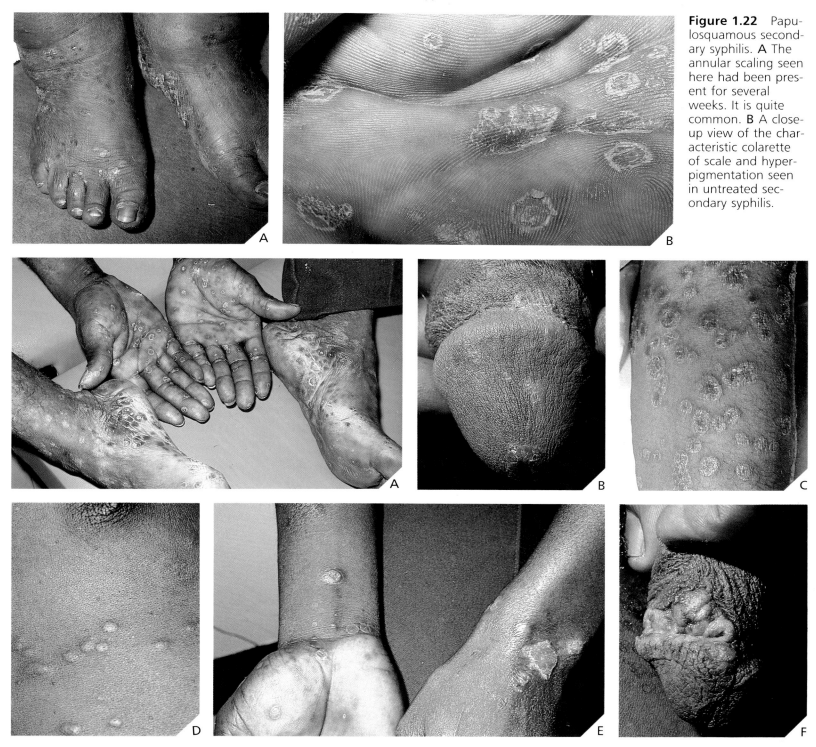

Figure 1.22 Papulosquamous secondary syphilis. **A** The annular scaling seen here had been present for several weeks. It is quite common. **B** A close-up view of the characteristic colarette of scale and hyperpigmentation seen in untreated secondary syphilis.

Figure 1.23 Varieties of papular syphilids. **A** Palmar and plantar papulosquamous secondary syphilis. **B** Papulosquamous syphilids are typically flat papules, which are red, indurated, and slightly scaly. Lesions may be limited to the genital region. **C** Annular syphilids are florid annular scaly plaques, some with a targetoid hyperpigmented center. **D** Smooth firm pea-sized brown papules characterize the lenticular form of secondary syphilis. **E** Large and small psoriasiform plaques with thick scale and an irregular shape in late secondary syphilis. **F** Verrucous and eroded (framboesiform) lesions of late secondary syphilis in the coronal sulcus.

Moist hypertrophic papular lesions, *condylomata lata*, occur in intertriginous areas, such as the genitals (Fig. 1.24) and gluteal folds (Fig. 1.25). Occasionally they may become hyperplastic or verrucous, and as such may very closely resemble condylomata acuminata (Fig. 1.26). These lesions also may be seen in extragenital areas (Fig. 1.27). Condylomata lata are usually covered with a grayish exudate containing numerous spirochetes, making them much more infectious than other secondary syphilids. Another variant of papular syphilis are the so-called "split papules" found in the postauricular area (Fig. 1.28) or in the oral commissures. Nonspecific superficial erosions of the oral or genital mucous membranes, called mucous

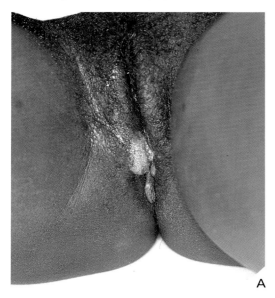
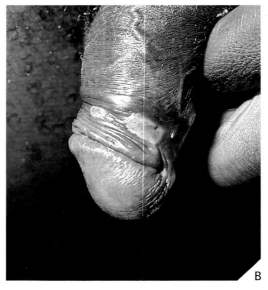
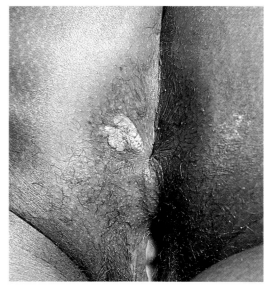

A

B

Figure 1.24   Condylomata lata. A Typical condylomata lata on the labia and perineum are moist gray plaques and papules.

B Flat, broad-based dark-field positive plaques are seen in the folds of the foreskin.

Figure 1.25   Condylomata lata. Perianal condylomata detected in a patient who sought help because of a palmar rash.

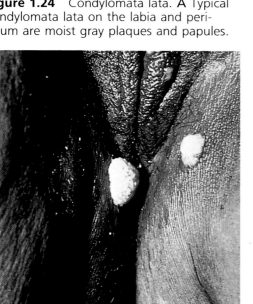
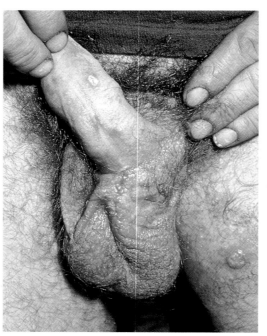
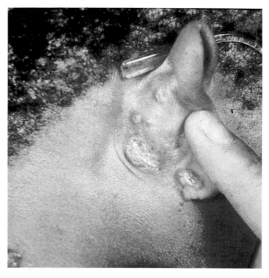

Figure 1.26   Condylomata lata. Unusually verrucous condylomata lata resembling condylomata acuminata in a patient who presented with a generalized macular eruption.

Figure 1.27   Broad-based moist, dark-field positive condylomata on the thigh. Note the other erosive lesions of secondary syphilis on the penile shaft.

Figure 1.28   Split papules, seen here on the posterior auricular fold, may also be present at the angles of the mouth.

patches, are another common manifestation of secondary syphilis. These round or oval lesions appear as grayish or denuded patches on the buccal or labial mucosa (Fig. 1.29A), on the tongue (Figs. 1.29B and C) or on the palate or tonsils.

Alopecia may occur during secondary syphilis as a patchy thinning (Fig. 1.30A) or as a more diffuse loss of hair (Fig. 1.30B).

Eyebrows, beard hair, or any other hairy body areas may be involved. The alopecia regrows in both treated and untreated patients.

The signs and symptoms of secondary syphilis usually last only a few weeks. Relapses may occur in the untreated patient, usually within the first year or two after infection, but are rare events after adequate penicillin therapy.

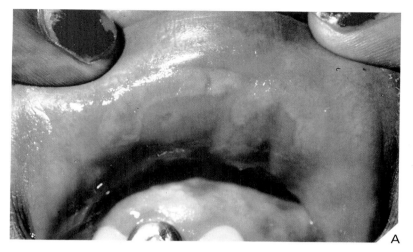

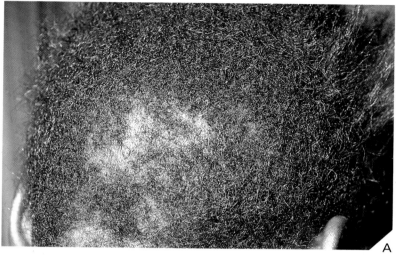

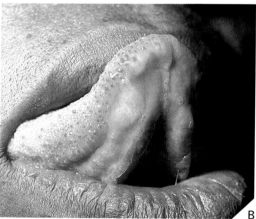

Figure 1.29 Mucous patches in secondary syphilis. **A** Serpiginous mucous patches on the labial mucosa and tongue were the presenting sign of syphilis in this patient. **B** and **C** Mucous patches are seen on the tongue.

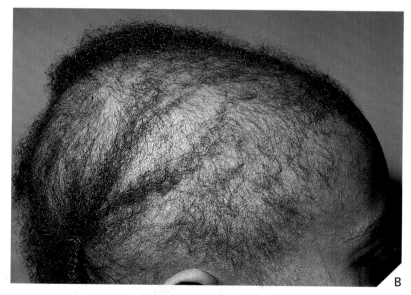

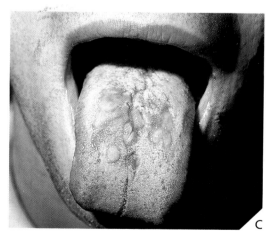

Figure 1.30 Alopecia in secondary syphilis. **A** The patchy or "moth-eaten" alopecia may not be noticed by the patient, but can be found by the alert examiner. **B** Occasionally a more diffuse alopecia accompanies secondary syphilis.

Differential Diagnosis

The eruptions of secondary syphilis are almost infinitely varied and mimic many common dermatoses. In this section, examples of common presentations of secondary syphilis are compared to the nonsyphilitic dermatoses that resemble them.

The brown-red hyperpigmentation and fine scale seen in cases of secondary syphilis (Fig. 1.31A) may closely resemble the characteristically oval, slightly scaly, brown-red eruptions of pityriasis rosea (Fig. 1.31B). However, generalized adenopathy is absent and serologic tests for syphilis are negative in pityriasis rosea.

The appearance of hyperpigmented oval plaques of secondary syphilis on the upper back (Fig. 1.32A) resembles a common form of hyperpigmented tinea versicolor. Tinea versicolor is usually found in this location and has adherent KOH-positive scales, which may not be readily visible (Fig. 1.32B).

The generalized macular and papular eruptions of syphilis (Fig. 1.33A) may at first glance resemble generalized scabies (Fig. 1.33B). However, the pruritus in scabies is pronounced, and the lesions frequently are excoriated. Lack of these signs and symptoms should suggest syphilis in eruptions of this sort.

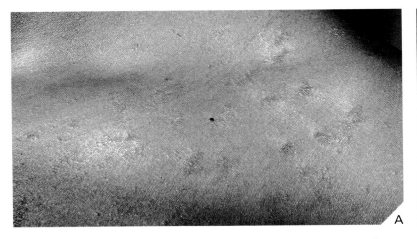

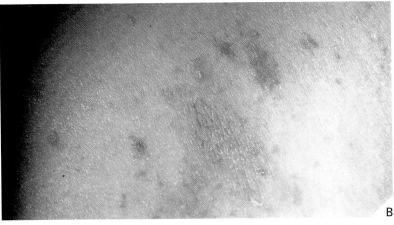

Figure 1.31 Differential diagnosis in secondary syphilis. **A** Early papulosquamous form of syphilis. **B** Pityriasis rosea.

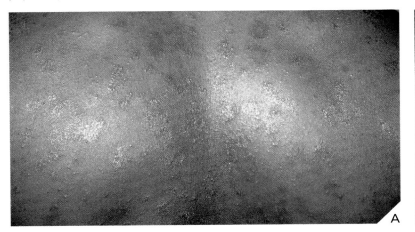

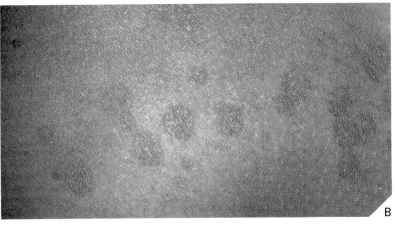

Figure 1.32 Differential diagnosis in secondary syphilis. **A** Hyperpigmented oval macules of secondary syphilis. **B** Tinea versicolor.

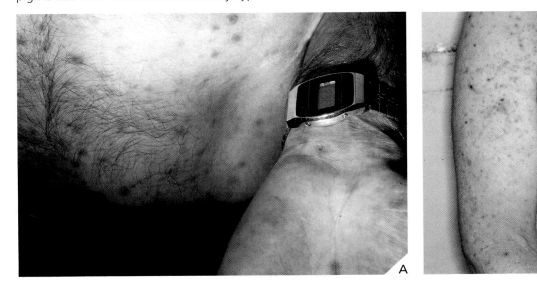

Figure 1.33 Differential diagnosis in secondary syphilis. **A** Generalized papular form of secondary syphilis. **B** Generalized scabies.

Occasionally the scattered papulosquamous eruptions of secondary syphilis (Fig. 1.34A) resemble the guttate variety of psoriasis (Fig. 1.34B). However, psoriatic scaling is frequently quite thick and adherent. In addition, involvement of the scalp and extensor surfaces in psoriasis may offer further clues to the correct diagnosis. Adenopathy and alopecia, common in syphilis, generally are absent in psoriasis. Involvement of the genitals may occur in either disorder (see Chapter 12).

Secondary syphilis may be the cause of fairly large erythematous plaques on the penis, which resemble fixed drug eruptions (Fig. 1.35A). The latter has a predilection for the genitals and hands. The erythematous plaques of early fixed drug erup-

tions (Fig. 1.35B), which later become scaly and hyperpigmented, can closely resemble the eruptions of secondary syphilis. Tetracycline, a commonly prescribed antibiotic in the STD clinic, is one of the drugs most frequently implicated as a causative agent of fixed drug eruptions (see Chapter 12).

Annular palmar or plantar macules or plaques in some cases of syphilis (Fig. 1.36A) may resemble the characteristic "target" or "iris" lesions of erythema multiforme (Fig. 1.36B). However, erythema multiforme usually is not scaly and may even become bullous. Bullae do not occur in acquired secondary syphilis. Serologic tests for syphilis help differentiate the two, in most cases.

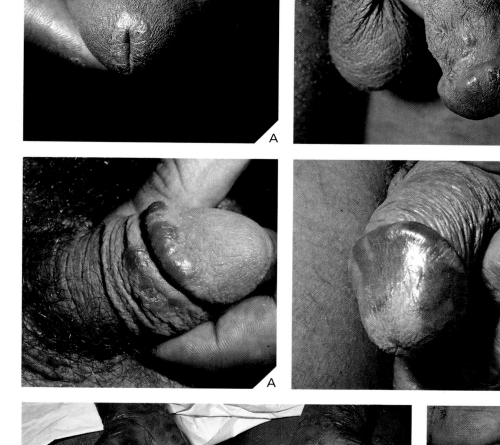

Figure 1.34 Differential diagnosis in secondary syphilis. **A** Papulosquamous secondary syphilis of the penis. **B** Psoriasis involving the genitals.

Figure 1.35 Differential diagnosis in secondary syphilis. **A** Erythematous penile plaques of secondary syphilis. **B** Fixed drug eruption.

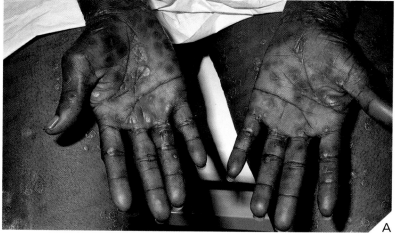

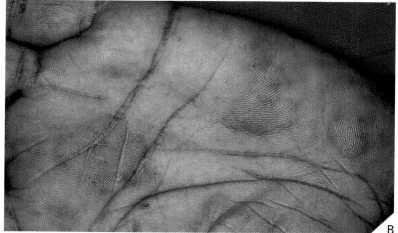

Figure 1.36 Differential diagnosis in secondary syphilis. **A** Targetoid annular papulosquamous secondary syphilis of the palms.

B Erythema multiforme on the palm.

Plantar or palmar eruptions of syphilis that have developed very little scale (Fig. 1.37A) may resemble entities such as pityriasis lichenoides chronica (Fig. 1.37B), a chronic, mildly scaly skin disorder, or even viral exanthems. If serologic testing is not definitive, biopsies may be necessary.

Annular syphilids with central hyperpigmentation on sun-exposed skin (Fig. 1.38A) resemble discoid lupus erythematosus (Fig. 1.38B). False-positive syphilis serologies in lupus may confuse the picture. However, rapid plasma reagin titers are generally of high titer in secondary syphilis (1:16 or greater) and low in lupus (1:8 or less).

LATENT SYPHILIS

Latent syphilis is the period of quiescence after completion of the secondary stage of disease, during which there are no clinical manifestations. An exposure history and a positive serologic test for syphilis is the only way of establishing the diagnosis. Not infrequently, no history of syphilis can be obtained, and, in such a case, a true-positive serology must be distinguished from a false-positive one (see laboratory section on interpretation of test results).

Latency is divided into early and late phases. Early latency encompasses the first year after secondary infection. It is during this period that relapses of secondary disease are most apt to occur in the untreated patient. Infection of a partner occasionally may occur during early latency, and the pregnant woman is at risk of transmitting the disease to her fetus. The patient in late latency (more than 1 year into the latent period) has a decreasing risk of transmission to partner or fetus as latency progresses.

LATE SYPHILIS

The late manifestations of syphilis fall into three main types: cardiovascular, gummatous, and meningovascular (neural). In general, these events occur decades after infection, but some of the meningeal and cerebrovascular forms can occur within a year after initial infection. The common underlying pathophysiologic event appears to be an endarteritis and periarteritis of small and medium-sized vessels (Fig. 1.39).

Cardiovascular Syphilis

This form of late syphilis is uncommon today, but still needs to be considered in the evaluation of aortic aneurysm and aortic valvular disease (Fig. 1.40). It has been estimated to occur in approximately 10% of cases of untreated syphilis, and may affect black patients more commonly than white ones.

The major pathologic changes in cardiovascular syphilis are dilatation of the aortic ring with incompetence of the valve, left ventricular hypertrophy, aortic root dilatation with aneurysm formation, and stenosis of the coronary artery ostia (Fig. 1.41).

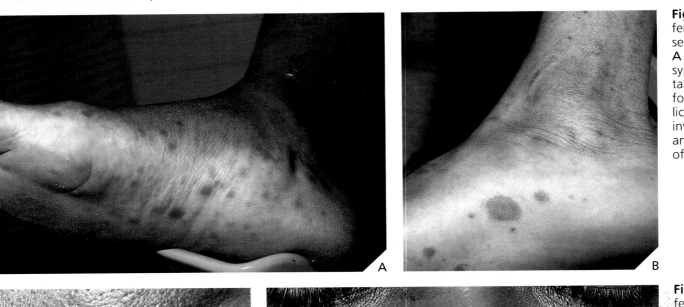

A B

Figure 1.37 Differential diagnosis in secondary syphilis. **A** Papular secondary syphilis of the plantar surface of the foot. **B** Pityriasis lichenoides chronica involving the leg and plantar aspect of the foot.

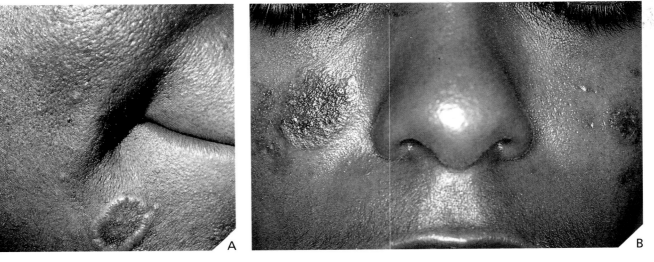

A B

Figure 1.38 Differential diagnosis in secondary syphilis. **A** Discoid secondary syphilis of the face. **B** Discoid lupus erythematosus.

Late Benign Syphilis

The gummatous lesion probably represents a severe inflammatory response to treponemal antigens, but the exact mechanism of pathogenesis is not known. Microscopically, the active lesions are granulomas. Older lesions show extensive fibrosis and the lesions heal with deep scarring and fibrosis. Treponemes are difficult to detect in gummata.

Virtually any organ system may be affected by this inflammatory process, but the skin and bones are affected most commonly. Skin lesions may be nodular, noduloulcerative, or gummatous. The nodules appear in groups, and usually are asymmetrical in distribution. They are chronic, painless and slowly progressive, and are found most often on the face, trunk, and extremities. Over time the nodules may break down into

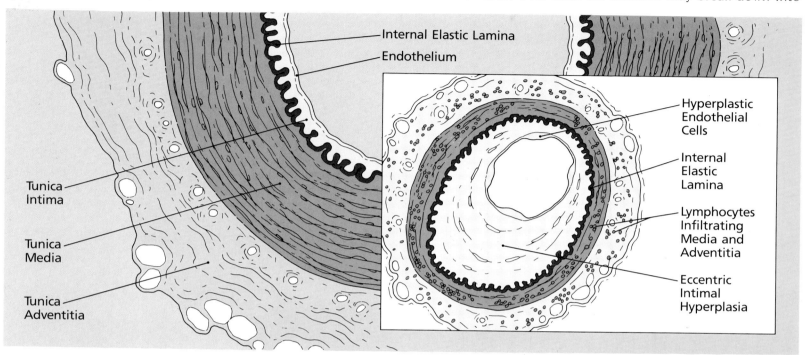

Figure 1.39   The primary pathologic lesions of neurosyphilis. Schematic diagram showing the endarteritis of cerebral blood vessels, with lymphocytic infiltration and obliteration of the vessel lumen.

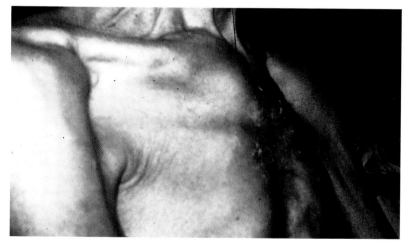

Figure 1.40   Cardiovascular syphilis. Syphilitic aortic aneurysm with erosion through the chest wall.

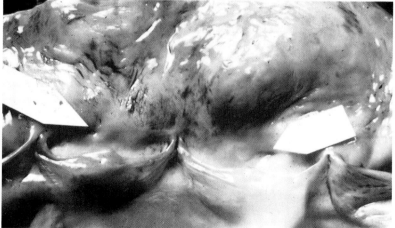

Figure 1.41   Cardiovascular syphilis. Narrowing of the coronary ostia in syphilitic aortitis.

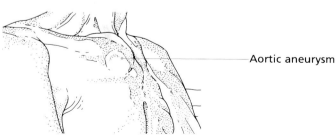

Aortic aneurysm

ulcers (Fig. 1.42), which heal slowly centrally, leaving a characteristic arciform scar. Gummata of the skin are usually deep in the dermis and are solitary. They evolve into a granulomatous ulcer, with areas of spontaneous healing and scar formation. The most common lesion in bone is an osteitis, usually with periosteal changes. Radiographically it may be indistinguishable from bacterial osteomyelitis. Characteristic areas of involvement are the hard palate, leading to perforation (Fig. 1.43), and the nasal bones and nasal septum. Any mucous membrane surface also may be affected (Fig. 1.44). The digestive system also may be involved, especially the stomach, liver, and esophagus. These lesions usually are initially misdiagnosed as carcinomas.

Neurosyphilis

T. pallidum invades meninges and neural tissue during the secondary stage of the disease. Spirochetes may be seen in CSF, and in ocular and middle ear fluid. There are basically two types of histopathologic lesions found in CNS syphilis:

1. A chronic, low-grade meningitis with lymphocytic infiltration of meninges
2. An endarteritis of small vessels of the brain and spinal cord

Most often, the two lesion types coexist, accounting for the complex constellation of signs and symptoms in the various forms of neurosyphilis. With suitable stains, spirochetes may be demonstrated in neural tissue of patients with neurosyphilis (Fig. 1.45). A general classification of neurosyphilis is presented in Figure 1.46.

CONGENITAL SYPHILIS

Infection of the fetus in utero occurs through hematogenous routes and results in clinical manifestations that may resemble acquired secondary syphilis eruptions. Other forms of congenital syphilis may affect development of bones, teeth, hearing or other organ systems, and will result in characteristic clinical presentations.

By definition, early congenital syphilis becomes manifest before 2 years of age. Some of the manifestations of early congenital syphilis include localized or generalized papulosquamous or bullous eruptions, condylomata lata, mucous patches, and an inflammatory rhinitis called *snuffles*. Manifestations of late congenital syphilis, which by definition occurs after 2 years of age, include interstitial keratitis, mulberry (first) molars, pegged (or Hutchinson's) incisors, saber shins, and Charcot joints.

The scope of this Atlas does not allow a full discussion of this protean disorder, and the reader is referred to other excellent texts for a more complete discussion of this disease.

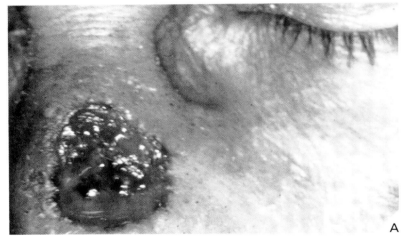

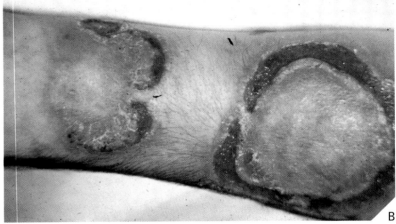

Figure 1.42 Benign tertiary or gummatous syphilis. **A** Ulcerating facial gummata such as these are now unusual in the United States although they are still common in other parts of the world. **B** Serpiginous gummata of the forearm. Note the active border and areas of partial spontaneous resolution, with scarring.

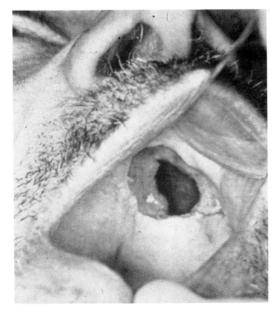

Figure 1.43 Old gummatous perforation of the hard palate. This is a common area of involvement in late syphilis and other treponematoses.

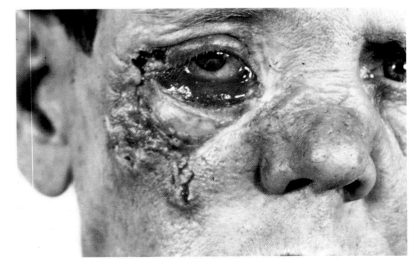

Figure 1.44 Gummatous involvement of conjunctiva. Note also a noduloulcerative gumma over the right malar surface.

Treatment

Penicillin is the mainstay of syphilotherapy. Although alternative drugs are listed, their efficacy has never been proven in clinical trials. The recommendations presented in Figure 1.47 are a synopsis of those provided by the Centers for Disease Control in Atlanta, Georgia.

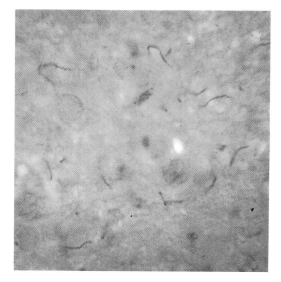

Figure 1.45 Spirochetes demonstrated in neural tissue (Dieterle's silver stain).

Laboratory Tests
COLLECTION OF SPECIMENS

Specimens for both dark-field microscopy and the direct immunofluorescent antibody test for T. *pallidum* (DFA-TP) can be collected from oral, genital, and anal lesions or from lymph nodes. The ideal specimen for direct examination is serous fluid

NEUROSYPHILITIC SYNDROMES

I. MENINGEAL SYPHILIS
   a. Acute syphilitic meningitis
   b. Spinal pachymeningitis

II. MENINGOVASCULAR SYPHILIS
   a. Cerebrovascular syphilis
   b. Meningovascular syphilis of the spinal cord

III. PARENCHYMATOUS NEUROSYPHILIS
   a. General paresis
   b. Tabes dorsalis

IV. CNS GUMMATA

V. ISOLATED NEURAL EVENTS
   a. Optic neuritis/atrophy
   b. Sensorineural hearing loss

VI. CONGENITAL NEUROSYPHILIS

Figure 1.46 Neurosyphilitic syndromes.

TREATMENT SCHEDULES FOR SYPHILIS*

A EARLY SYPHILIS

(primary, secondary, latent < 1 year's duration)

1. Benzathine penicillin G: 2.4 million U, IM stat.

2. For the penicillin-allergic patient: a) tetracycline HCl: 500 mg PO, QID for 15 days, or b) erythromycin: 500 mg PO, QID for 15 days.

B SYPHILIS OF MORE THAN ONE YEAR'S DURATION

(latent syphilis of indeterminate or > 1 year's duration, cardiovascular, or late benign syphilis, NOT neurosyphilis)

1. Benzathine penicillin G: 2.4 million U, IM once a week for 3 successive weeks (7.2 million U total).

2. Penicillin-allergic patients: Same as early syphilis (A), except the duration of therapy is 30 days.

C CSF EXAMINATION

Cerebrospinal fluid examination should be done for patients with clinical symptoms or signs consistent with neurosyphilis. This examination is desirable in all patients with syphilis of indeterminate age to rule out asymptomatic neurosyphilis. However, this is not always practical. Patients who are treated without spinal fluid examination should be followed carefully.

D NEUROSYPHILIS

1. Aqueous crystalline penicillin G: 12 million U every 4 hours for 10 days + benzathine penicillin G: 2.4 million U IM weekly for 3 consecutive weeks.

2. Aqueous procaine penicillin G: 2.4 million U IM daily for 10 days + 3 weeks of benzathine penicillin as above.

3. Benzathine penicillin G: 2.4 million U IM, weekly for 3 doses. (This is the least desirable regimen.)

4. Regimen for penicillin-allergic patients: there are no recommended regimens. Consult with an infectious diseases specialist.

E SYPHILIS DURING PREGNANCY

1. For the nonpenicillin-allergic woman, penicillin prescribed in the doses recommended for nonpregnant patients appropriate for the stage of syphilis should be administered.

2. Erythromycin in the same doses described above should be prescribed for the penicillin-allergic patient.

3. If compliance and serologic follow-up cannot be assured, the patient should be hospitalized for therapy.

4. Patients should have monthly quantitative nontreponemal serologic tests for the remainder of the pregnancy. Women with a fourfold rise in titer should be retreated.

*Specimens for dark-field examination and blood for serologic tests for syphilis should always be collected and preferably interpreted together with clinical findings prior to instituting therapy for syphilis.

Figure 1.47 A through E Treatment schedules for syphilis.

with few red blood cells. To collect serous material from the chancre, any scab or crust should first be gently removed using a scalpel blade, a tongue blade, or a needle. A gauze sponge, soaked in 0.9% nonbacteriostatic saline, should be used to remove tissue debris and superficial bacteria from the lesion. The first few drops of exudate, which may contain blood, are then wiped away. Relatively clear fluid should be collected, either by applying a clean microscope slide or coverslip to the lesion, or by transferring the fluid, using a bacteriologic loop, to the microscope slide. The coverslip is then pressed onto a clean glass slide and examined on a dark-field microscope. The steps for properly collecting this material are demonstrated in Figure 1.48. Specimens for DFA-TP may be collected in capillary tubes as well. Material collected from the depths of the lesion is more likely to contain motile treponemes than surface material. Healing skin lesions merit examination as well. They should be abraded with a sharp instrument, or fluid may be collected from the lesion by injecting a drop of sterile saline into the base of the lesion and aspirating with a small-gauge needle and syringe.

Collection of lesional material in the cervix or vaginal vault for direct examination follows the same principles, but must always be by direct visualization through a speculum. Aspiration of lymph nodes is done by injecting 0.2 mL or less of sterile saline into the node through sterilized skin, followed by aspiration of the tissue material. This material should be examined immediately by dark-field microscopy, but may be held at 2 to 8°C for DFA-TP.

For all serologic tests for syphilis, blood is collected into dry tubes without anticoagulant, allowed to clot, and the serum separated by centrifugation (Fig. 1.49). If the test is not to be performed immediately, sera should be removed from the clots and either stored at refrigerator temperature (4°C) or frozen.

DIRECT DIAGNOSIS

The most specific method for the diagnosis of the early stages of syphilis is direct microscopy of material taken from the lesion or lymph node aspirates. These tests are usually the first to become positive. The demonstration of treponemes with characteristic morphology and motility or staining with a fluorescent-labeled conjugate specific for T. *pallidum* is diagnostic of primary, secondary, and congenital syphilis, and of relapses during early latent syphilis, if yaws, bejel, and pinta are excluded.

Direct microscopy is useful in establishing a diagnosis of reinfection as well. Additionally, direct microscopy is frequently used to rule out syphilis as the cause of lesions associated with other sexually transmitted diseases. When specimens are properly collected, the direct methods are at least 95% sensitive.

Dark-field Microscopy

In dark-field microscopy, light rays strike organisms or particles at such an oblique angle that no direct light enters the microscope, except that reflected from the organisms or particles. Thus anything in the light path appears luminous against a dark background (Fig. 1.50). The nonpathogens T. *refringens* and

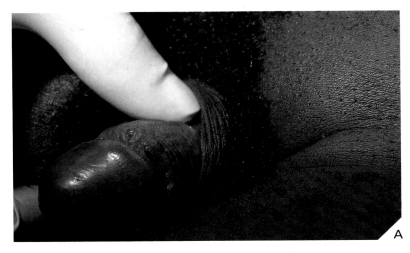

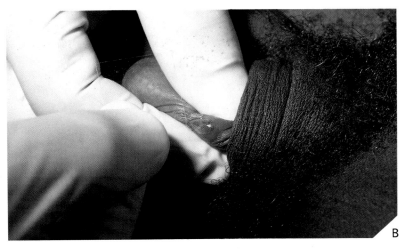

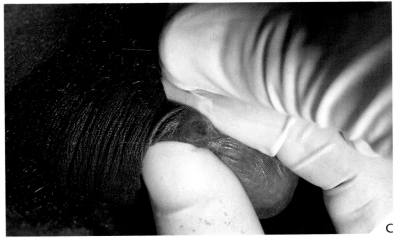

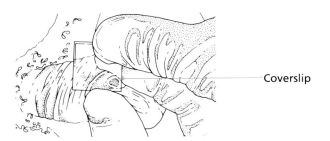

Figure 1.48 Collection of specimen for dark-field or DFA-TP test. **A** Penile ulcer after cleaning with gauze. **B** Squeezing the ulcer to obtain exudate. **C** Touching coverslip to ulcer to obtain fluid for dark-field examination.

Coverslip

T. denticola are usually found in the gastrointestinal tract and are easily confused with *T. pallidum* on dark-field examination.

Direct Fluorescent Antibody Test for T. *Pallidum* (DFA-TP)

The DFA-TP is an immunofluorescent antibody test in which an anti-*T. pallidum* globulin is labeled with a fluorochrome dye (fluoroscein-isothiocyanate—FITC) to identify the organism specifically.

Body fluids, suspensions of macerated tissues, or other materials are smeared onto slides, air-dried, and perhaps fixed in methanol or acetone, and then reacted with the FITC conjugate. Treponemes can be located in the positive specimens using a fluorescence microscope (Fig. 1.51).

INDIRECT DIAGNOSIS USING NONTREPONEMAL SEROLOGIC TESTS

The serologic tests for syphilis are divided into screening tests and confirmation tests, based on the specific antigen used.

Nontreponemal antigens are used in screening tests to measure both IgG and IgM antilipid antibodies. These antibodies are formed by the host, in response to lipoidal material released from damaged host cells early in the infection and most likely to lipids from the treponeme.

In primary syphilis, reactivity in these tests does not develop until 1 to 4 weeks after the chancre first appears. For this reason, patients with suspect lesions and nonreactive nontreponemal tests should have repeat tests performed at 1-week, 1-month, and 3-month intervals from the time of initial testing. Nonreactive tests during the 3-month period exclude the diagnosis of syphilis.

The nontreponemal tests are reactive in secondary syphilis almost without exception, and usually in titers of 1:16 or greater regardless of the test method used. Less than 2% of sera will exhibit a prozone (Fig. 1.52). Nontreponemal test titers in early latent syphilis are similar to those of secondary syphilis. However, as the duration of the latent stage increases the titer decreases.

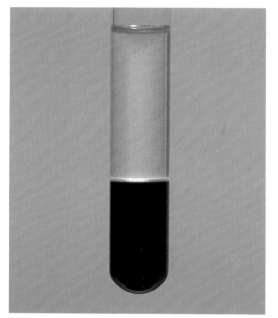

Figure 1.49 Centrifuged blood clot ready for removal of serum after centrifugation. Serum is collected by venipuncture into a "red top" vacutainer tube without anticoagulant, centrifuged, and, if necessary, separated from clot for storage.

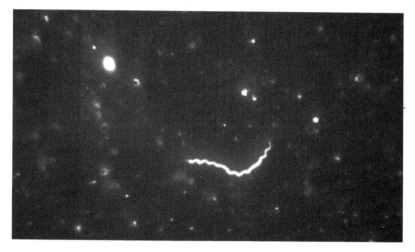

Figure 1.50 Positive dark-field examination. Treponemes are recognized by their characteristic corkscrew shape and deliberate forward and backward movement with rotation about the longitudinal axis.

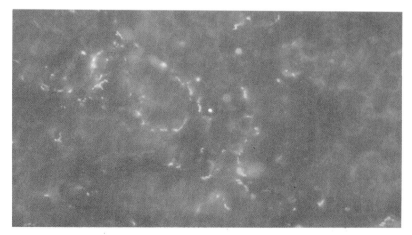

Figure 1.51 DFA-TP positive tissue section. The DFA-TP has the following advantages over the dark-field examination: (1) motile organisms are not required, (2) pathogenic treponemes can be differentiated from nonpathogenic treponemes in oral lesions, and (3) tissue sections for biopsy can be examined as well as autopsy material.

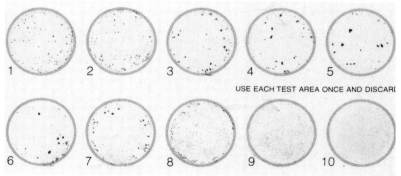

USE EACH TEST AREA ONCE AND DISCARD

Figure 1.52 The prozone phenomenon. Some high-titered sera, such as this one at 1:256, when tested undiluted may appear to give rough nonreactive or minimally reactive (circle 1) results. However, upon dilution, the flocculation intensifies (circle 5) and then progressively decreases to become nonreactive (circle 10). The prozone phenomenon may be due not only to an antibody excess, but also to blocking or incomplete antibody formation.

The nontreponemal CSF VDRL test (see Fig. 1.53) is the only serologic test recognized as a standard test for the diagnosis of neurosyphilis. Asymptomatic neurosyphilis should not be diagnosed by a reactive CSF VDRL alone. CSF criteria for the diagnosis of neurosyphilis are:

Reactive CSF VDRL
Reactive serum treponemal test
5 or more lymphocytes/mm^3 CSF
CSF total protein of $\geq$ 45 mg/dL

Symptomatic neurosyphilis is diagnosed by clinical symptoms and signs, supplemented with positive results in the above diagnostic procedures.

Serial quantitative nontreponemal tests can be used to measure the adequacy of therapy. Titers should be obtained at 3-month intervals for at least 1 year. A fourfold drop in titer should be noted by 3 months, in adequately treated early syphilis.

In congenital syphilis, the role of nontreponemal tests is to monitor the antibody titer. A rising titer in monthly tests from an infant over a 6-month period is diagnostic for congenital syphilis. If the infant was not infected in utero, by 3 months passively transferred antibodies should no longer be detected by nontreponemal tests.

All nontreponemal tests will occasionally give false-positive results. In general populations, this occurs in 1 to 2% of tests. **Acute false-positive** reactions lasting less than 6 months usually occur after febrile diseases, immunizations, or during pregnancy. However, false-positive rates may exceed 10% in populations with a high prevalence of intravenous drug use. The titers of false-positive reactions are usually less than 1:8. Since titers are also low in latent syphilis, not all low titers are false positives. In addition, not all high titers are true positives. In intravenous drug users, approximately 12% of false-positive titers are 1:8 or greater. **Chronic false-positive** reactions are more often associated with autoimmune disorders, such as rheumatoid arthritis and systemic lupus erythematosus, or with chronic infections such as leprosy. Titers in chronic false-positive reactions also are low, usually less than 1:8.

Specific Nontreponemal Serologic Tests
Standard nontreponemal tests for syphilis are listed in Figure 1.53. All four tests use the VDRL antigen (cardiolipin, cholesterol, and lecithin). The VDRL slide test is the only test using an antigen that has not been stabilized by the addition of EDTA, and which does not contain choline chloride to eliminate the need for heat-inactivation of the serum. The RPR is the most widely used test. The VDRL CSF slide test is the only recognized procedure for the serodiagnosis of neurosyphilis. All four tests use similar equipment (Fig. 1.54).

VDRL SLIDE TEST This test is based on an antigen-antibody reaction, but it differs from most other serologic tests in that the antigen-antibody complex remains suspended, and, rather than agglutination or precipitation, flocculation occurs (Fig. 1.55), which necessitates use of a microscope to read results.

USR This test is a microscopic test like the VDRL. The principle of the USR is identical to that of the VDRL, although the antigen for the USR has been stabilized. The USR has two advantages over the VDRL: firstly, the antigen is ready for use once it reaches room temperature, and secondly, the sera do not require heating before testing. In all other aspects, the test is performed and read like the VDRL slide test (see Fig. 1.55). The antigen should be checked with control sera prior to testing specimens.

RPR CARD TEST The principle of the RPR card test is the same as that of the VDRL slide test. However, in this test, charcoal particles are added to the USR antigen. The particles become entrapped within the antigen-antibody lattice of a positive reaction, yielding a clumping that is visible to the naked eye (Fig. 1.56). No microscope or water bath is needed, which makes this test much more convenient than either the VDRL or USR, accounting for its present popularity.

RST The test antigen for the RST is identical to that for the USR, except a lipid-soluble dye is added, which actually stains the antigen to aid in the visualization of the antigen-antibody reaction (Fig. 1.57). The test is performed much like the RPR card test.

INDIRECT DIAGNOSIS USING TREPONEMAL SEROLOGIC TESTS
In contrast to the nontreponemal tests, the treponemal tests should be reserved for confirmatory testing when the clinical signs and/or history disagree with the reactive nontreponemal test results. Treponemal tests are based on the detection of

STANDARD NONTREPONEMAL TESTS
MICROSCOPIC TESTS
Venereal Disease Research Laboratory (VDRL) Slide Test
Unheated Serum Reagin (USR) Test
MACROSCOPIC TESTS
Rapid Plasma Reagin (RPR) Test
Reagin Screen Test (RST)

Figure 1.53 Standard nontreponemal tests.

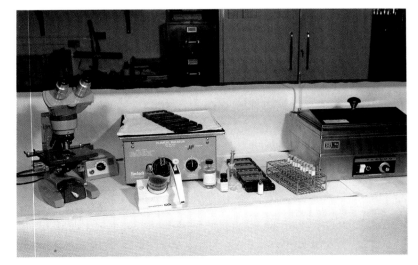

Figure 1.54 This is an example of equipment required to perform the nontreponemal tests for syphilis. Shown here are a mechanical rotator, a water bath, a microscope, a safety pipetter, and reagents.

antibodies formed specifically to the antigenic determinants of the treponemes. They are qualitative procedures, which therefore cannot be used to monitor the efficacy of treatment. About 10% of patients treated during early syphilis will become nonreactive within 2 years of treatment. Like the nontreponemal tests, treponemal tests are almost always reactive in secondary and latent syphilis. For most cases, once the treponemal tests are reactive, they remain so for the patient's lifetime. In fact, in some patients with late syphilis, a reactive treponemal test may be the only means of confirming the suspected diagnosis. Currently, none of the treponemal tests are recommended for use with CSF.

Reactivity in infants may be due to antibodies that are passively transferred to the fetus from the maternal circulation or to infection of the fetus. Passively transferred treponemal antibodies should become undetectable in the noninfected infant by 6 months of age. This is about 3 months longer than the expected time period for the detection of antilipid antibodies.

The greatest value of the treponemal tests is to differentiate true-positive nontreponemal test results from false-positive results. However, false-positive treponemal test results do occur with about the same frequency (1%) as false-positive nontreponemal test results. Although some false-positive results in the treponemal tests are transient and of unknown cause, they have been associated with connective tissue diseases. When unexplained reactive tests occur in elderly patients, attempts should be made to rule out acquired or congenital syphilis, or infections with other treponemes, before a diagnosis of false-positive serology is made.

Specific Treponemal Serologic Tests

Standard treponemal tests for syphilis are listed in Figure 1.58.

FTA-ABS AND FTA-ABS DS Both of these indirect immunofluorescence tests are based on the same principle. The patient's serum, which has been diluted with sorbent, is layered

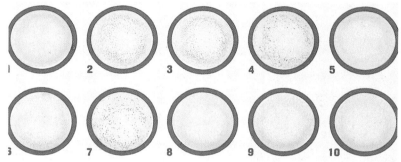

Figure 1.56 Qualitative RPR card test. Specimens exhibiting medium to large flocculation are reported as reactive (circles 4 and 7). Specimens with definite but small flocculation are read as reactive minimal (Rm) (circles 2 and 3). Specimens with an even dispersion of antigen particles (circles 1, 5, 8 and 10) or specimens that are slightly rough (circle 6) are reported as nonreactive.

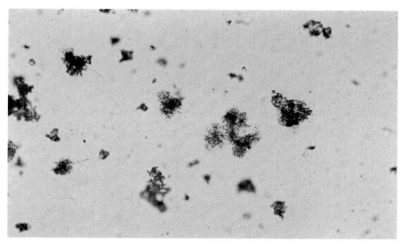

Figure 1.55 Reactive VDRL or USR result. Specimens exhibiting medium and/or large flocculation particles are reported as reactive (R). Those with small particles are reported as weakly reactive (W) while those with complete dispersion of antigen particles or slight roughness are reported as nonreactive (NR). Sera exhibiting slight roughness should be quantitated to check for the prozone phenomenon.

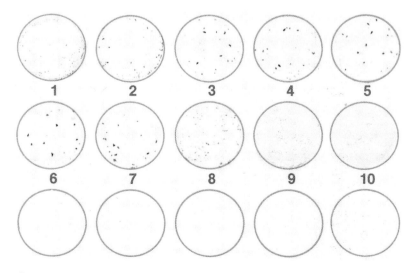

Figure 1.57 Quantitative RST. The reading of the RST is identical to that of the RPR card test. The prozone phenomenon, shown in Figure 1.52 with the RPR card test, is again demonstrated, with the same serum tested with the RST instead.

STANDARD TREPONEMAL TESTS

Fluorescent Treponemal Antibody Absorption (FTA-ABS) Test

FTA-ABS double-staining (DS) Test (FTA-ABS DS)

Microhemagglutination Assay for Antibodies to *T. pallidum* (MHA-TP)

Hemagglutination Treponemal Test (HATTS)

Figure 1.58 Standard treponemal tests.

on a microscope slide to which T. *pallidum* has been fixed. If the patient's serum contains antibody, it will coat the treponeme. The double-stain test employs a fluorescein isothiocyanate (FITC)-labeled conjugate as the direct stain and a tetramethyl rhodamine isothiocyanate (TMRITC)-labeled antihuman immunoglobulin conjugate for antibody detection (the indirect stain). This eliminates the need for having to use dark-field microscopy on the smear first, to find treponemes (Figs. 1.59 and 1.60). Both tests are reported as shown in Figure 1.61.

MHA-TP AND HATTS   Both of these microhemagglutination tests are virtually identical in principle. The major difference is in the erythrocyte carrier employed for the T. *pallidum* subspecies *pallidum* antigen. In the HATTS, turkey erythrocytes are used for both the sensitized and unsensitized cells, whereas in the MHA-TP, sheep erythrocytes are used. In both tests, patients' sera are diluted in an absorbing diluent that is similar, and in the HATTS, identical, to the sorbent of the FTA-ABS test. In the MHA-TP, unheated sera are used in the test, although previously heated sera may be used. Sera are absorbed at a

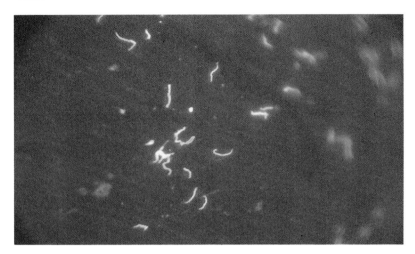

Figure 1.59   Example of the FTA-ABS DS. In reading the FTA-ABS DS, the treponemes are easily located, since the antigen is counterstained with the direct-staining FITC-labeled antitreponemal globulin component. If the patient's serum does not contain anti-T. *pallidum* antibodies, when the slide is read using the rhodamine filter set, no treponemes will be observed.

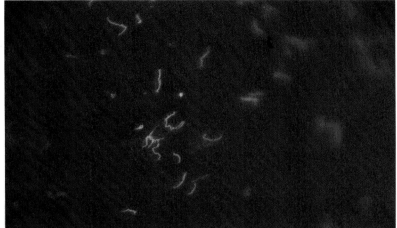

Figure 1.60   Reactive FTA-ABS DS test. If the patient's serum contains antibodies to T. *pallidum,* when the rhodamine filters are used the treponemes will appear reddish-orange, due to the TMRITC-labeled anti-human IgG globulin used as the indicator stain or indirect component of the system.

Figure 1.61   Interpretation and reporting of FTA-ABS and FTA-ABS DS tests.

INTERPRETATION AND REPORTING OF FTA-ABS AND FTA-ABS DS TESTS

INTERPRETATION OF FLUORESCENCE

INITIAL TEST	REPEAT TEST	REPORT
2+ to 4+		Reactive
1+	> 1+	Reactive
1+	= 1+	Reactive minimal*
< 1+		NR
−		NR

*In the absence of historical or clinical evidence of treponemal infection, this test result should be considered equivocal. A second specimen should be submitted for serologic testing.

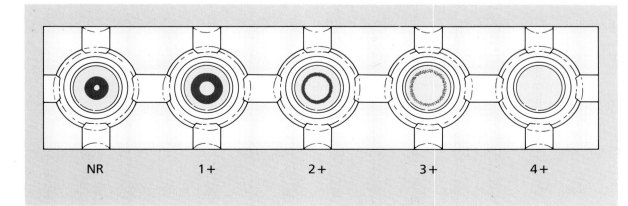

NR   1+   2+   3+   4+

Figure 1.62   Hemagglutination test results. Results for the MHA-TP and HATTS are reported as reactive (1+, 2+, 3+, 4+) or nonreactive (±, −). Completely negative readings vary in pattern from a solid compact button of cells to a circle of cells with a small central hole, as seen in this drawing.

1:20 dilution prior to testing. In the HATTS, heated sera are usually used. The diluted sera are placed in a microtitration plate and sensitized cells are added. Incubation of the test is at 22° to 25°C (room temperature) for 4 hours or overnight. The sera, which contain treponemal antibodies, react with the antigen on the erythrocytes, and agglutination occurs (Figs. 1.62 and 1.63).

SENSITIVITY AND SPECIFICITY OF SEROLOGIC TESTS

While the overall sensitivity of the nontreponemal tests (Fig. 1.64) is approximately 90%, up to 28% of patients with early primary syphilis will have nonreactive nontreponemal test results on the initial visit. In addition, patients will present with nonreactive nontreponemal tests in about 30% of cases of late

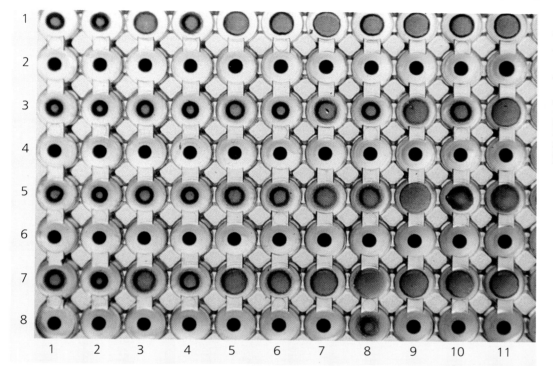

Figure 1.63 Example of a HATTS test result. (Rows are vertical and wells are horizontal.) Agglutination patterns vary from 1+ (well 5, row 3) to 4+ (well 5, row 1). An example of a 2+ is seen in well 7, row 5, while an example of a 3+ appears in well 7, row 7. A ± reading appears in well 3 of row 3. Heterophil reactions occur in both the MHA-TP and HATTS procedures; an example of a heterophil reaction is seen in well 8, row 8.

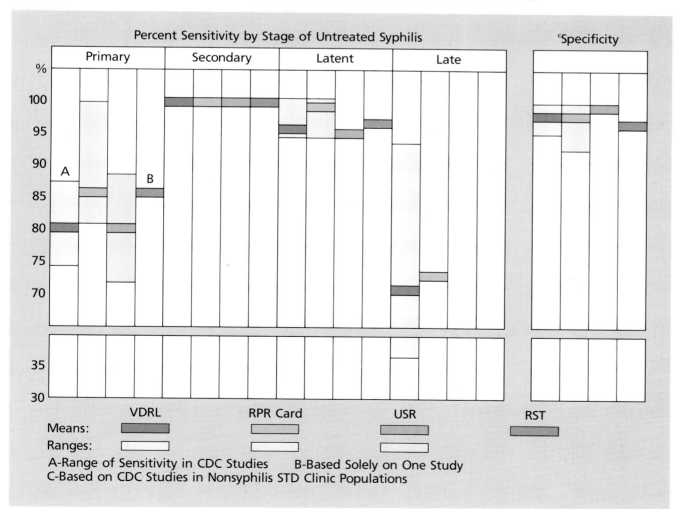

Figure 1.64 Sensitivity and specificity of nontreponemal tests.

untreated syphilis. Specificity for the nontreponemal tests is 98%. However, the specificity of the test is greatly influenced by the population being tested. In intravenous drug users, the specificity may be as low as 79% for the VDRL slide test, to approximately 89% for the RPR test. The VDRL CSF test is 90% sensitive in symptomatic cases of neurosyphilis and 100% specific, but it is only about 10% specific in asymptomatic neurosyphilis.

The overall sensitivity of the FTA-ABS test, around 98%, is greater than that of the other three major treponemal tests (each of which has a sensitivity of approximately 95%) (Fig. 1.65). The major difference in the sensitivities of these tests is found in primary syphilis. However, if data are analyzed with the diagnosis of primary syphilis based on dark-field positive lesions alone, and primary cases are separated into those with reactive nontreponemal test results, then the sensitivities of the four treponemal tests are almost identical and are greater than 99%. False positives can occur in the treponemal tests, but only rarely do false positives occur in both treponemal and nontreponemal tests for the same patient. Individuals with connective tissue diseases may present difficult serodiagnostic problems.

Serologic tests must be interpreted according to the disease stage, possible underlying disease conditions, and the possibility of false-positive test results. Ideally all sera in suspected cases of syphilis should be tested first with a nontreponemal procedure and reactive results verified with a second specimen and quantification. Cases in which clinical or epidemiologic evidence is counter to the diagnosis of syphilis should be confirmed with a treponemal test. With the proper use of serologic

tests, a reactive nontreponemal test with a reactive treponemal test gives a positive predictive value of approximately 97%, or only a 3% error factor. In contrast, if any one test is used, the positive predictive value, regardless of the method, is less than 50% in a low-prevalence disease such as syphilis.

Misinterpretation of test results for nontreponemal tests most often results from:

1. The failure to recognize the variation of plus or minus one dilution inherent in most serologic tests
2. The failure to establish the true positivity of test results
3. The failure to recognize reactivity due to nonvenereal treponematoses

In summary, serologic testing for syphilis often plays a crucial role in making a diagnosis of syphilis. Many tests are commercially available and are of high quality. All tests require rigid standardization with negative and positive control sera before being used to test sera from patients. Finally, the serologic tests should be interpreted carefully by an experienced clinician, in light of a thorough history, physical, and, if possible, dark-field examination, before a diagnosis of syphilis is made.

Picture credits for this chapter are as follows: Figs. 1.5 and 1.6 adapted from the unpublished work of Hans Ristow, MD; Fig. 1.23D courtesy of Heidi Watts; Fig. 1.39 adapted from a drawing by Karlene Hewan-Lowe, MD; Fig. 1.50 courtesy of Ralph Ramsey; Figs. 1.10, 1.11, 1.14–1.16, 1.28, 1.40–1.45, 1.49, 1.51, 1.52, 1.54–1.57, 1.59, 1.60, and 1.63 from the collection of the Centers for Disease Control in Atlanta, Georgia.

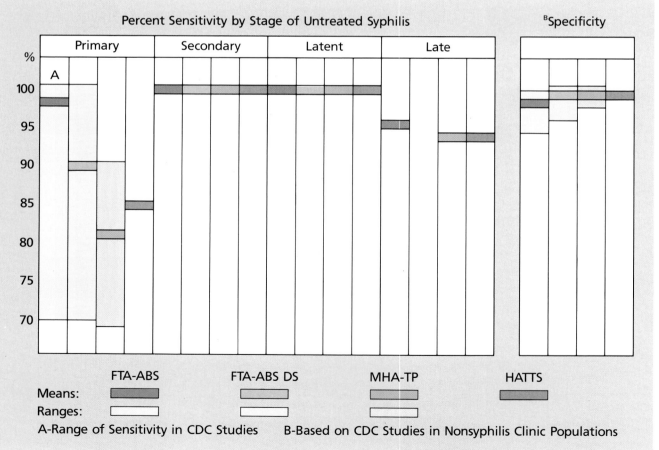

Figure 1.65 Sensitivity and specificity of treponemal tests.

BIBLIOGRAPHY

Bayne LL, Sidley JW, Goodin DS: Acute syphilitic meningitis: Its occurrence after clinical and serologic cure of secondary syphilis with penicillin G. *Arch Neurol* 43:137, 1986.

Brown ST, Zaidi A, Larsen SA, Reynolds GH: Serological response to syphilis treatment: A new analysis of old data. JAMA 253:1296, 1985.

Clark EG, Dunbolt N: The Oslo study of the natural course of untreated syphilis: An epidemiologic investigation based on a re-study of the Boeck–Bruusgaard material. *Med Clin North Am* 48:613, 1964.

Fiumara NJ: Treatment of primary and secondary syphilis: Serologic responses. JAMA 243:2500, 1980.

Heggtveit HA: Syphilitic aortitis: A clinicopathologic autopsy study of 100 cases, 1950 to 1960. *Circulation* 29:346, 1964.

Hooshmand H, Escobar MR, Kopf SW: Neurosyphilis: A study of 241 patients. JAMA 219:726, 1972.

Kampmeier RH: The late manifestations of syphilis: Skeletal, visceral and cardiovascular. *Med Clin North Am* 48:667, 1964.

Larsen SA, Hambie EA, Pettit DE, Perryman MW, Kraus SJ: Specificity, sensitivity and reproducibility among the fluorescent antibody absorption test, the microhemagglutination assay for *Treponema pallidum* antibodies, and the hemagglutination treponemal test for syphilis. J *Clin Microbiol* 14:441, 1981.

Larsen SA, Hunter EF, McGrew BE: Syphilis, in *Laboratory Methods for the Diagnosis of Sexually Transmitted Diseases*. Washington, DC, American Public Health Association, 1985.

Manual of Tests for Syphilis, US Dept of Health, Education and Welfare publication No. (PHS) 411. Atlanta, National Communicable Disease Center, 1969.

Olansky S: Late benign syphilis. *Med Clin North Am* 48:653, 1964.

Schroeter AL, Lucas JB, Price EV, Falcone VH: Treatment of early syphilis and reactivity of serologic tests. JAMA 221:471, 1972.

Stokes JH, Beerman H, Ingraham NR: *Modern Clinical Syphilology: Diagnosis, Treatment, Case Study*, ed 3. Philadelphia, WB Saunders Co, 1944.

World Health Organization: *Treponemal Infections*. Technical Report Series No. 674. Geneva, WHO, 1982.

Genital Herpes 2

A.A. MORELAND, J.A. BRYAN, S.D. SHAFRAN

Introduction

Genital herpes is a common, often painful disease that has serious consequences for certain populations. Medical research in this century has significantly expanded our knowledge of the infection and its treatment. Prior to the 19th century, the term *herpes* was used in medical literature for a variety of skin eruptions. Gradually, the meaning of the term narrowed to mean primarily the classic grouped vesicles on an erythematous base. The viral etiology was eventually suggested by transmission experiments in the early 1900s, and was confirmed and classified in relation to other viral diseases by the 1950s.

Genital herpes infections are caused by the herpes simplex virus (HSV), which is a large (150 to 200 nm) virus consisting of viral DNA surrounded by layers of viral proteins and covered

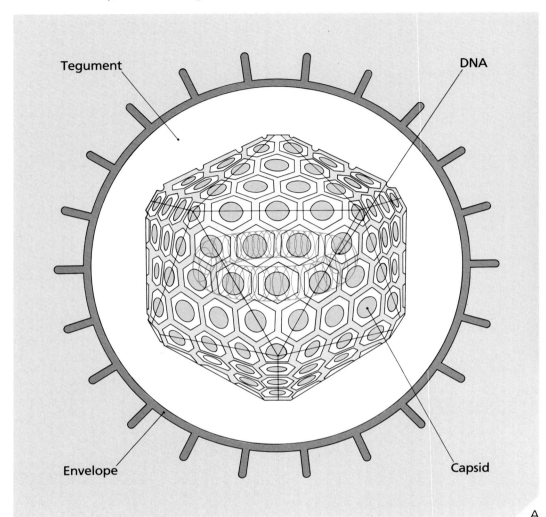

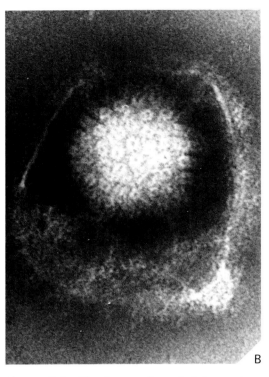

Figure 2.1 The herpesvirus. **A** Schematic representation. **B** Electron micrograph.

Figure 2.2 Human herpesviruses.

HUMAN HERPESVIRUSES

VIRUS	PRINCIPAL DISEASES
Herpes simplex virus type 1 (HSV-1)	Skin and mucosal vesicles and ulcers, especially oral
Herpes simplex virus type 2 (HSV-2)	Skin and mucosal vesicles and ulcers, especially genital
Varicella-zoster virus (VZV)	Chickenpox, shingles
Epstein-Barr virus (EBV)	Infectious mononucleosis
Cytomegalovirus (CMV)	Serious disease in immunosuppressed patients and congenital infection
Human herpesvirus-6 (HHV-6)	Roseola infantum (suspected)

by a trilaminar envelope derived from the host cell (Fig. 2.1). Two types of herpes simplex virus exist—HSV type 1 and HSV type 2; these constitute two of the six known human herpesviruses (Fig. 2.2). The two types of HSV share approximately 50% of their genomic content. HSV-1 is responsible for more than 90% of orolabial herpes and herpes keratitis. HSV-2 is responsible for approximately 90% of genital herpes. The infection is characterized by viral shedding from affected skin or mucous membranes and production of several types of specific humoral antibodies. The neutralizing antibodies, which are produced early in the course of infection and persist for variable lengths of time, do not appear to prevent recurrence of the active phase of disease, perhaps because extracellular virus is inactivated by these antibodies while intracellular viral replication and direct cell-to-cell transfer of new infectious virus still occur. The exact role of humoral antibodies in the reactivation of the infection is not fully understood; however, antibodies appear to attenuate the severity of the disease since recurrences generally are less severe than primary infection. Cell-mediated immune responses undoubtedly play an important role in the manifestation of herpes infections as evi-denced by severe, prolonged, and frequently recurring infections in patients who have impaired cell-mediated immunity.

Epidemiology

Accurate data regarding the incidence and prevalence of genital herpes are not available, although several estimates have been made. Seroprevalence studies from several Western countries have found that 7 to 20% of adults possess HSV-2-specific antibodies. The results of one such study are depicted in Figure 2.3. A Canadian study, which found a seroprevalence of 15.5%, observed that only 22% of seropositive individuals reported a history of genital herpes. In addition, asymptomatic genital shedding of HSV has been demonstrated in 0.25 to 3.0% of women without a history of herpes infections. These data suggest that asymptomatic genital herpes is more prevalent than symptomatic cases.

Genital herpes accounted for 2% of visits to STD clinics in the United Kingdom in 1979 and 4% of visits to an STD clinic in Seattle in 1980. There is a widely held belief that the prevalence of genital herpes increased dramatically in the 1960s

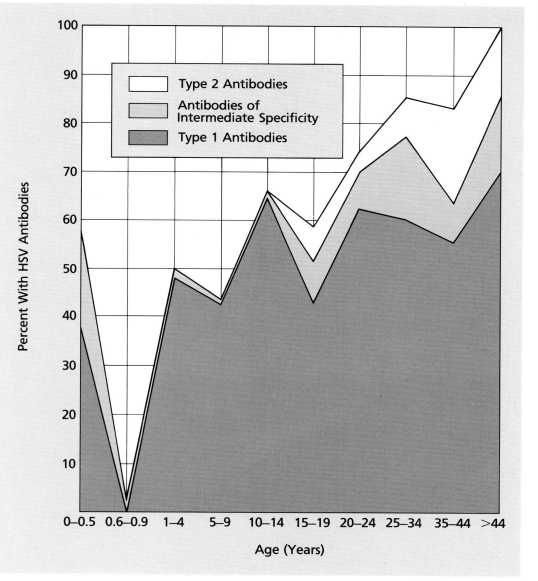

Figure 2.3 Distribution, by age, of antibodies to HSV.

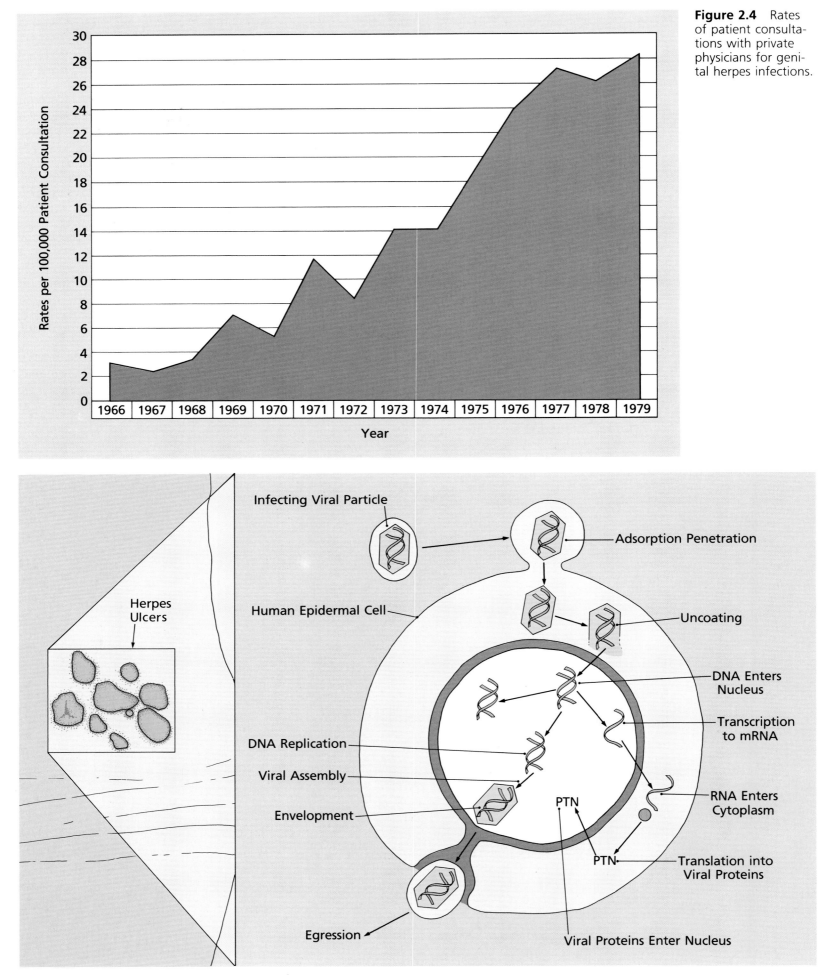

Figure 2.4 Rates of patient consultations with private physicians for genital herpes infections.

Figure 2.5 Transmission of herpes.

and 1970s. Data supporting this view were analyzed by the Centers for Disease Control in 1982 and are shown in Figure 2.4.

In developed countries, genital herpes, like nongonococcal urethritis, is more prevalent among economically advantaged individuals. This contrasts with gonorrhea, which is more prevalent in the economically disadvantaged.

Spread of the infection occurs when viral particles enter the skin or mucous membranes through traumatic microscopic openings or fissures. Genital mucosal surfaces commonly are subjected to friction during intercourse, which results in a favorable environment for passage of the virus into keratinocytes. There the virus replicates inside the nucleus and spreads to surrounding cells (Fig. 2.5). The infected epidermal cells are destroyed, resulting in damage to the involved epidermis. The virus then enters the peripheral sensory or autonomic nerve endings and ascends to sensory or autonomic root ganglia, where it becomes latent. Subsequently, viral reactivation may occur, causing the virus to descend along the involved nerve root back to, or very close to, the original site of infection on the skin or mucous membrane. Clinically, this is called a recurrence. Recurrences may be either symptomatic or asymptomatic. Transmission of the infection can occur readily by contact with open vesicles, but can also occur in persons who are asymptomatically shedding the virus. Approximately one-third of individuals with newly diagnosed genital herpes do not give a history of contact with an infected individual, supporting the epidemiologic importance of asymptomatic HSV shedding.

ASSOCIATION WITH CERVICAL NEOPLASIA

Since 1969, many studies have shown an association between genital herpes and cervical carcinoma in women. Both conditions appear to be STDs and therefore patients have common risk factors. More recently, a much stronger association between cervical cancer and human papillomavirus (HPV) has been demonstrated. Several recent studies have found no relationship between genital herpes and cervical neoplasia when multivariate analysis accounted for HPV and sexual experience. Nevertheless, HSV-2 genetic material has been demonstrated in cervical tissue from women with cervical neoplasia. The precise role of HSV in cervical neoplasia remains to be determined, but it appears to be less well linked to cervical neoplasia than is HPV.

Clinical Manifestations

TYPES OF GENITAL HERPES

There are four types of genital herpes: (1) first episode primary, (2) first episode nonprimary, (3) recurrent, and (4) asymptomatic (Figs. 2.6 and 2.7). *First episode primary genital herpes* is a true pri-

Figure 2.6   Types of genital herpes.

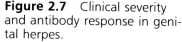

TYPES OF GENITAL HERPES

First episode genital herpes Primary Nonprimary	Recurrent genital herpes Asymptomatic genital herpes

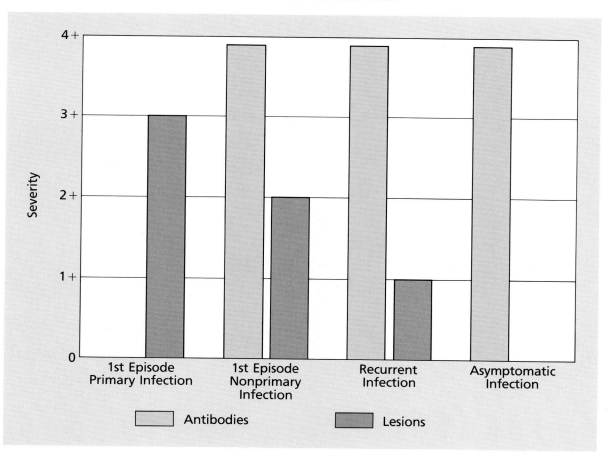

Figure 2.7   Clinical severity and antibody response in genital herpes.

mary infection. The affected individual has no history of previous genital herpetic lesions and is seronegative for HSV antibodies. In general, this type of genital herpes is the most severe clinically.

First *episode nonprimary genital herpes* refers to the first recognized episode of genital herpes in individuals whose sera contain HSV antibodies. In general, first episode nonprimary genital herpes is less severe than first episode primary genital herpes but more severe than recurrent disease. The preexisting antibody is thought to attenuate the severity of disease. The distinction between first episode primary and first episode nonprimary genital herpes in any one individual cannot be made clinically.

Recurrent genital herpes refers to repeated episodes of genital herpes in the same individual. It has been demonstrated that the recurrence rate for genital infections is higher with HSV-2 than with HSV-1. A comparison of the mean duration of symptoms and signs in patients with first episode primary, first episode nonprimary, and recurrent genital herpes is shown in Figure 2.8.

Asymptomatic genital herpes refers to episodes in which individuals shed HSV at genital sites in the absence of symptoms. Some of these individuals have genital lesions that they do not notice, but many do not; many do not know that they have genital herpes. While the quantity of virus shed by these individuals is much less than is found in clinical lesions, asymptomatic shedders can transmit infection and thus are important epidemiologically.

PRIMARY GENITAL INFECTION

After intimate contact with an infected person and an incubation period of approximately one week (2 to 12 days), painful,

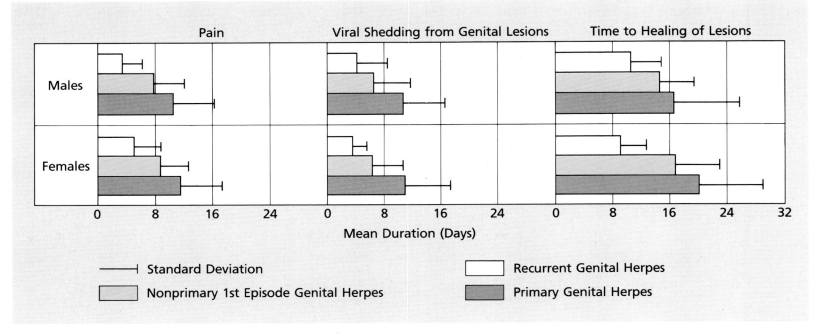

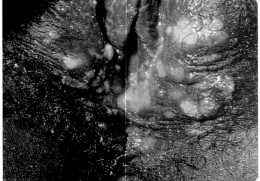

Figure 2.8 Comparison of symptoms and signs in different types of genital herpes.

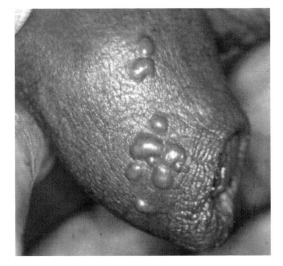

Figure 2.9 Early lesions of primary genital herpes. Clear, grouped vesicles appear on an erythematous base. Some vesicles are discrete and some coalesce, which frequently results in a scalloped border.

Figure 2.10 Vulvar herpes of several days' duration. Several stages in the natural evolution of the eruption are apparent here: clear vesicles, pustules, and grayish exudate cover plaques where the roofs of blisters have eroded.

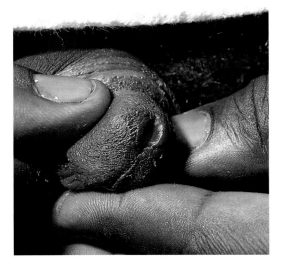

Figure 2.11 Herpes erosion in the urethral meatus. Dysuria resulted from this erythematous and painful erosion. Urethral involvement is less common than lesions on the shaft or the foreskin of the penis.

grouped, discrete vesicles appear (Fig. 2.9). The vesicles usually evolve into pustules, which then erode, creating an ulcer. The remaining grayish plaques crust before healing takes place (Fig. 2.10). This process takes 15 to 20 days before reepithelialization occurs. The lesions shed infectious particles of virus for at least 10 to 12 days, and new lesions may appear until the tenth day. Typical lesions in men occur on the glans penis, coronal sulcus, urethra (Fig. 2.11), shaft of the penis, or perianal region. Less frequently, lesions occur on the scrotum, mons area, thighs, or buttocks. In women, lesions usually occur around the introitus, the urethral meatus, or the labia (Fig. 2.12), but can also occur in extragenital sites such as the perineal or perianal regions or on the thighs and buttocks. Cervicitis is common, occurring in 70 to 90% of women with the first episode of genital herpes.

Cervicitis occurs less frequently in recurrent genital herpes. The appearance of the cervix is usually normal, although it may have ulcerations and appear red and friable (Fig. 2.13).

Because of individual differences in immunity, environmental factors, or other skin diseases, the presentation of primary genital herpes may be unusual or may differ significantly from this classical picture. Immunosuppression, because of either medications or disease (Fig. 2.14) is sometimes a contributing factor in more severe or prolonged infections. Chronic tinea cruris is characterized by scaling, vesicles or pustules, excoriations, and erosions in the folds of the groin. Exposure of this skin to fresh genital herpes lesions may lead to a superinfection with herpes (Fig. 2.15). Chronic eczema may also render the skin susceptible

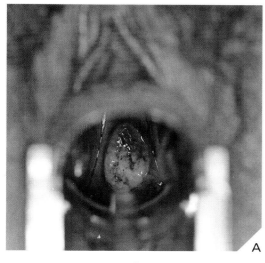

A

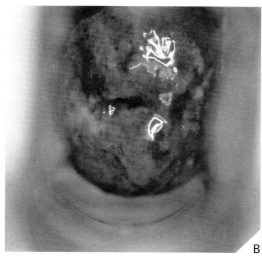

B

Figure 2.12 Primary vulvar herpes. **A** The linear appearance of these painful herpetic erosions on the labia is a result of coalescence of several closely grouped vesicles, which have subsequently shed the vesicle roof. **B** These painful ulcers were present on the vulva of the patient in Fig. 2.13A.

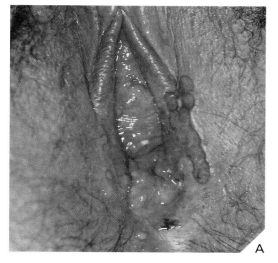

A

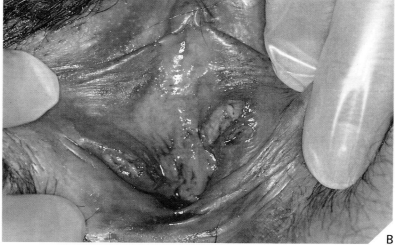

B

Figure 2.13 Herpetic cervicitis. **A** Erosive cervicitis was present in this case of primary herpes presenting with vulvar ulcers (see Fig. 2.12B). **B** Erythema, purulent exudate, and erosions present on the cervix of this patient with genital herpes.

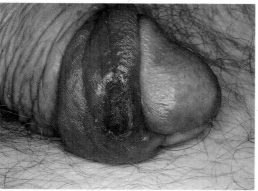

Figure 2.14 Herpes in a patient with leukemia in whom edema is notable around a large herpetic erosion on the penis. The duration of the lesions was much longer than in healthy individuals.

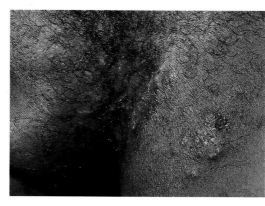

Figure 2.15 Primary herpes arising in chronic tinea cruris infection. Hyperpigmentation and scaling in inguinal folds are signs of a chronic dermatitis. Tzanck smears from moist erosions and vesicles in the inguinal fold and at the border on the thigh showed characteristic multinucleated giant cells.

to infection by herpesvirus (eczema herpeticum) (Fig. 2.16), which can involve the genitals.

Associated genitourinary symptoms in primary genital herpes include dysuria in the majority of cases in both women and men. Vaginal discharge, urethral discharge, and inguinal adenopathy are not uncommon. Pain occurs frequently in men and women with primary symptomatic genital herpes infections. Pain is usually present for at least 1 week; sometimes it persists for 2 weeks.

In addition, patients with primary genital herpes often have other associated systemic symptoms, including headache, fever, malaise, and myalgia. These symptoms appear to be more common in women than in men. Pharyngitis, aseptic meningitis, transverse myelitis, and radiculitis are also associated with genital herpes infections in some patients. Neurologic complications occur in about 13 to 35% of patients. Complaints of a stiff neck, headache, or photophobia ordinarily occur about 3 to 12 days after the onset of genital lesions. Sacral radiculitis may result in urinary retention. Serious neurologic sequelae are rare but have been reported. Herpetic autoinoculation of extragenital sites—most frequently the fingers—is another complication of genital herpes, which probably occurs during primary infection. Such infections occur more commonly in women (Fig. 2.17).

RECURRENT GENITAL HERPES

Recurrent genital herpes may vary in individual patients from completely asymptomatic episodes of viral shedding to mild episodes (Fig. 2.18A and B) or may cause severe discomfort (Fig. 2.19A and B). Although the recurrence rate is highly variable in any one individual, most individuals experience five to eight recurrences per year. In the majority of cases, however, the symptoms and signs are milder and of shorter duration than in primary infection and there frequently is a prodrome of itching (Fig. 2.20), burning, or tingling at the affected site a few hours to a day before the lesions appear. Dysuria is less common and viral shedding is shorter, lasting only about four days. The duration of lesions is approximately 10 days to reepithelialization in recurrent herpes. In immunocompromised patients, recurrences may be atypical in appearance or have a prolonged duration (Fig. 2.21). Some individuals experience "trigger factors," which seem to precipitate a recurrence. Com-

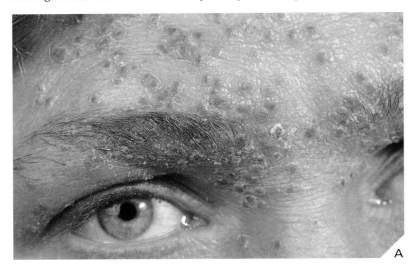
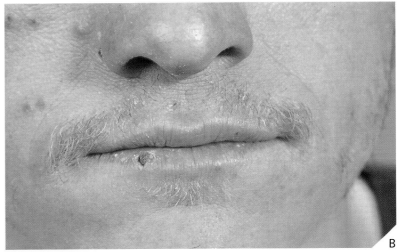

Figure 2.16 Eczema herpeticum. Generalized herpes simplex (A) in this case started with an oral lesion (B) in a patient with atopic dermatitis. Genital eruptions may also be the source of a generalized infection in predisposed individuals.

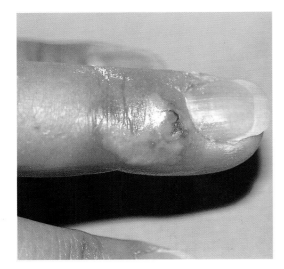
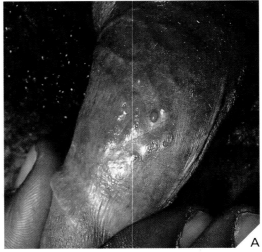
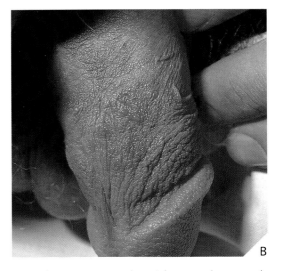

Figure 2.17 Autoinoculation. Commonly called a herpetic whitlow, these herpes blisters are extremely painful and can be recurrent, but heal spontaneously.

Figure 2.18 Recurrent genital herpes. A Many vesicles have eroded and are healing quickly in this mildly symptomatic case.

B Erythema, grouped vesicles, erosions, and edema seen on shaft of penis.

monly noted trigger factors include stress, fatigue, and menses. Erythema multiforme occasionally occurs in conjunction with recurrences and may become more troublesome than the herpetic lesions (see Figs. 12.55 to 12.57).

Nearly half of all individuals with recurrent genital herpes with lesions will also experience some prodromes without lesions wherein a typical herpetic prodrome is not followed by the development of lesions. Prodromes without lesions are also known as false prodromes or aborted prodromes, and are probably due to better immunologic control than occurs when lesions develop.

GENITAL HERPES AND PREGNANCY
The manifestations of genital herpes do not differ between pregnant and nonpregnant women. Nevertheless, the consequences of maternal genital herpes infection for the fetus can be very severe. Maternal–fetal transmission almost always occurs during parturition, but rarely can occur in utero. The rate of transmission depends primarily on whether the mother is experiencing primary or recurrent infection. In primary maternal infection, the rate of fetal transmission is about 50%. In contrast, the rate of fetal transmission is less than 8% in recurrent ma-

ternal disease. The major factor accounting for the marked discrepancy in the rate of fetal transmission between primary and recurrent maternal infection is that in recurrent disease, maternal HSV antibodies are transferred to the fetus and prevent or attenuate fetal infection. In addition, primary genital herpes is associated with larger quantities of virus and a much greater likelihood of cervicitis. Despite the lower fetal transmission rate of recurrent herpes, transmission at this stage is epidemiologically significant since recurrent maternal infection is much more prevalent than primary infection.

Pregnant women with a history of genital herpes should be examined very carefully for genital lesions under good light early in labor. If any lesions are detected, the infant probably should be delivered by cesarean section, preferably before membrane rupture, to prevent direct exposure of the infant to maternal virus. A small percentage of transmission occurs in utero and will not be prevented by cesarean delivery.

NEONATAL INFECTION
Unfortunately, 50 to 60% of infants with neonatal herpes simplex infection are born to mothers with no history of genital herpes, so that careful monitoring of women with such a history

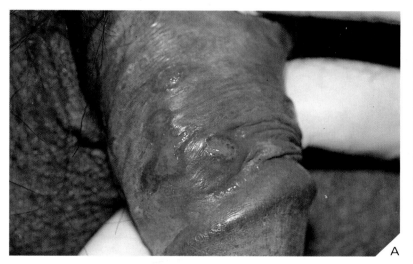
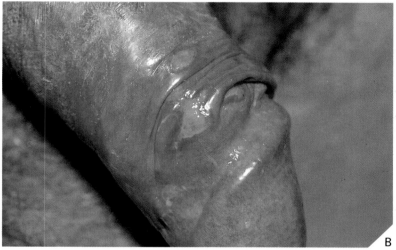

Figure 2.19 A and B Recurrent penile herpes. These discrete and confluent well-demarcated shallow ulcerations on the shaft of the penis were extremely painful in this 32-year old diabetic patient.

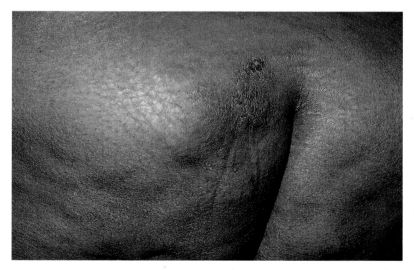

Figure 2.20 Extragenital HSV of the buttocks. Pruritus and irritation were the first symptoms in this recurrent episode. (Black circle is the site chosen for biopsy.)

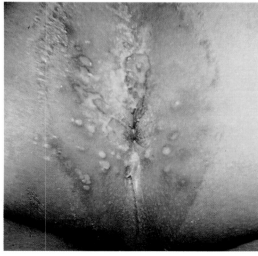

Figure 2.21 Chronic perianal herpes in an AIDS patient. This infection was very difficult to control even with acyclovir therapy.

will fail to prevent many cases of neonatal herpes infection.

Neonatal herpes simplex infection (Fig. 2.22) is very serious. It is associated with prematurity, but is seldom clinically manifested at birth. Clinical disease usually manifests at 3 to 30 days of age, with mucocutaneous disease, visceral disease, or both. Visceral illness frequently involves the central nervous system and is associated with considerable morbidity and mortality. The diagnosis of neonatal herpes is particularly challenging when mucocutaneous lesions are absent, as it may resemble bacterial sepsis or other congenital infections (e.g., rubella or toxoplasmosis). Neonatal herpes infection should be diagnosed as early as possible since treatment with either acyclovir or vidarabine reduces morbidity and mortality.

Any vesicle, bulla, or erosion on the skin of a neonate should be cultured for herpes in addition to routine bacterial cultures. Rapid information can be obtained by a Tzanck smear (see Figs. 2.28 and 2.29), electron microscopy, or direct immunofluorescence, but viral cultures are desirable for confirmation. Confirmed and highly suspected cases should be treated as soon as possible with intravenous acyclovir or vidarabine.

DIFFERENTIAL DIAGNOSIS

When painful grouped vesicles with an erythematous base appear on the genital skin, the diagnosis is almost certainly herpes, but other STDs besides herpes also cause erosions that may be painful. Of these, chancroid (Fig. 2.23) most closely resembles herpes in the clinical presentation, frequently with multiple, painful erosions that develop an exudate similar to that seen in the postvesicular stages of genital herpes (see Chapter 3, Chancroid).

Syphilis also causes erosions on the genitals (Fig. 2.24), but a primary chancre of syphilis that is not secondarily infected with bacteria is usually solitary and not painful. In primary syphilis, dark-field examination of lesion exudate is positive if the area has not been recently treated with topical agents and the patient has not been taking oral antibiotics. In adults, secondary syphilis rarely is erosive, but never is vesicular. Serologic tests invariably are positive in secondary syphilis and should be done in any erosive genital lesions since STDs frequently coexist in such patients (see Chapter 1, Syphilis).

Traumatic genital ulcers are painful but ordinarily are not multiple or grouped. They have angular borders rather than the scalloped edge seen in herpes erosions (see Chapter 12, Nonvenereal Genital Dermatoses).

Contact dermatitis of the genitals usually is itchy and results in vesicles, crusting, and erosions. Secondary infection may result in tenderness. Because contact with the offending allergen may occur as long as two weeks before the dermatitis appears, diagnosis may be difficult. Vesicles and erosions should be

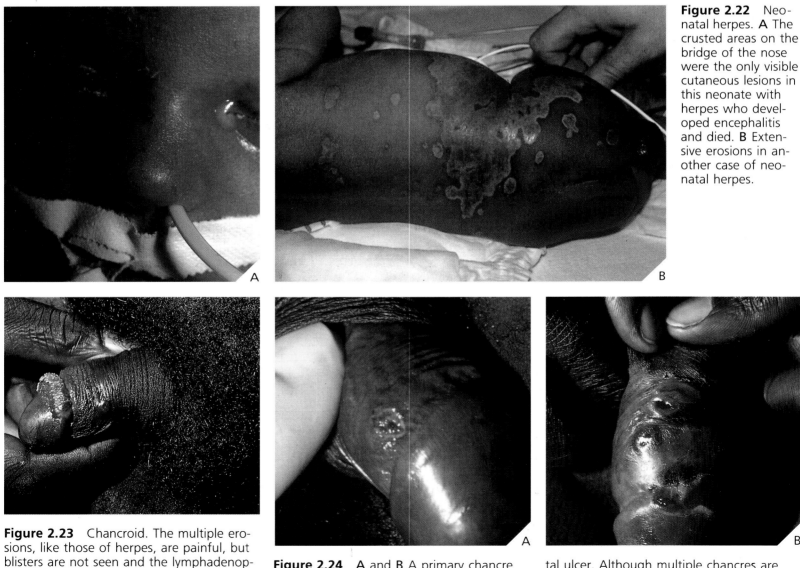

Figure 2.22 Neonatal herpes. **A** The crusted areas on the bridge of the nose were the only visible cutaneous lesions in this neonate with herpes who developed encephalitis and died. **B** Extensive erosions in another case of neonatal herpes.

Figure 2.23 Chancroid. The multiple erosions, like those of herpes, are painful, but blisters are not seen and the lymphadenopathy is more prominent than in comparable herpes eruptions.

Figure 2.24 **A** and **B** A primary chancre of syphilis is usually solitary and painless, but syphilis should be ruled out in any genital ulcer. Although multiple chancres are not common, the appearance may closely resemble that of genital herpes.

sampled for cytology (Tzanck smears), and viral cultures should be done to rule out herpes before the patient is treated for contact dermatitis (see Chapter 12).

Other bullous or erosive diseases, such as impetigo, pemphigus, pemphigoid, Hailey-Hailey disease (benign familial pemphigus) (Fig. 2.25), Darier's disease, Behcet's disease, and Crohn's disease, either may resemble herpes because of bullae or erosions or may become secondarily infected with the virus. Clinical history and diagnostic tests, including Tzanck smears, Gram stains, and cultures, usually clarify the problem, but biopsies occasionally may be necessary.

Laboratory Tests

Direct examination of clinical materials for virus or viral antigens and isolation and identification of viruses from clinical specimens provide the most commonly used specific and clinically useful techniques in the diagnosis of genital herpes.

DIRECT EXAMINATION OF CLINICAL SPECIMENS
Direct examination of clinical specimens permits the most rapid recognition and identification of HSV. Direct methods include

histopathology, cytopathology (CP), electron microscopy (EM), immunofluorescence (FA) and immunoenzyme (IE) techniques, enzyme immunoassay (EIA), and nucleic acid probes (NAPs). Histopathology and cytopathology permit identification of nuclear–cytoplasmic inclusions and other cellular alterations by light microscopy, while EM permits direct ultrastructural visualization of viral particles. With FA, IE, and EIA, the specimen is incubated with an antibody that is specific for the virus (viral antigen) to be identified and examined for the presence of specific fluorescence (FA) or color development (IE, EIA). NAPs use segments of RNA or DNA to detect and identify viral pathogens.

HISTOPATHOLOGY
Early herpes simplex infections are characterized by intracellular edema, suprabasal intraepidermal vesicles (Fig. 2.26), ballooning degeneration, and homogenization and margination of nuclear chromatin. Intranuclear inclusions and multinucleated giant cells are seen at the periphery of the lesions (Fig. 2.27). In later ulcerative stages, keratinocyte necrosis and lysis predominate. Inflammatory cells such as polymorphonuclear leukocytes and lymphocytes appear within the vesicle and der-

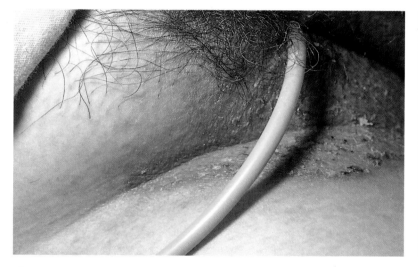

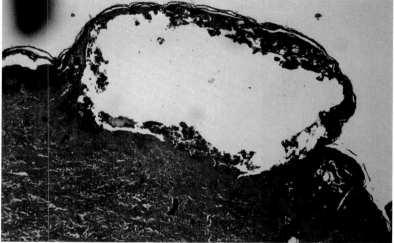

Figure 2.26 Intraepidermal vesicle of HSV infection.

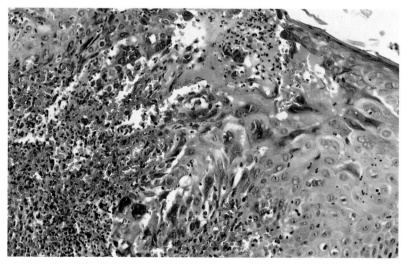

Figure 2.25 Benign familial pemphigus (Hailey-Hailey disease). Multiple fragile vesicles and bullae are seen at the edge of these characteristic erosive plaques. Clinical history and biopsies are diagnostic.

Figure 2.27 Periphery of HSV erosion showing single and multinucleated epithelial cells with "ground-glass" nuclei.

mis. As the lesion progresses, the epidermis sloughs; the remaining erosion reepithelializes as it heals. Cervical herpes infections are characterized by multinucleated giant cells and intranuclear "ground-glass" viral inclusions visualized on Papanicolaou smears. Biopsies are usually not performed, but show changes similar to those described above.

CYTOPATHOLOGY

Cytopathology is useful in identifying HSV infections because characteristic cytopathic effects occur in infected cells. Specimens from vesicular skin and mucosal lesions may be obtained by scraping the edge of the "unroofed" lesion with a sterile swab or scalpel blade and fixing the prepared slide in 95% ethanol, Zenker's solution, or Bouin's solution (Tzanck smear). HSV-infected cells usually exhibit a combination of virus-induced and degenerative changes. The virus predominantly in-

fects immature epithelial cells. Early manifestations of infection include (1) nuclear hypertrophy; (2) disappearance of nucleoli; (3) progressive increase in deoxyribonuclear protein (DRNP), which imparts a distinct, homogeneous, "ground-glass" appearance to the nucleus; and (4) displacement of the nuclear chromatin to the periphery, where it adheres and imparts a "thicker" appearance to the nuclear membrane (Fig. 2.28). Multinucleated giant cells, produced by fusion of cytoplasmic membranes of individual infected cells, frequently are observed; the nuclei vary in size and shape and usually mold against one another (Fig. 2.29).

Later in the course of HSV infection, the DRNP condenses, moves to the center of the nucleus, and forms a single, coarsely granular, acidophilic, intranuclear inclusion surrounded by a prominent halo (Fig. 2.30). Degenerative changes (not HSV-specific) also occur in infected cells; these include increased

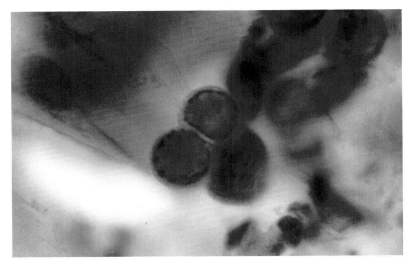

Figure 2.28 HSV-infected cells in a cytology specimen exhibiting homogeneous, "ground-glass"-appearing nuclei and peripheral chromatin margination imparting an irregular and more distinct appearance to the nuclear membrane.

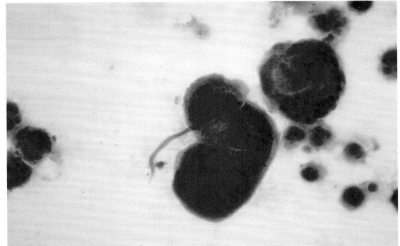

Figure 2.29 Multinucleated giant HSV-infected cell showing variation in nuclear size and shape and molding of individual nuclei against one another.

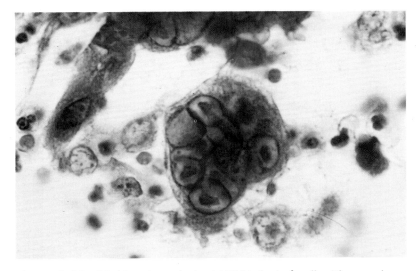

Figure 2.30 Multinucleated giant HSV-infected cell with prominent intranuclear inclusions surrounded by distinct halos.

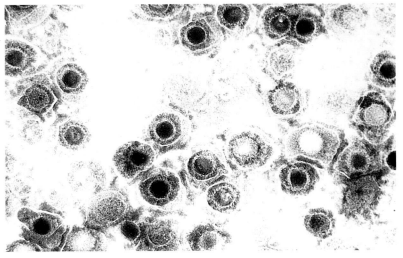

Figure 2.31 HSV particles detected by direct EM. Defective or damaged particles have dark centers due to penetration of phosphotungstic acid stain into the viral nucleocapsid.

cytoplasmic and nuclear vacuolization, loss of normal cell shape, and, in later stages of infection, breakage of cytoplasmic and nuclear membranes. Cytologic changes alone cannot serve to differentiate primary HSV infections from recurrent HSV and, similarly, do not distinguish HSV-2 infections from those due to HSV-1. Most cytologists do not attempt to differentiate infection caused by HSV from that due to varicella-zoster virus on cytologic morphology alone.

ELECTRON MICROSCOPY

Electron microscopy (EM) is most applicable for investigating viral infections in which the concentration of viral particles in the clinical specimen is greater than 10^6 to 10^7 particles/mL. To permit detection and definitive identification of virus morphology, the specimen also must be free of background debris. Types of specimens examined usually include biopsies or fluid and scrapings from vesicles.

Following appropriate preparation, clinical specimens are negatively stained with 2 to 4% phosphotungstic acid and are examined directly for the presence of virus (Fig. 2.31). En-

hancement techniques can be used to increase the sensitivity of EM when examining clinical specimens with virus titers lower than 10^6 particles/mL. Pseudoreplica and agar gel diffusion, which can be used to concentrate and purify clinical specimens, are useful procedures for identifying HSV in vesicle or body fluids. Since all viruses in the herpes group have an identical ultrastructural morphologic appearance, the technique of immune EM (IEM) must be used for specific identification. IEM provides direct observation of the interaction of the virus with homologous antibody (Fig. 2.32).

IMMUNOFLUORESCENCE METHODS

Immunofluorescence (FA) techniques are time-honored, reliable methods for the diagnosis of HSV. They can be used to detect viral antigens in clinical specimens (Fig. 2.33) or to confirm the presence of HSV in cell cultures inoculated with clinical materials (Fig. 2.34).

Clinical specimens or viral cultures can be evaluated for HSV by either direct (DFA) or indirect (IFA) methods. With DFA staining, fluorescein isothiocyanate (FITC)-labeled HSV-specific

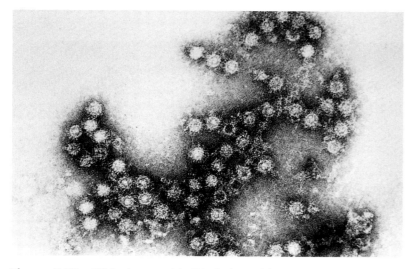

Figure 2.32 IEM of coxsackie B4 viral particles. An aggregate is formed of individual particles linked together by specific antibody (anti-coxsackie B4).

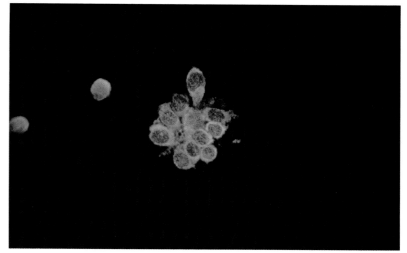

Figure 2.33 DFA of HSV-infected cells obtained from scraping an ulcerated genital lesion.

Figure 2.34 FA of HSV-infected cells in a cell culture monolayer previously inoculated with a clinical specimen from a genital lesion.

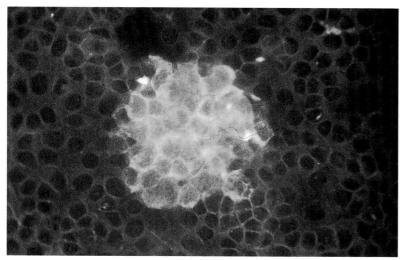

immunoglobulin (anti-HSV) binds directly to HSV-infected cells present in the specimen (Figs. 2.35 and 2.36A). With IFA staining, the anti-HSV is not FITC-labeled (Fig. 2.36B); rather, a FITC-labeled antispecies immunoglobulin is used to detect the anti-HSV bound to the HSV-infected cells. IFA methods are more sensitive than DFA methods; however, DFA has several advantages over IFA, including greater specificity, cleaner background (less nonspecific fluorescence), fewer necessary manipulations and reagents, and less time required for incubation (one step instead of two). DFA permits detection of viral antigens only, whereas IFA can be used for detection of either anti-HSV or HSV antigens. Most commercially available reagents for detection of HSV are monoclonal antibody products intended for use with DFA methodology (Fig. 2.35). Most of these products are also licensed for use in "typing" HSV present in clinical specimens, although this procedure is not always necessary. Specimens that can be used for FA diagnosis include frozen sections of tissue, impression smears, lesion scrapings, or resuspended cells from centifuged sediment. After preparation, the slides are air-dried completely and fixed (usually in acetone or methanol) prior to staining with anti-HSV. If needed, slides can be stored for long periods of time at −70°C.

Strict criteria and appropriate positive and negative controls must be used in interpreting FA results. Fluorescence must be bright, apple green in color (with FITC conjugates), and appropriate in cellular location. To diagnose HSV infection, nuclear fluorescence must be observed; cytoplasmic fluorescence may also occur. False-positive fluorescence can be encountered with leukocytes, mucus, and yeasts; leukocytes possess immunoglobulin Fc receptors that can nonspecifically bind conjugates (Fig. 2.37). False-negative tests can occur when an insufficient number of viral particles (antigens) are present or when reagents do not perform optimally.

IMMUNOENZYME METHODS

Immunoenzyme (IE) methods are now being widely used as a substitute for FA procedures to examine smears of clinical lesions for the presence of HSV. The general principles of specimen handling and preparation are similar. However, the ability to identify a colored final reaction product that can be visualized with an ordinary bright-field microscope offers great advantages for diagnostic histopathology and cytology. The enzyme, which is attached to the specific antibody to be used, substitutes for the FITC that was used as the detector system in FA meth-

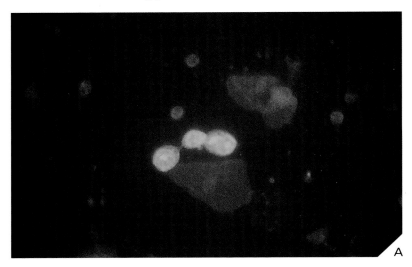

Figure 2.35 DFA test. **A** Positive result for HSV-2 with monoclonal antibody. **B** Negative result for HSV-2 with monoclonal antibody.

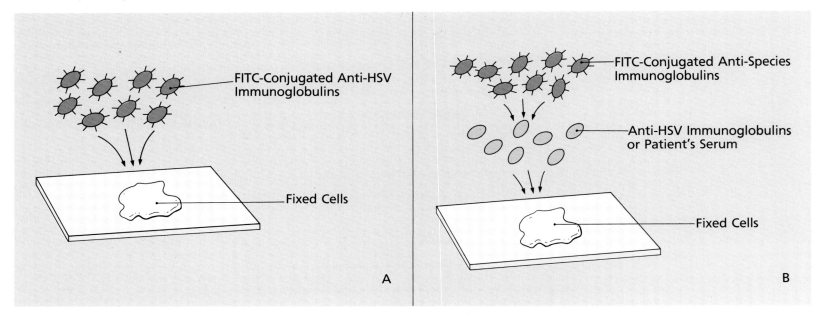

Figure 2.36 **A** The direct immunofluorescence test. **B** The indirect immunofluorescence test.

odology. The enzyme, when reacted with its specific chromogenic substrate, yields a colored product. Enzyme-conjugate methods are generally more sensitive than fluorochrome-conjugate ones because the former produce a higher signal, the intensity of which is determined by the length of the enzyme reaction time. New designs in methodology and the introduction of monoclonal antibodies and the avidin–biotin amplification system have greatly increased the sensitivity and specificity of these immunocytochemical methods. These procedures are easy to perform, do not require a fluorescence microscope, and constitute a permanent record since the color of the chromogenic product remains stable for indefinite periods.

ENZYME IMMUNOASSAYS (SOLID PHASE)

Enzyme immunoassay (EIA), including enzyme-linked immunosorbent assay (ELISA), also detects viral antigens by using as an indicator the action of an enzyme on its specific substrate. However, EIA methods detect viral antigens that are present in solution, usually contained in a small cylindrical tube or in microtiter plate wells. Specimens appropriate for detecting HSV

antigens by EIA are swabs of vesicular fluid or genital tract lesions. Several EIA systems currently are available for detection of HSV.

NUCLEIC ACID PROBES

Nucleic acid probes (NAPs) (Fig. 2.38) are discrete segments of single-stranded RNA or DNA that can bind covalently (hybridize) with their specific complementary strand of nucleic acid. Hybridization can occur between complementary DNA strands (DNA–DNA duplex), complementary RNA strands (RNA–RNA duplex), or complementary RNA and DNA strands (RNA–DNA hybrid). NAP technology can detect and identify viral pathogens in only a few hours. The probe is mixed with the clinical specimen under proper conditions so that denaturation (separation of double-stranded DNA) can occur; if the specimen contains a nucleic acid segment complementary to the labeled nucleic acid sequence of the probe, hybridization will take place and a double-stranded structure containing the probe will be formed. The labeled probe (radioactive tag, enzyme label) then can be treated to allow visualization. Biotin–avidin labeling often is used to increase the sensitivity of the reaction. At pres-

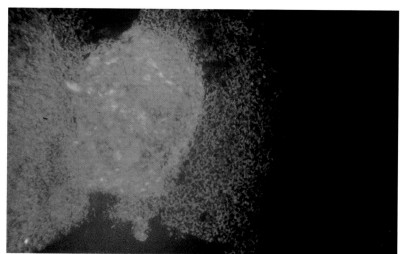

Figure 2.37 Nonspecific FA due to binding of labeled antibody via the Fc portion of the molecule to leukocyte Fc receptors.

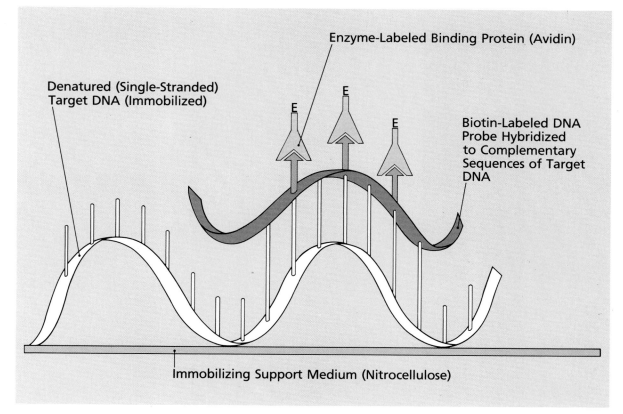

Figure 2.38 Nucleic acid probe. DNA probes bind to viral DNA to form a visible reaction product indicating the presence of HSV DNA sequences in clinical specimens or viral isolates.

Enzyme-Labeled Binding Protein (Avidin)

Denatured (Single-Stranded) Target DNA (Immobilized)

Biotin-Labeled DNA Probe Hybridized to Complementary Sequences of Target DNA

Immobilizing Support Medium (Nitrocellulose)

ent, most materials to be tested (clinical specimens, viral isolates) need to be affixed to a solid matrix (usually some type of filter or glass microscope slide); however, newer techniques and probes are under development that will not require a solid matrix for testing. NAPs presently are available commercially for use in detecting DNA sequences of HSV-1 and HSV-2.

IDENTIFICATION OF VIRUSES FROM CLINICAL SPECIMENS

Virus Isolation

In general, virus isolation takes longer than direct methods to detect viruses in clinical specimens. Yet isolation is a more sensitive technique (except, perhaps, for NAPs) because clinical specimens usually contain only small numbers of viral particles and amplification in host systems is necessary for detection. Moreover, virus isolation has the added advantage of permitting recovery of additional viral agents (other than the one primarily being considered) from clinical specimens. Host systems for isolating HSV from clinical specimens include cell cultures and embryonated hens' eggs. Most diagnostic virology laboratories that perform isolation for HSV utilize cell monolayers.

The likelihood of recovery of HSV in culture relates to the clinical phase of the lesion; the yield is generally higher from vesicular (94%) than from pustular (87%), ulcerated (70%), or crusted (27%) lesions. HSV-1 and HSV-2 replicate well in many primary or established cell lines of human or primate origin. However, Vero cells (a continuous African monkey kidney cell line) and human diploid lines (such as foreskin fibroblasts or embryonic lung fibroblasts) (Fig. 2.39) are especially recommended.

When a specimen contains a high titer of HSV particles, cytopathic effect (CPE) may be detected as early as 24 hours after inoculation. In most cases, visible CPE usually develops within two to four days. HSV-infected cells in the monolayer develop a cytoplasmic granularity and become enlarged, ballooned, and, eventually, round and refractile (glassy) (Fig. 2.40). Individual lesions grow in size as cell-to-adjacent-cell spread of virus oc-

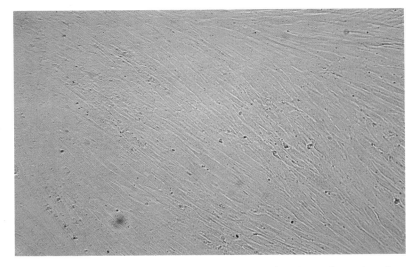

Figure 2.39 Human diploid fibroblast monolayer—uninoculated.

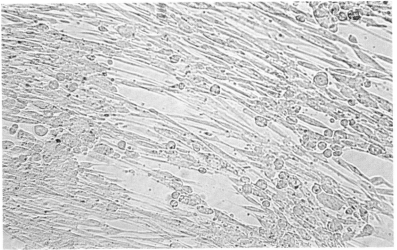

Figure 2.40 Human diploid fibroblasts infected with HSV and showing cytopathic effects. There is extensive cell rounding, and many degenerated cells have fallen off the glass surface.

Figure 2.41 One-dram shell vial containing cell media and coverslip with cell monolayer.

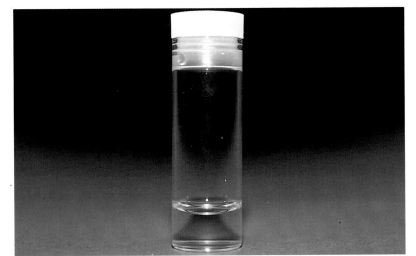

curs; eventually, the entire monolayer becomes infected. Multinucleated giant cells usually are identified. If typing of the HSV isolates is desired, isolates of HSV-1 may be distinguished from isolates of HSV-2 by a variety of procedures, most commonly FA or IE.

Rapid detection of HSV in cell culture as early as 16 hours following inoculation and prior to the development of visible CPE, usually requiring two to four days, can be accomplished using coverslip monolayers in shell vials (Fig. 2.41). Centrifugation of the specimen onto the monolayer and the use of monoclonal antibodies specifically directed against HSV early antigens, expressed on cell membranes within a few hours following HSV attachment and penetration, are key elements in this procedure. Positive reactions may be visualized using a fluorochrome-labeled antibody or by immunoenzymatic reactions that generate a visible color. This methodology offers the advantages of (1) increased sensitivity (due to host amplification of the number of virus particles) compared with rapid methods performed directly on clinical specimens and (2) reduction in the time required to detect viral agents in cell culture (16 to 24 hours) compared with conventional methods (two to four days).

Serology

A variety of serologic techniques have been developed to detect HSV antibodies. Such assays have shown that the seroprevalence of HSV antibodies in adults exceeds 50%. Very few clinical laboratories performing HSV serology use assays that discriminate between HSV-1 and HSV-2. In individuals presenting with a first episode of genital herpes, serologic studies can differentiate between primary and nonprimary infection, but such knowledge will have no effect on management. In recurrent genital herpes, less than 10% of individuals will develop a significant rise in antibody titer. Serology is therefore not recommended in the diagnosis of genital herpes.

Treatment

Perhaps the most important aspect in the management of genital herpes is educating patients regarding their condition. Such education includes advising patients to abstain from sexual contact if prodromal symptoms or lesions are present. Some patients will require extensive counseling. Women should be advised to inform their obstetric care provider(s) of their condition if they are pregnant.

Presently, acyclovir is the only drug of proven efficacy in the treatment of genital herpes (Fig. 2.42). Acyclovir is an acyclic derivative of the nucleoside guanosine. Acyclovir is actually a "prodrug," which must be phosphorylated by a virus-specified enzyme, thymidine kinase, to acyclovir monophosphate. Cellular enzymes further phosphorylate the compound into the active drug, acyclovir triphosphate, which is a potent inhibitor of viral DNA polymerase. Additionally, some acyclovir triphosphate gets incorporated into new viral DNA and functions as a DNA chain terminator. Many individuals with genital herpes do not require acyclovir since (1) lesions will heal spontaneously, (2) acyclovir

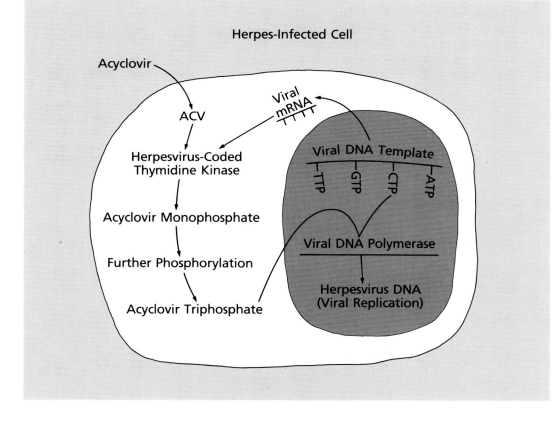

Figure 2.42 Mechanism of action of acyclovir in infected cell.

is expensive, and (3) the benefits of acyclovir are modest, except in immunosuppressed patients. Acyclovir is contraindicated during pregnancy. Recommendations regarding treatment of genital herpes are discussed below and summarized in Figure 2.43.

FIRST EPISODE GENITAL HERPES
Individuals with severe first episode herpes occasionally require hospitalization, particularly when serious neurologic complications occur. This small subset of individuals should be treated with intravenous acyclovir, 5 mg/kg over 60 min every eight hours for five days, in addition to supportive care, which frequently includes analgesics. Some women will require a urinary catheter either for urinary retention or because voiding is extremely painful due to spillage of urine onto herpetic lesions (external dysuria). Most other individuals with first episode genital herpes should be treated with oral acyclovir, 200 mg five times daily for 10 days. Occasional individuals with first episode genital herpes do not require acyclovir therapy. These include pregnant women, individuals with mild manifestations, and individuals presenting later in their course with most or all lesions in the crust stage.

The benefit of acyclovir therapy in first episode genital herpes is greater in primary than in nonprimary infection, but such a distinction is available only retrospectively. Acyclovir treatment of first episode genital herpes has no effect on the subsequent recurrence pattern.

RECURRENT GENITAL HERPES
Four strategies of management can be used in the management of recurrent genital herpes: (1) no specific therapy, (2) episodic oral acyclovir, (3) chronic suppressive oral acyclovir, or (4) episodic suppressive oral acyclovir. No antiviral therapy is required for many individuals with recurrent genital herpes, particularly those with mild and/or infrequent episodes.

Oral acyclovir, 200 mg five times daily for five days, may be given for each episode. Such episodic therapy will accelerate healing by about 1½ days with little pain reduction and is particularly suited for individuals with infrequent severe episodes, particularly with a long prodrome.

Chronic suppressive oral acyclovir is highly effective, suppressing about 90% of recurrences. Many individuals will respond to 200 mg twice daily, but the dose frequency may need to be increased to three or four times daily in a few patients. Suppressive therapy is safe and effective for at least a year at a time. Chronic suppressive therapy is particularly suited to individuals with frequent recurrences (more than about eight per year). It is recommended that a temporary "drug holiday" be given after a year of continuous therapy to reevaluate the natural recurrence frequency. In some individuals, the recurrence frequency diminishes sufficiently that chronic prophylaxis is no longer required. Thus far, some individuals have safely and effectively been treated with chronic suppressive acyclovir therapy for over 3½ years, except for brief drug holidays.

Episodic suppressive oral acyclovir refers to the administration of suppressive doses of oral acyclovir to individuals with recurrent genital herpes over short periods of time when a recurrence would be particularly distressing. Such occasions would include honeymoons, holidays, and important school examinations.

TOPICAL ACYCLOVIR
Topical acyclovir is ineffective in recurrent genital herpes and shows only trivial benefit in primary genital herpes. It is less effective than oral acyclovir, and its use is not recommended.

Picture credits for this chapter are as follows: Fig. 2.1 courtesy of McKendrick GDW, Sutherland S: An Introduction to Herpes Infections. London, Gower Medical Publishing Ltd, 1983; Fig. 2.3 adapted from Nahmias AJ, Josey WE, Naib ZM, et al: Antibodies to Herpesvirus hominis types 1 and 2 in humans: 1. Patients with genital herpetic infections. Am J Epidemiol 91:539, 1970; Fig. 2.4 adapted from Straus SE (moderator): Herpes simplex virus infection: Biology, treatment, and prevention. Ann Intern Med 103:404, 1985; Fig. 2.5 courtesy of Milton Tam, MD; Figs. 2.12 and 2.13 courtesy of Barbara Romenowski, MD; Fig. 2.16 courtesy of David Mandeville and Peter Lane, MD; Fig. 2.22 courtesy of Mary Spraker, MD; Fig. 2.42 adapted from Mertz GJ, Corey L: Genital herpes simplex virus infections in adults. Urol Clin N Am 11:107; 1983.

Figure 2.43 Treatment of genital herpes.

TREATMENT OF GENITAL HERPES

PRESENTATION	TREATMENT
First episode Severe, requiring hospitalization	Acyclovir 5 mg/kg IV over 60 min q8h × 5 days
Presentation when lesions are already crusted	No antiviral treatment
All others	Acyclovir 200 mg PO five times daily × 10 days
Recurrent episodes Infrequent and/or mild	No antiviral treatment
Infrequent and moderate to severe	Episodal acyclovir 200 mg PO five times daily × 5 days
Frequent	Chronic suppressive oral acyclovir 200 mg two to four times daily
Pregnant women	Acyclovir is contraindicated in pregnancy, but may be considered for severe neurologic complications of primary disease

BIBLIOGRAPHY

Bryan JA: Laboratory diagnosis of viral infections, in Conn RB (ed): *Current Diagnosis*, ed 7. Philadelphia, W.B. Saunders, 1985, pp 174–182.

Corey L, Adams HG, Brown ZA, et al: Genital herpes simplex virus infection clinical manifestations, course, and complications. *Ann Intern Med* 98:958, 1983.

Corey L, Holmes KK: Genital herpes simplex virus infections: Current concepts in diagnosis, therapy, and prevention. *Ann Intern Med* 98:973, 1983.

Drew WL, Rawls WE: Herpes simplex viruses, in Lennette EH, Balows A, Hausler Jr WJ, Shadomy HJ (eds): *Manual of Clinical Microbiology*, ed 4. American Society of Microbiology, 1985, pp 705–710.

Genital herpes infection—United States, 1966–1979. MMWR 31:137, 1982.

Gill MJ, Arlette J, Buchan K: Herpes simplex virus infection of the hand: A profile of 79 cases. *Am J Med* 84:89, 1988.

Guinan ME, Wolinsky SM, Reichman RC: Epidemiology of genital herpes simplex infections. *Epidemiol Rev* 7:127, 1985.

Keyserling HL, Nahmias A: Herpes simplex viral infections, in Conn RB (ed): *Current Diagnosis*, ed 7. Philadelphia, W.B. Saunders, 1985, pp 197–203.

Lafferty WE, Coombs RW, Benedetti J, et al: Recurrences after oral and genital herpes simplex virus infections: Influence of site of infection and viral type. *N Engl J Med* 316:1444, 1987.

Nahmias AJ, Josey WE, Naib ZM, et al: Antibodies to *Herpesvirus hominis* types 1 and 2 in humans: I. Patients with genital herpetic infections. *Am J Epidemiol* 91:539, 1970.

Prober CG, Sullender WM, Yasukawa LL, et al: Low risk of herpes simplex virus infections in neonates exposed to the virus at the time of vaginal delivery to mothers with recurrent genital herpes virus infections. *N Engl J Med* 316:240, 1987.

Rooney, JF, Felser JM, Ostrove JM, Straus SE: Acquisition of genital herpes from an asymptomatic sexual partner. *N Engl J Med* 314:1561, 1986.

Sacks SL: Frequency and duration of patient-observed recurrent genital herpes simplex virus infection: Characterization of the nonlesional prodrome. *J Infect Dis* 150:873, 1984.

Sacks SL: The role of oral acyclovir in the management of genital herpes simplex. *Can Med Assoc J* 136:701, 1987.

Stavraky KM, Rawls WE, Chiavetta J, et al: Sexual and economic factors affecting the risk of past infections with herpes simplex virus type 2. *Am J Epidemiol* 118:109, 1983.

Straus SE (moderator): Herpes simplex virus infection: Biology, treatment, and prevention. *Ann Intern Med* 103:404, 1985.

Straus SE, Croen KD, Sawyer MH, et al: Acyclovir suppression of frequently recurring genital herpes: Efficacy and diminishing need during successive years of treatment. JAMA 260:2227, 1988.

Whitley RJ, Nahmias AJ, Visintine AM, et al: The natural history of herpes simplex virus infection of mother and newborn. *Pediatrics* 66:489, 1980.

Chancroid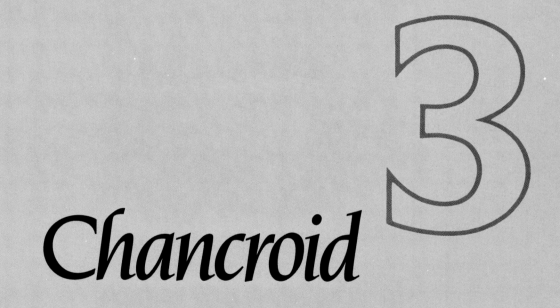

G.P. SCHMID, W.O. SCHALLA, W.E. DeWITT

Introduction

Chancroid, or soft chancre (ulcus molle), is characterized by one or more genital ulcers (chancres) and often by painful inguinal lymphadenopathy. The disease was differentiated clinically from syphilis by Bassereau in France in 1852. In 1889, Ducrey in Italy showed the infectious origin of the disease by inoculating the forearm skin of human volunteers with purulent material from their own genital ulcers. At weekly intervals, he inoculated a new site with material from the most recent ulcer and, following the fifth or sixth reinoculation in each patient, he found a single microorganism in the ulcer exudate. The organism described was a short, compact, streptobacillary rod. Ducrey could not, however, isolate the causative bacterium that now bears his name, *Haemophilus ducreyi*. Isolation was accomplished by other workers by 1900.

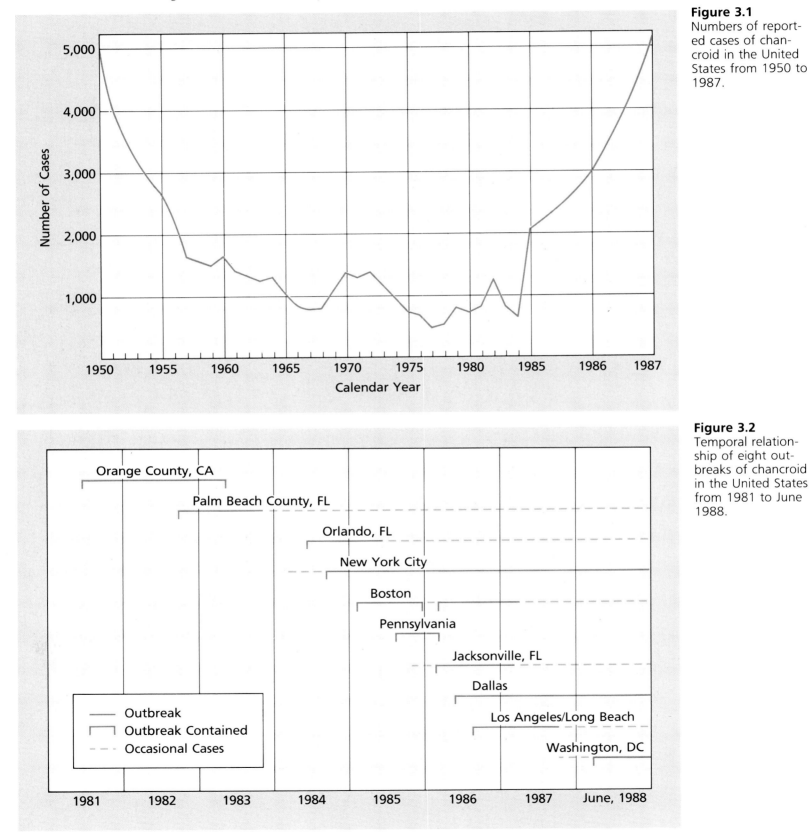

Figure 3.1
Numbers of reported cases of chancroid in the United States from 1950 to 1987.

Figure 3.2
Temporal relationship of eight outbreaks of chancroid in the United States from 1981 to June 1988.

Epidemiology

Although chancroid is an uncommon disease in the United States and other developed countries, it is quite common in developing parts of the world. In many countries, it is the most common cause of genital ulcers, and its global incidence is said to exceed that of syphilis. In general, the incidence of chancroid is related to poor living conditions and is often prominent during times of war.

In the United States, the number of reported cases of chancroid peaked in 1947, when over 10,000 cases were reported (Fig. 3.1). The number of cases then declined, reaching a mean level of 878 cases annually between 1971 and 1980. Since 1981, however, the numbers have begun to rise. In 1985, the number of reported cases rose above 2,000 for the first time since 1956 in 1987, 5,047 cases were reported.

The recent increase in number of cases is the result of increasingly frequent outbreaks of disease that began in 1981 and have occurred in a number of cities with increasing frequency (Fig. 3.2). Some outbreaks have distinct dates of onset, probably related to the entrance of infected, highly sexually active individuals into a previously nonendemic area. Other outbreaks have had indistinct dates of onset and probably represent escalation of already endemic disease. It is known that individuals have become infected in outbreak areas and have sought treatment outside these areas, thus probably spreading disease to additional areas. Only the outbreaks in Orange County, California, and southeastern Pennsylvania have been successfully terminated. The outbreak in Boston was originally thought to have been terminated, only to subsequently recur. In other areas, small numbers of cases have continued.

The outbreaks share many epidemiologic features. Disease is occurring predominantly in black and Hispanic males. Prostitution has been important in many of the outbreaks outside of Florida; in Florida, however, disease appears to be occurring among sexually active individuals not associated with prostitution. In addition, other areas have reported cases of chancroid. We have concluded that this disease appears to be highly localized (Fig. 3.3). Because individuals may be infected in one area and travel to another, however, individuals with chancroid may be seen anywhere.

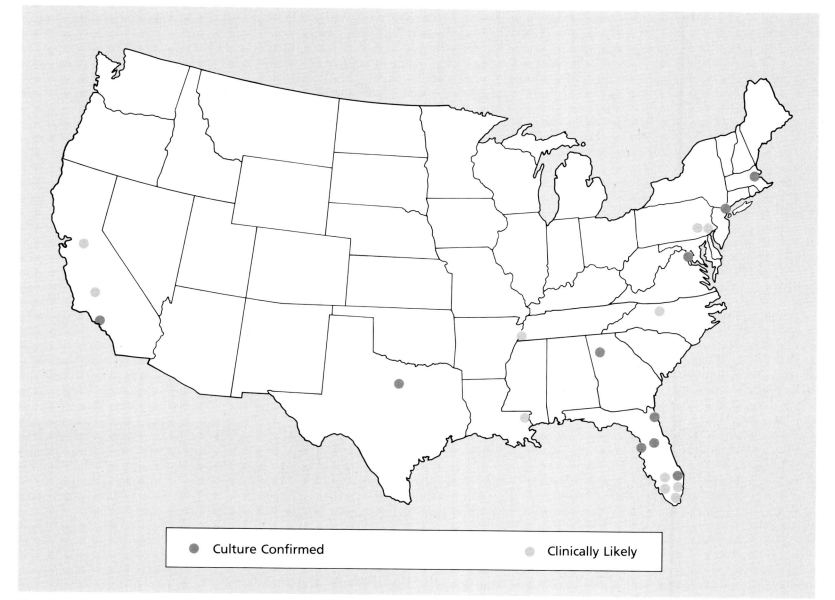

Figure 3.3 Cities in the United States where at least three culture-confirmed or clinically diagnosed cases of chancroid were reported in one calendar year from 1983 to June 1988.

The majority of cases occurs in males (Fig. 3.4). This is probably the result of a combination of factors: more easily visible male anatomy, small numbers of infected prostitutes having sexual relations with many men, women with cervical ulcers who are asymptomatic, and possibly infected women without symptoms or signs of disease.

Clinical Manifestations

The incubation period is usually 4 to 10 days, but longer incubation periods are not uncommon. The chancre begins as a tender, erythematous papule at the site of inoculation (Fig. 3.5); some patients do not recall a papule but describe an initial erythematous, shallow ulcer. The early lesion may be described simply as a "sore." Over the next one to two days, the papule erodes into a painful ulcer. Some ulcers may be quite superficial (Fig. 3.6), but most are deep (Figs. 3.7 to 3.9); the ulcers are excavated into the skin and often have a beefy, granular base. The edge of the ulcer is usually irregular, has a red margin, and

is not indurated. The tenderness of the ulcer often makes examination difficult. The ulcer is sometimes masked by dried or crusted exudate that, when gently removed by saline-soaked gauze, will reveal the ulceration. In men, ulcers often occur on the prepuce, resulting in phimosis, a painful inability to retract the prepuce (Figs. 3.10 and 3.11).

As the disease progresses, as many as one-half of the cases develop unilateral or bilateral inguinal lymphadenopathy, which is characteristically painful even though nodes may be small (Fig. 3.12). Adenopathy ranges from being barely palpable—yet quite painful—to quite large. Buboes (large, fluctuant lymph nodes) may occur, a finding that is not seen with syphilis or genital herpes. In the absence of effective treatment and prophylactic needle drainage, buboes frequently suppurate, leaving fistulas or secondary ulcers at the drainage site (Fig. 3.13). A variant form of ulcer known as chancre mou volant (transient chancre) has been described, which involutes spontaneously after four to six days but may be followed by diagnostically puzzling inguinal adenopathy.

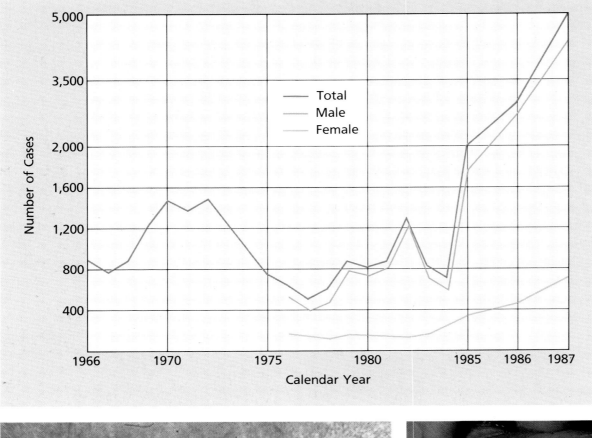

Figure 3.4 Reported cases of chancroid by sex in the United States from 1966 to 1987.

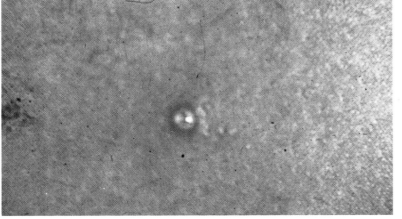

Figure 3.5 Papule, the first sign of infection, at site where ulcer will appear.

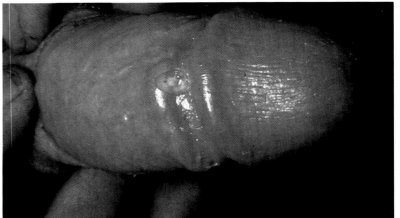

Figure 3.6 Superficial ulcer in coronal sulcus.

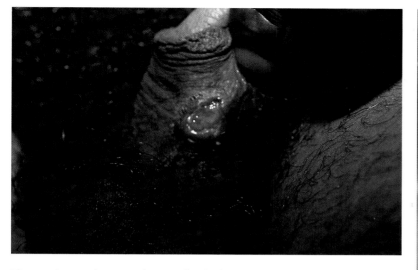

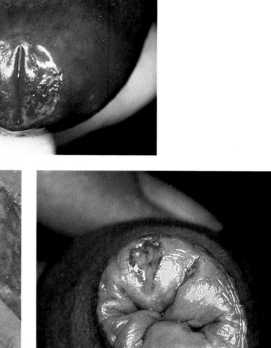

Figure 3.8
Although most ul-
cers in men occur
on the foreskin or
shaft, ulcers can oc-
cur on the glans.

Figure 3.7   Ulcer on the penile shaft, with beefy red base.

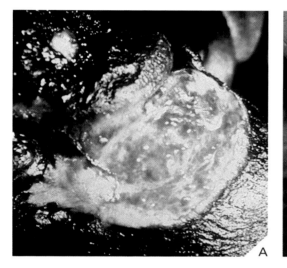

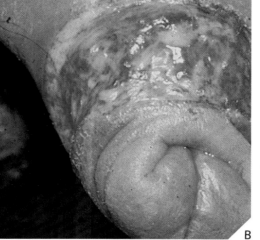

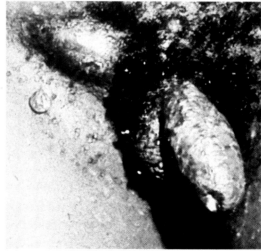

Figure 3.9   Extensive ulceration may occur.
A and **B** The base of the ulcer in both lesions is granular and friable.

Figure 3.10   Lesions occurring on the prepuce are commonly associated with swelling of the prepuce; retraction of the foreskin may be impossible.

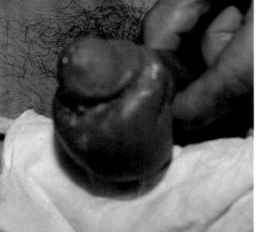

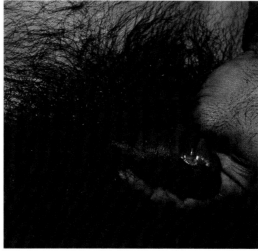

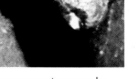

Figure 3.11   Ulcer on the retracted prepuce (not visible) with secondary edema.

Figure 3.12   Ulcer on the prepuce, with
visibly enlarged inguinal lymph nodes showing overlying erythema of the skin.

Figure 3.13   Buboes may spontaneously
suppurate and subsequently form draining,
chronic fistulas.

Ulcers in women usually occur in the vulvar area; carriage of H. *ducreyi* without any sign of infection appears to be very uncommon (Figs. 3.14 to 3.16).

There are several differences in disease expression between men and women (Fig. 3.17). In about one-half of individuals, there is more than one ulcer. In men, it is unusual to have more than four ulcers. Men are invariably symptomatic, but an occasional woman may not be symptomatic due to the presence of asymptomatic ulcers on the cervix or in the vagina. Anal ulcers in women are thought to be the result of drainage or autoinoculation and not necessarily anal intercourse. The relative infrequency of adenopathy in women is presumably due to differences in lymphatic drainage between males and females.

Ulcers may occur in the mouth as a result of oral intercourse and, rarely, elsewhere on the body because of autoinoculation (Fig. 3.18). Colonization of the mouth, cervix, and penis in the absence of signs or symptoms has been described.

DIFFERENTIAL DIAGNOSIS

The two diseases that most commonly must be differentiated from chancroid are syphilis and genital herpes; one of these diseases coexists with chancroid in about 10% of chancroid cases. In contrast to the ulcers of syphilis, the ulcers of chancroid almost invariably are tender and, in contrast to the ulcers of genital herpes, they tend to be deeper and not grouped (Fig. 3.19). A dark-field examination of the lesion and a serologic test for syphilis should always be performed. Ideally, a follow-up serologic test for syphilis should be performed, as current therapy for chancroid cannot be relied upon to successfully treat syphilis. Lymphogranuloma venereum may occasionally need to be differentiated from chancroid, particularly when lymphadenopathy is the prominent feature of the clinical presentation. The ulcer sometimes associated with lymphogranuloma venereum, however, is not a prominent part of the illness, is transitory, and precedes the appearance of lymphadenopathy. Granuloma inguinale, although causing destructive lesions in the genital area, is not associated with acute, painful ulcerations or lymphadenopathy (although lesions in the inguinal area can occur).

Laboratory Tests
HISTOPATHOLOGY

Biopsy of ulcers, although not studied in recent years, was formerly described as being diagnostically useful. A biopsy specimen 3 mm in diameter from the ulcer base or bubo wall, obtained without the necessity of anesthesia, is adequate for

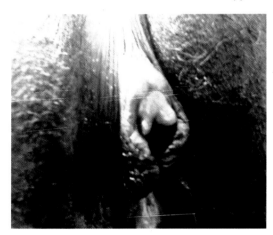
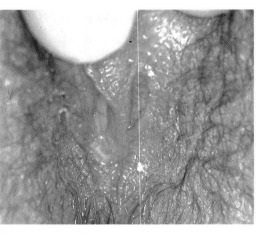
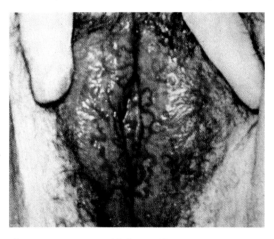

Figure 3.14 Single, erythematous ulcer of the vaginal introitus.

Figure 3.15 Single ulcer with granular base of the vaginal fourchette; ulcers are commonly found also in the perineum.

Figure 3.16 Multiple shallow, erythematous, serpiginous ulcers of the labia.

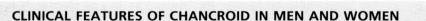

CLINICAL FEATURES OF CHANCROID IN MEN AND WOMEN

FEATURES	MEN	WOMEN
Genital ulcer(s)	1 to 4 in number Usually on prepuce (uncircumcised) or coronal sulcus (circumcised) Painful ulcers	1 to 7 in number Usually vulvar, but anal and cervical ulcers may occur Painful ulcers on vulva or anus; cervical ulcers asymptomatic
Inguinal lymphadenopathy	Up to 50% of cases Painful Large nodes suppurate May be bilateral	Occasionally Painful Suppuration not common May be bilateral

Figure 3.17 Clinical features of chancroid in men and women.

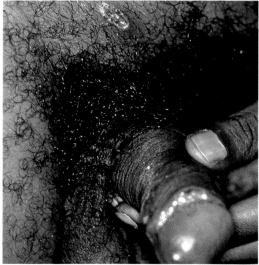

Figure 3.18 Ulcers at areas distant from the site of initial inoculation may be formed by autoinoculation.

study. Three histologic zones occur in lesions of 2 to 3 weeks' duration (Fig. 3.20). The first, from the base of the ulcer, is shallow and consists of polymorphonuclear leukocytes, fibrin, red blood cells, and necrotic tissue. Below this surface zone is a wide cellular zone in which the predominant cells are proliferating endothelial cells, both within existing vessels and by cells involved in new vessel formation. Near the surface zone, vessels may be infiltrated with neutrophils and may be undergoing necrosis. The supporting connective tissue is edematous and, in contrast to the endothelial cell proliferation, there is a marked lack of fibroblast proliferation. The interstitium is infiltrated by neutrophils near the surface zone and deeper by lymphocytes and plasma cells. Finally, the deep zone of the ulcer is characterized by a marked infiltration of plasma

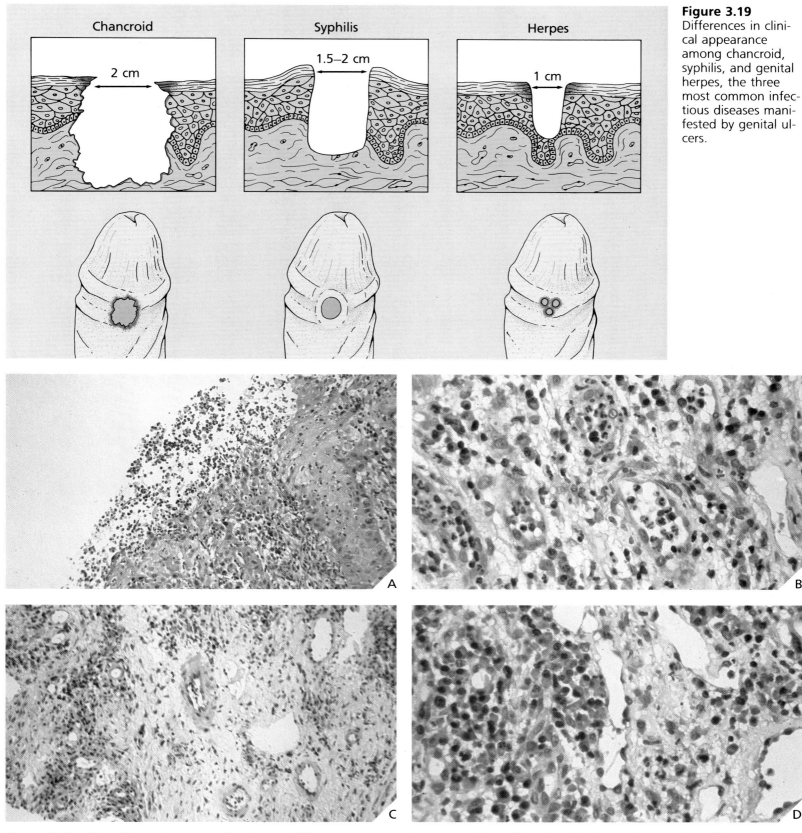

Figure 3.19 Differences in clinical appearance among chancroid, syphilis, and genital herpes, the three most common infectious diseases manifested by genital ulcers.

Figure 3.20 Ulcer biopsy demonstrating three cellular zones. **A** At the surface is an inflammatory exudate with partial ulceration of the skin (hematoxylin and eosin). **B** Below the base is a wide cellular zone, with proliferating blood vessels. **C** In the cellular zone there is granulation tissue with edema of the connective tissue. **D** Deeper cellular zone, composed of plasma cells and lymphocytes.

cells and, less so, by lymphocytes. Some endothelial proliferation within the vessel lumen may be seen, but there is neither infiltration of the vessel walls by inflammatory cells nor endothelial necrosis. Occasionally, organisms morphologically compatible with H. ducreyi may be seen in the first or the upper middle zone.

SPECIMEN COLLECTION

Before obtaining Gram stain and culture material, the ulcer base should be exposed and free of pus. If necessary, crusted pus can be removed by gentle soaks with sterile saline; it is otherwise unnecessary to clean the ulcer. Gram stain material should be obtained from the base or margins with a cotton or calcium alginate swab and rolled over the slide to preserve cellular morphology, which might be disturbed by smearing the material. Material for culture should be obtained from the base or margins of the ulcer with either a swab or a wire loop. The ability of transport media to maintain H. ducreyi has not been well studied, and it is best to directly inoculate culture plates with the swab or loop. Also, primary isolation plates frequently have only small numbers of colonies; it is conceivable that the dilution effect of liquid transport media might cause some cultures to be falsely negative.

GRAM STAIN CHARACTERISTICS

H. ducreyi is a small, gram-negative, nonmotile rod, 0.5 to 0.6 μm in width by 1.6 to 2.0 μm in length. Examination of Gram-stained smears of human genital lesion material reveals groups or clumps of H. ducreyi cells with occasional short streptobacillary chains among the lesion debris (Fig. 3.21). Sometimes organisms forming long trails within mucous strands are seen, the so-called "railroad tracks," which are felt to be characteristic of H. ducreyi (Fig. 3.22). The utility of the Gram stain in diagnosing chancroid is unclear. A sensitivity of 40 to 60% has been generally accepted, but the specificity has not been well defined,

as organisms with a similar morphology that might be mistaken for H. ducreyi may be found in genital secretions. Thus, the Gram stain from lesion material should be used as a presumptive means of diagnosis only (Fig. 3.23). Gram stains of material aspirated from buboes are more specific, but the organism is difficult to find in such smears.

GROWTH CHARACTERISTICS

H. ducreyi is a fastidious organism that requires microbiologists experienced in working with H. ducreyi to obtain optimal isolation rates. The isolation of H. ducreyi as the primary means of diagnosis has been a difficult task. Most isolation rates of H. ducreyi from patients who are suspected of having chancroid have been less than 60%, although studies in Kenya have reported higher rates. Isolation of H. ducreyi from buboes, for reasons that are unclear, is even less successful than isolation from ulcers.

Growth temperatures of 33 to 35°C are recommended, but 33°C may be preferable. Inoculated plates are incubated in a humid atmosphere (about 100%) with 5% CO_2; these conditions are often met by the use of a candle jar with a moist, but not dripping, paper towel in the bottom of the jar.

H. ducreyi can be cultivated on an enriched medium containing supplements such as IsoVitaleX (BBL), Vitox (Oxoid), or CVA (Gibco); the organism requires the X (hemin) factor, but not the V (NAD) factor for growth. A variety of media have been devised for the cultivation of H. ducreyi, but no one medium appears able to support the growth of all strains from clinical material (Fig. 3.24). To increase isolation rates, most workers recommend that two media be used; a blood agar and a chocolated agar plate are usually chosen. The addition of vancomycin (3 μg/mL) greatly enhances the ability to recover H. ducreyi from clinical specimens by suppressing the growth of other microorganisms, and its effect can be quite dramatic (Fig. 3.25).

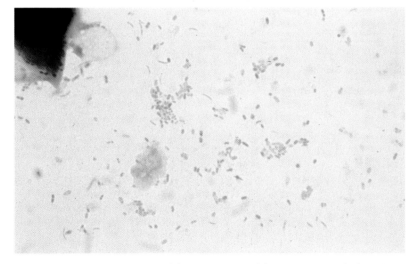

Figure 3.21 Gram-stained human genital lesion material showing groups of organisms (oil immersion, × 1000).

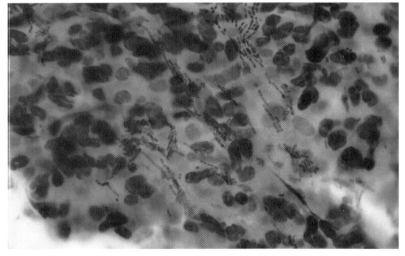

Figure 3.22 Gram-stained human genital lesion material showing the "railroad track" appearance (oil immersion, × 1000).

Figure 3.23 Diagnostic methods in chancroid.

DIAGNOSTIC METHODS IN CHANCROID	
PRESUMPTIVE	DIAGNOSTIC
Gram stain of material from genital lesion	Culture
Immunofluorescence of organisms in ulcer smears using monoclonal antibody	

MEDIUM[†]	COMMENTS	CULTURE SENSITIVITY
GC agar base (Difco)[‡] + 1% hemoglobin + 1% IsoVitaleX (BBL)	Relatively low sensitivity.	56%
Heart infusion agar (BBL) + 10% fetal bovine serum (FBS)	The addition of FBS resulted in an increase in colony size; medium has not been extensively evaluated.	81%
GC agar base (Gibco)[‡] + 1 or 2% hemoglobin + 5% FBS + 1% CVA enrichment (Gibco) (GcHbFBS)	Best medium when only a single medium is used to isolate *H. ducreyi*.	67–84%
Mueller Hinton agar + 5% chocolatized horse blood + 1% CVA enrichment (MH-HB)	Not as sensitive as GcHbFBS. However, some isolates will grow on MH-HB that do not grow on GcHbFBS.	53–65%
GcHbFBS and MH-HB	Can be used in a single biplate.	75–81%
Modified Bieling agar[§]	More complicated to prepare than either GcHbFBS or MH-HB if a commercial source of yeast dialysate is not available. *H. ducreyi* colonies are easily recognized on this medium.	77%
GcHbFBS (2 cultures, 48 h apart)	A 48-h delay in initiating therapy may preclude use of this technique.	85%

*Most of the cited studies were performed on patient populations having a high prevalence of chancroid.
[†]All media contained vancomycin (3μg/ml).
[‡]The manufacturer is given where the composition of the medium may vary with the manufacturer.
[§]Modified Bieling agar is comprised of Columbia agar base (2 parts) and hemolized horse blood (1 part) that is supplemented with 2.5% yeast dialysate and 1% CVA enrichment.

Figure 3.24 Isolation of *H. ducreyi* on selective media from patients with a clinical diagnosis of chancroid.

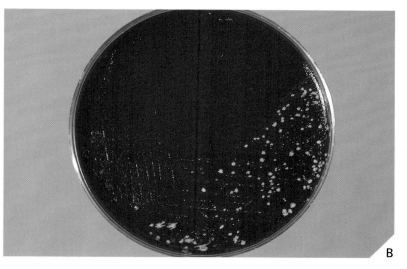

Figure 3.25 Growth of microorganisms from human genital lesion material. **A** Heart infusion agar containing 5% rabbit blood, 1% IsoVitaleX, and 10% fetal bovine serum. **B** The same medium but with vancomycin (3.0 μg/mL). On the left side of this plate, there is almost pure growth of *H. ducreyi*.

Colonies growing on rabbit blood agar are semiopaque, translucent, and yellow–light gray (Fig. 3.26). The colonies are nonmucoid and can easily be pushed intact across the agar surface with an inoculating loop. The removal of colonies may show slight pitting of the agar surface.

PRESERVATION
H. *ducreyi* can be removed from the agar surface with a swab, suspended in one of several freezing solutions, and stored at varying temperatures (Fig. 3.27). All solutions can be used in liquid nitrogen storage at −70, −35, or −20°C. The latter two temperatures should be used only for short-term storage since marked losses in viability may occur.

CULTURE CHARACTERIZATION
On primary isolation media, growth may be visible at 24 hours, but identifiable colonies of H. *ducreyi* may not be seen until 48 to 72 hours of incubation. Plates should not be discarded as negative, however, until after at least five days of incubation.

Colonies of H. *ducreyi* are almost invariably smaller than colonies of other bacteria isolated from the genital tract. A unique characteristic of colonies of H. *ducreyi* is that they can be pushed along the agar surface with a wire loop, a useful diagnostic clue. A Gram stain should be performed on colonies suspected of being H. *ducreyi*. Various arrangements of gram-negative bacilli may be present, depending upon the age of the culture and the media from which a colony is isolated. These include individual organisms, "school-of-fish" arrangements (cells lined up parallel with one another, suggesting a school of fish swimming in one direction), "fingerprint" swirls (a variation of the "school-of-fish" pattern), and short streptobacillary chains (Fig. 3.28).

Gram-negative bacilli from colonies compatible with H. *ducreyi* should be biochemically tested. Carbohydrate fermentation tests are not useful in identifying H. *ducreyi*, and differentiation from other *Haemophilus* species depends upon biochemical testing. H. *ducreyi* requires hemin (X factor) for growth and thus is negative in the porphyrin test (Fig. 3.29). H. *ducreyi* is also negative in the catalase test (Fig. 3.30). Positive reactions are obtained from alkaline phosphatase (Fig. 3.31) and nitrate reductase (Fig. 3.32) tests. In the oxidase test, a positive reaction is observed only using tetramethyl-p-phenylenediamine; it is important not to use the dimethyl reagent, which will result in a negative test (Fig. 3.33).

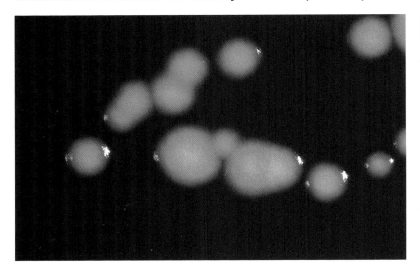

Figure 3.26 Colonies of *H. ducreyi* growing on heart infusion agar, 5% rabbit blood, 1% IsoVitaleX, and 10% fetal bovine serum.

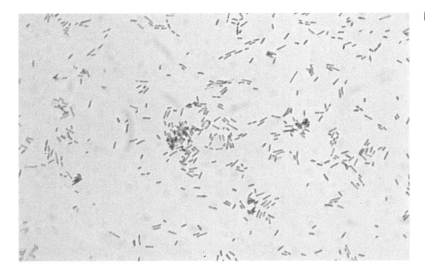

METHODS OF PRESERVING *H. DUCREYI*

SOLUTIONS
Heart infusion broth, trypticase soy broth, or bovine serum albumin, containing 10% glycerol and 10% fetal bovine serum (filter sterilized)
Skim milk, with or without 10% glycerol (filter sterilized)
Defibrinated rabbit blood
Serum–inositol (for lyophilization)

STORAGE CONDITIONS
Liquid nitrogen
−70°C
−35°C
−20°C
Lyophilization

Figure 3.27 To preserve *H. ducreyi*, growth is removed from the agar surface, mixed into any one of the listed freezing solutions, and then immediately frozen.

Figure 3.28 Gram stain of *H. ducreyi* from agar medium.

PATHOGENICITY

The virulence of H. *ducreyi* has been studied by injecting pus from human genital lesions into the skin of rabbits. Within 48 hours, a lesion 1 to 2 cm in diameter occurred. After 24 hours, the lesions subsided, and healing was complete within 1 week. Some strains of H. *ducreyi* failed to produce lesions after serial passage on laboratory media, suggesting that these strains may have lost one or more as yet unidentified virulence factors. H. *ducreyi* produces lesions that appear more rapidly and are larger than lesions produced by *Treponema pallidum*, subspecies *pallidum* in the rabbit model (Fig. 3.34).

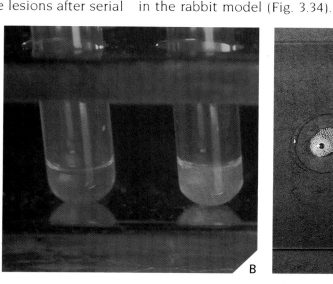

Figure 3.29 Porphyrin test. A negative result with H. *ducreyi* is shown on the left.

A Room light. **B** Viewed with a Wood's lamp.

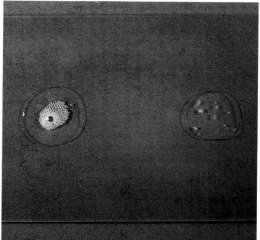

Figure 3.30 Catalase test. A negative result with H. *ducreyi* is shown on the right.

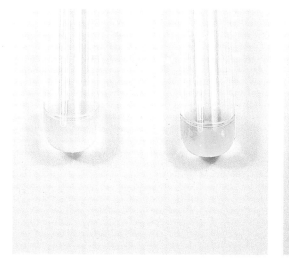

Figure 3.31 Alkaline phosphatase test. A positive result with H. *ducreyi* is shown on the right.

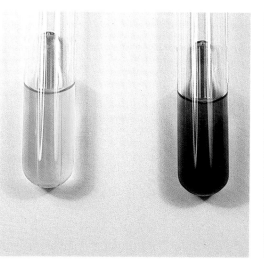

Figure 3.32 Nitrate reductase test. A positive result with H. *ducreyi* is shown on the right.

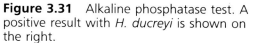

Figure 3.33 Oxidase test. A positive result with H. *ducreyi*, showing dark colonies where oxidase reagent has been placed.

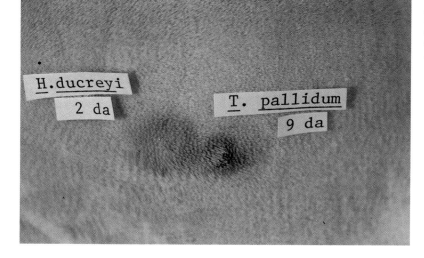

H. ducreyi 2 da

T. pallidum 9 da

Figure 3.34 Induction of skin lesions in a normal rabbit by injection of H. *ducreyi* and *T. pallidum*. The *T. pallidum* lesion is shown as a smaller pustule requiring nine days for induction, compared with the larger lesion of H. *ducreyi*, which requires only 48 hours for lesion formation.

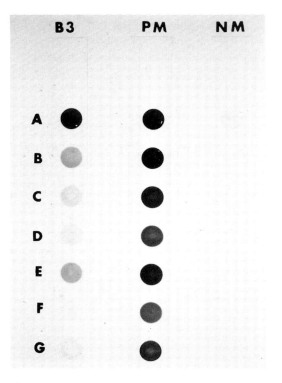

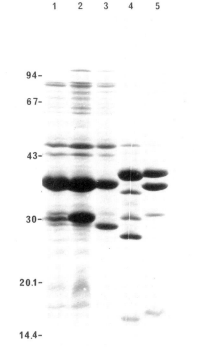

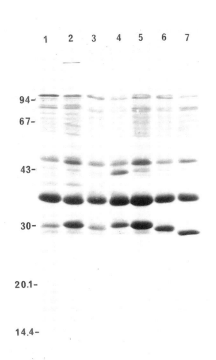

Figure 3.35 Dot-immunobinding assay of a monoclonal antibody directed against *H. ducreyi,* incubated with outer membrane preparations (OMP) from other *Haemophilus* species. Row A, *H. ducreyi* OMP; row B, *H. influenzae* OMP; row C, *H. parainfluenzae* OMP; row D, *H. aphrophilus* OMP; row E, *H. paraphrophilus* OMP; row F, *H. pleuropneumoniae* OMP; row G, *H. parasuis* OMP. Vertically: B3, monoclonal antibody to *H. ducreyi*; PM, polyvalent sera from mice; NM, normal sera from mice.

Figure 3.36 SDS-PAGE of outer membrane preparations of two strains of *H. ducreyi* isolated in the United States (lanes 1 and 2), *H. ducreyi* strain CIP 542 (lane 3), *H. influenzae* ATCC 8143 (lane 4), and *H. parainfluenzae* ATCC 7857 (lane 5).

Figure 3.37 SDS-PAGE of U.S. *H. ducreyi* outer membrane preparations (lanes 1 to 6) and an outer membrane preparation of *H. ducreyi* strain CIP 542 (lane 7).

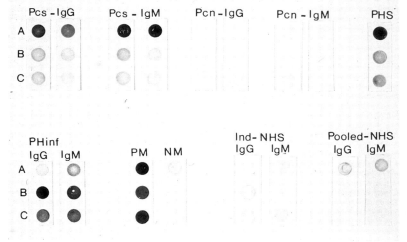

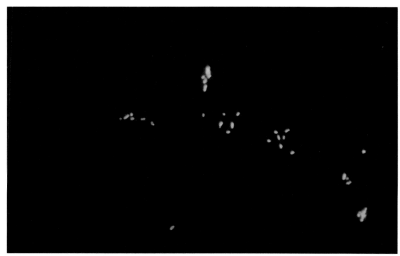

Figure 3.38 Representative results of a dot-immunobinding assay of sera from patients and controls with outer membrane preparations from *H. ducreyi* (row A), *H. influenzae* (row B), and *H. parainfluenzae* (row C). Pcs, sera from patients; Pcn, sera from control subjects; PHS, *H. ducreyi*-positive human sera; PHinf, *H. influenzae*-positive human sera; PM, polyvalent mouse sera; NM, normal mouse sera; Ind-NHS, individual sera from human volunteers (control); Pooled-NHS, pooled sera from normal human volunteers (control).

Figure 3.39 Indirect immunofluorescence assay of human genital lesion material with a monoclonal antibody directed against *H. ducreyi.*

IMMUNOCHEMISTRY

There is considerable serologic cross-reactivity among *Haemophilus* species, making the development of a serologic test capable of distinguishing among the various species difficult. Consequently, no serologic test is commercially available. Mouse antisera produced against H. *ducreyi* outer membrane preparations cross-react with outer membrane preparations from several other *Haemophilus* species (Fig. 3.35) The outer membrane protein profile of H. *ducreyi* can be differentiated from the outer membrane protein profiles of *Haemophilus influenzae* or *Haemophilus parainfluenzae* using sodium dodecyl-sulfate polyacrylamide gel electrophoresis (SDS-PAGE) (Fig. 3.36). Similar, but not identical, outer membrane protein profiles of H. *ducreyi* strains isolated from different geographic locations in the United States may provide a useful epidemiologic tool (Fig. 3.37).

Although serologic tests have not been useful in the diagnosis of chancroid, recent developments may provide a useful adjunct to clinical diagnosis. A dot-immunobinding assay using nitrocellulose-bound outer membrane preparations of H. *ducreyi*, H. *influenzae*, and H. *parainfluenzae* can be used to examine the serum from patients in whom chancroid is suspected for the presence of IgG and IgM immunoglobulins specifically directed against H. *ducreyi* (Fig. 3.38). An enzyme-linked immunosorbent assay (ELISA) test appears promising.

Monoclonal antibodies have been developed and used in immunofluorescence assays to detect H. *ducreyi*. The organism has been detected in human genital lesion material by an indirect immunofluorescence assay. The test is performed by incubating a slide containing lesion material with mouse monoclonal antibody. After washing, the bound antibody is detected by adding fluorescein-labeled anti-mouse immunoglobulin and examining the slide (Fig. 3.39).

ULTRASTRUCTURE

H. *ducreyi* ultrastructure viewed by transmission electron microscopy shows the typical streptobacillary chains with cells adhering to each other end to end (Fig. 3.40). Organisms also appear to adhere at the sides or from end to side, which may explain the appearance of clumps of cells that are frequently

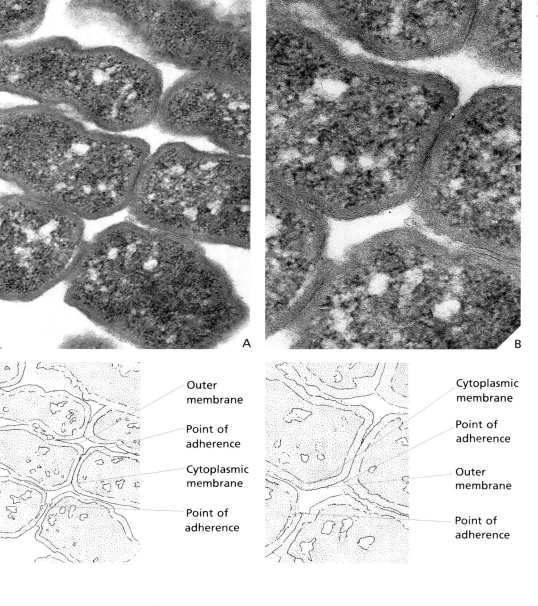

Figure 3.40 Thin-section electron micrographs of H. *ducreyi* from agar medium. **A** ×90,000. **B** ×175,000.

Outer membrane

Point of adherence

Cytoplasmic membrane

Point of adherence

Cytoplasmic membrane

Point of adherence

Outer membrane

Point of adherence

observed in Gram-stained smears (Fig. 3.41). The cell envelope is typical of gram-negative bacteria and is bordered on the outside by an outer membrane and on the inside by a cytoplasmic membrane, between which is a layer of medium electron-dense material (peptidoglycan). Regions of distinct nuclear material are not evident.

Treatment

Over the past decade, H. *ducreyi* has developed resistance to penicillins, sulfonamides, and tetracyclines by acquiring plasmids encoding resistance to these drugs; resistance to tetracycline in some cases is chromosomally mediated (Fig. 3.42). The plasmids in H. *ducreyi* have varying functions (Fig. 3.43).

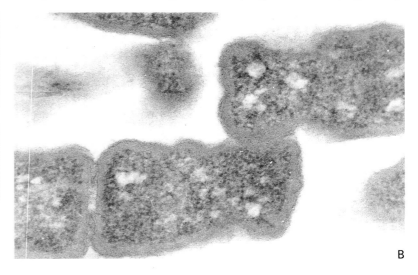

A

B

Figure 3.41 A and B Thin-section electron micrographs of H. *ducreyi* showing side-by-side and end-to-end adherence (×120,000).

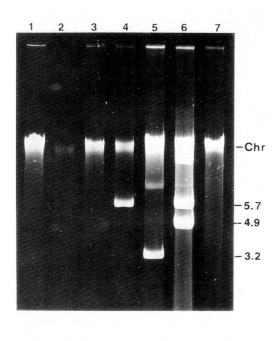

Figure 3.42 Electrophoresis of plasmid DNA (0.7% agarose) of H. *ducreyi* strains isolated in the United States in 1956 (lanes 1 and 2), H. *ducreyi* strain CIP 542 (American Type Culture Collection 33940) (lanes 3 and 7), and H. *ducreyi* strains isolated in the United States after 1980 (lanes 4 to 6).

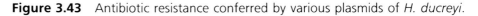

ANTIBIOTIC RESISTANCE CONFERRED BY VARIOUS PLASMIDS OF H. DUCREYI

SIZE (MDAL)	CONJUGATIVE	ANTIBIOTIC	COMMENTS
7.0	−	Ampicillin	Related to 4.4 Mdal gonococcal Pc^r plasmid which only contains right-hand 40% of TnA sequence
5.7	−	Ampicillin	Differs from 3.2 Mdal gonococcal Pc^r plasmid by 1.3 Mdal insertion element
3.2	−	Ampicillin	Identical to 3.2 Mdal gonococcal Pc^r plasmid
4.9	−	Sulfonamide	Related to enteric Str^r Sul^r plasmid RSF1010 (79%)
30	+	Tetracycline	Related to other Tet^r plasmids in *Haemophilus* spp.
34	+	Tetracycline and chloramphenicol	Related to plasmid from H. *influenzae*
23.5	+	None	Will transfer small plasmids from *Haemophilus* spp.

Figure 3.43 Antibiotic resistance conferred by various plasmids of H. *ducreyi*.

The 3.2- and 5.7-megadalton plasmids encode for beta-lactamase, conferring resistance to penicillins, while the 4.9-megadalton plasmid encodes for sulfonamide resistance. Many strains from East Africa contain a 7.0-megadalton plasmid that encodes for beta-lactamase. The 3.2-, 5.7-, and 7.0-megadalton beta-lactamase plasmids are related to one another as well as to the beta-lactamase plasmids found in *Neisseria gonorrhoeae*. Plasmid analysis with *H. ducreyi*, as with other microorganisms, may offer an epidemiologic tool for distinguishing similarities among strains isolated in varying geographic areas. Geographic variation in plasmids has been reported (Fig. 3.44).

Little variability in minimum inhibitory concentrations to currently recommended antimicrobials occurs in isolates from around the world (Fig. 3.45). Ceftriaxone, cefotaxime, erythromycin, and members of the quinolone family are highly active in vitro.

Currently, treatment with erythromycin or ceftriaxone is recommended by the U.S. Public Health Service, although therapy with the combinations of amoxicillin and clavulanic acid or trimethoprim and sulfamethoxazole may be effective as well (Fig. 3.46). A subjective response to eventually successful therapy is almost always present within 48 hours of starting treat-

PLASMID PROFILES OF SELECTED *H. DUCREYI* ISOLATES, WORLDWIDE FROM 1952 TO 1985

LOCATION	YEAR	N	3.2	4.9 + 5.7	5.7	7.0	NONE
United States							
Atlanta, GA	1952–58	8	—	—	—–	—	8
Atlanta, GA	1980–81	10	1	5	4	—	—
Orange County, CA	1982	32	32	—	—	—	—
Palm Beach County, FL	1983	12	—	—	12	—	—
Orlando, FL	1985	2	—	—	2	—	—
Boston, MA	1985	4	—	—	4	—	—
New York, NY	1985	26	—	—	24	2	—
Winnipeg, Canada	1978	19	—	—	3	—	16
Nairobi, Kenya	1980–82	274	—	—	110	157	7

(header over columns 3.2–NONE: PLASMIDS (MDAL))

Figure 3.44
Plasmid profiles of selected *H. ducreyi* isolates, worldwide from 1952 to 1985.

SUSCEPTIBILITY OF STRAINS OF *H. DUCREYI* TO CLINICALLY USEFUL ANTIMICROBIALS FROM 1980 TO 1987

COUNTRY	N	ERYTHROMYCIN	CEFTRIAXONE/CEFOTAXIME	TRIMETHOPRIM
United States				
Orange County, CA	38	0.004–0.016 (0.004)[†]	≤0.001	0.032–16(4)
New York City, NY	22	<0.008–0.064 (<0.064)	≤0.001–0.008 (0.004)	0.25–4 (2)
Kenya	35	Not tested	Not tested	0.125–2.0 (2)
Thailand	100	0.007–0.06 (0.03)	0.0007–0.007 (0.003)	0.12–>16 (4)
France	29	0.002–0.032 (0.016)	0.004–0.016 (0.008)	Not tested

(header over the three antimicrobial columns: ANTIMICROBIAL*)

*Expressed as µg/mL.
[†] Figure in parentheses indicates minimum inhibitory concentration of 90% of strains.

Figure 3.45
Susceptibility of strains of *H. ducreyi* to clinically useful antimicrobials from 1980 to 1987.

THERAPEUTIC REGIMENS RECOMMENDED BY THE U.S. PUBLIC HEALTH SERVICE

RECOMMENDED

Erythromycin, 500 mg, orally, four times a day for 7 days
or
Ceftriaxone, 250 mg, IM, once

ALTERNATIVES

Trimethoprim/sulfamethoxazole, one double-strength tablet (160/800 mg), orally, twice a day for 7 days
or
Ciprofloxacin, 500 mg, orally, twice a day for 3 days
or
Amoxicillin, 500 mg, plus clavulanic acid, 125 mg, three times a day for 7 days

Figure 3.46
Therapeutic regimens recommended by the U.S. Public Health Service.

ment, and complete healing usually takes 10 to 11 days. The response of lymph nodes generally parallels that of ulcers, although some nodes progress to fluctance in spite of otherwise successful therapy, and this is not a sign of treatment failure. Fluctuant nodes should be aspirated by needle through normal skin. Sexual partners of affected persons should be examined and treated whether or not lesions are present.

Picture credits for this chapter are as follows: Fig. 3.5 courtesy of the Centers for Disease Control; Figs. 3.10, 3.15, and 3.18 courtesy of The American Academy of Dermatology; Figs. 3.35, 3.38, and 3.39 courtesy of The University of Chicago Press; Fig. 3.20 courtesy of Bhagirath Majmudar, MD.

BIBLIOGRAPHY

Blackmore CA, Limpakarnianarat K, Rigau-Perez JC, et al: An outbreak of chancroid in Orange County, California: Descriptive epidemiology and disease control measures. J Infect Dis 151:840, 1985.

Hammond GW, Lian CJ, Witt JC, Ronald AR: Comparison of specimen collection and laboratory techniques for the isolation of Haemophilus ducreyi. J Clin Microbiol 7:39, 1978.

Hammond GW, Slutchuk M, Scatliff J, Sherman E, Wilt JC, Ronald AR: Epidemiologic, clinical, laboratory and therapeutic features of an urban outbreak of chancroid in North America. Rev Infect Dis 2:867, 1980.

Kaplan W, Deacon WE, Olansky S, Albritton DC: VDRL Chancroid Studies II: Experimental chancroid in the rabbit. J Invest Dermatol 26:407, 1956.

Kilian M, Theilade J: Cell wall ultrastructure of Haemophilus ducreyi and Haemophilus piscium. Int J System Bacteriol 25:351, 1975.

Kinghorn GR, Hafiz S, McEntegart MG: Oropharyngeal Haemophilus ducreyi infection. Br Med J 287:650, 1983.

McNicol PJ, Ronald AR: The plasmids of Haemophilus ducreyi. J Antimicrob Chemother 14:561, 1984.

Museyi K, Van Dyck E, Vervoort T, Taylor D, Hoge C, Piot P: Use of an enzyme immunoassay to detect serum IgG antibodies to Haemophilus ducreyi. J Infect Dis 157:1039, 1988.

Nsanze H, Plummer FA, Maggwa ABN, Martha G, Dylewski J, Piot P, Ronald AR: Comparison of media for the isolation of Haemophilus ducreyi. Sex Transm Dis 11:6, 1984.

Oberhofer TR, Back AE: Isolation and identification of Haemophilus ducreyi. J Clin Microbiol 15:625, 1982.

Plummer FA, D'Costa LJ, Nsanze H, Karasira P, Maclean IW, Piot P, Ronald AR: Clinical and microbiologic studies of genital ulcers in Kenyan women. Sex Transm Dis 12:193, 1985.

Ronald AR, Plummer FA: Chancroid and Haemophilus ducreyi. Ann Intern Med 102:705, 1985.

Schalla WO, Sanders LL, Schmid GP, Tam MR, Morse SA: Use of dot-immunobinding and immunofluorescence assays to investigate clinically suspected cases of chancroid. J Infect Dis 153:879, 1986.

Schmid GP, Sanders LL Jr, Blount JH, Alexander ER: Chancroid in the United States: Reestablishment of an old disease. JAMA 258:3265, 1987.

Sheldon WH, Heyman A: Studies on chancroid: Observations on the histology with an evaluation of biopsy as a diagnostic procedure. Am J Pathol 22:415, 1945.

Sottnek FO, Biddle JW, Kraus SJ, Weaver RE, Stewart JA: Isolation and identification of Haemophilus ducreyi in a clinical study. J Clin Microbiol 12:170, 1980.

Taylor DN, Duangmani C, Suvongse C, O'Connor R, Pitarangsi C, Panikabutra K, Echeverria P: The role of Haemophilus ducreyi in penile ulcers in Bangkok, Thailand. Sex Transm Dis 11:148, 1984.

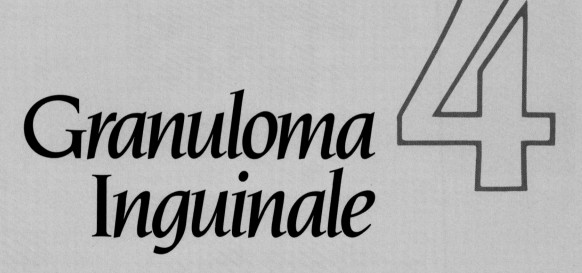

Granuloma Inguinale

4

D. KELLOGG, B. MAJMUDAR

Introduction

Donovanosis (granuloma inguinale, granuloma venereum) was first described in India (1882) as "serpiginous ulcer." Donovanosis is a progressive inflammatory disease of the skin and subcutaneous tissues of the genital and anal regions. Although the disease has been considered a sexually transmitted disease, nonvenereal transmission has been documented. Diagnosis relies on clinical findings and the demonstration of intracellular "Donovan bodies" in cytologic and tissue preparations. These bodies are generally not seen unless special stains are employed. This requirement could be partly responsible for the reported low incidence and the paucity of information regarding this disease. Once the diagnosis is established, the treatment usually is simple and effective.

The etiologic agent is *Calymmatobacterium granulomatis*, a coccobacillus (0.5 to 1.5 μm by 1 to 2 μm) that is gram-negative, nonmotile, asporogenic, and encapsulated. It is classified as an unassigned genus associated with the family *Enterobacteriaceae*. Morphologically and antigenically, it resembles members of the genus *Klebsiella*, in particular *K. rhinoscleromatis*. It has been cultured only under microaerophilic to anaerobic conditions. It will not grow on the surface of ordinary laboratory media, simple or complex. It has been grown in special liquid media, egg yolk slant fluid and yolk sacs of 5-day-old chicken embryos. Optimal growth temperature is 37°C. There are no cultures of this microorganism. Electron microscopy confirms ultrastructural characteristics similar to all gram-negative rods. It has also demonstrated possible bacteriophage-like particles in the Donovan bodies. *C. granulomatis* may be a normal intestinal organism that can be modified by a bacteriophage into a pathogenic organism.

Epidemiology

Donovanosis is found primarily in tropical and subtropical countries, most commonly in India, Brazil, West Indies, South China, and the west coast of Africa. Case reporting is incomplete in some areas and nonexistent in others. In the United States fewer than 100 cases are reported annually (STD Summary). It is considered a venereal disease because there is a preponderance of cases in the 20-to-30-year-old group, coinciding with the peak ages for sexually transmitted diseases. However, only 1 to 50% of marital partners of infected patients contract the disease and, although infrequently, it is also found in the very young and the elderly. The male-to-female ratio is 2.5:1. Most cases in the United States occur in the black population of the Southeast and among immigrants from the West Indies. No resistance to the disease has been documented and no spontaneous regressions of well-developed lesions have occurred without therapy even in the presence of high levels of circulating antibodies.

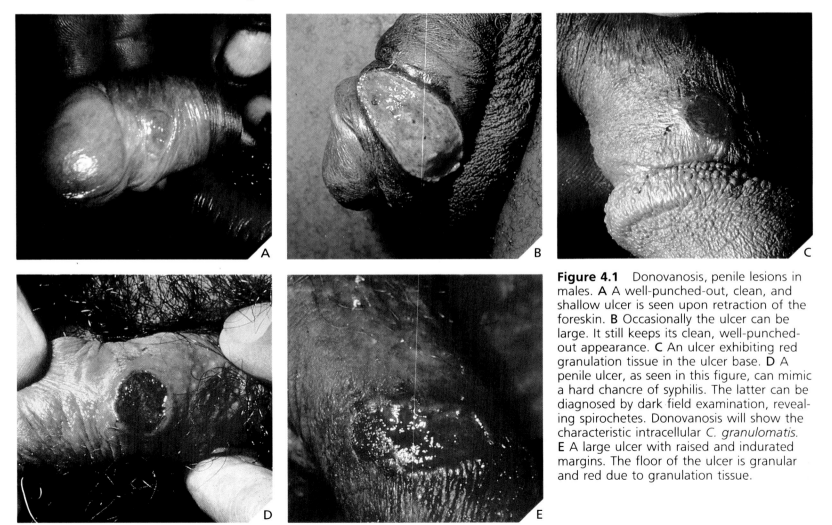

Figure 4.1 Donovanosis, penile lesions in males. **A** A well-punched-out, clean, and shallow ulcer is seen upon retraction of the foreskin. **B** Occasionally the ulcer can be large. It still keeps its clean, well-punched-out appearance. **C** An ulcer exhibiting red granulation tissue in the ulcer base. **D** A penile ulcer, as seen in this figure, can mimic a hard chancre of syphilis. The latter can be diagnosed by dark field examination, revealing spirochetes. Donovanosis will show the characteristic intracellular *C. granulomatis*. **E** A large ulcer with raised and indurated margins. The floor of the ulcer is granular and red due to granulation tissue.

A bacterium resembling *C. granulomatis* has been isolated from feces, suggesting *C. granulomatis* might be a member of the family *Enterobacteriaceae* normally residing in the intestine. Presumably, as a result of minor trauma such as a break in the skin or mucosa, the organisms are inoculated subcutaneously and produce the clinical lesions of donovanosis. This suggests the possibility of transmission by either intercourse or close physical contact to the anogenital region.

Two possible modes of transmission of this disease are:

1. Direct contact during rectal intercourse
2. Indirect contact through vaginal contamination by feces or fecal organisms

The latter might explain the rarity of the disease in prostitutes, most of whom douche regularly, which would tend to reduce any fecal contamination of the vaginal tract. In addition, those who develop clinical donovanosis, particularly the disseminated form, possibly are in some way deficient in their cellular immune response.

Clinical Manifestations

Donovanosis is an acute or chronic infection manifested by ulcerating necrotizing lesions of the skin and subcutaneous tissues in the genitoanal areas. In most patients the period from exposure to lesion is between 7 and 30 days. The initial lesion is a small papule that erodes the skin surface, breaking down to ulcers that progressively enlarge. Similar lesions are seen in both males (Fig. 4.1) and females (Fig. 4.2). Late lesions appear as hypertrophic, velvety, beefy red, indurated granulation tissue (Figs. 4.1E and 4.2B and D). Uncomplicated lesions are

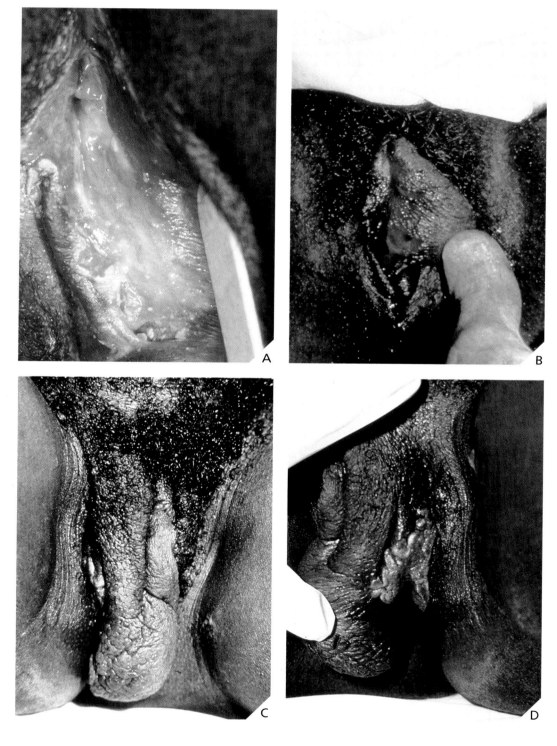

Figure 4.2 Donovanosis lesions in females. The morphology of the ulcers is similar in males and females. **A** In this figure, retraction of the left labium shows a shallow, clean ulcer. **B** Retraction of left edematous labium partially demonstrates a beefy red, ulcerating lesion. **C** and **D** Images from a patient showing a large ulcer partially obscured by markedly edematous labium majus. The patient was pregnant. Association of pregnancy and donovanosis can cause considerable therapeutic problems due to the contraindication of chloramphenicol and streptomycin in pregnancy.

painless, but secondary infection induces pain and an exudate (Fig. 4.3). Lesions most commonly occur on the inner aspect of the labia or the fourchette in the female (Fig. 4.4) and on the penis in the male (Fig. 4.1). The disease progresses by extension to adjacent skin and frequently spreads by autoinoculation and lymphatic or systemic dissemination.

In women, massive swelling of the labia is common. The lymphatics are widely dilated but unobstructed since dye injected into the tissues rapidly reaches the regional lymph nodes. Even in extensive donovanosis, the regional lymph nodes are not enlarged, painful, or tender. Absence of lymphadenopathy is a diagnostic characteristic; however, secondary infection produces inguinal adenopathy. These inguinal swellings appear as indurated masses or fluctuant abscesses, which eventually break down to be replaced by ulcers. They are called "pseudobuboes" because they represent subcutaneous granulation tissue and not enlarged lymph nodes (Fig. 4.5). Large and massively destructive lesions (Figs. 4.6 and 4.7) may be mistaken for malignancy. A combination of biopsy and cytology

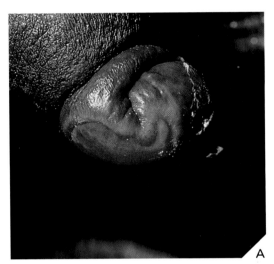
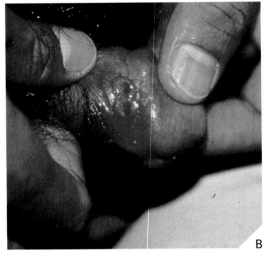
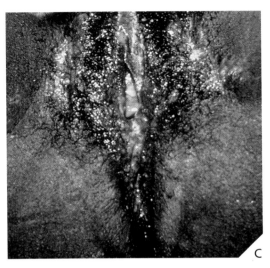

Figure 4.3 Secondary infections in donovanosis. **A** An irregular penile ulcer with an angry, red border and purulent floor suggesting a secondary infection. The lesion of donovanosis becomes painful when infected. Also note the marked edema of the surrounding skin. **B** Secondary infection of penile donovanosis makes it painful, red, and vascular. **C** Multiple, shallow ulcers seen on the vulvar skin. Secondary infection made them painful. Multiple lesions usually are caused by autoinoculation.

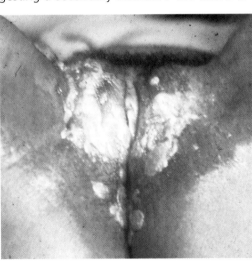

Figure 4.4 Labia and fourchette are the common sites of donovanosis in the female.

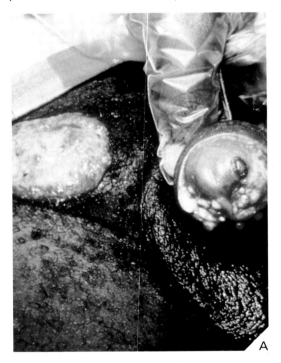
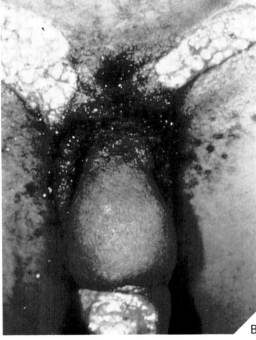

Figure 4.5 Pseudobuboes. **A** Penile donovanosis seen as an ulcerating, nodular lesion with marked tissue destruction. There is a large, inguinal ulcer indicating soft tissue breakdown in that area secondary to donovanosis. This is known as a "pseudobubo." **B** A large necrotic ulcer is seen in the glans penis. Note the secondary edema of the penile shaft. Bilateral inguinal pseudobuboes are also seen.

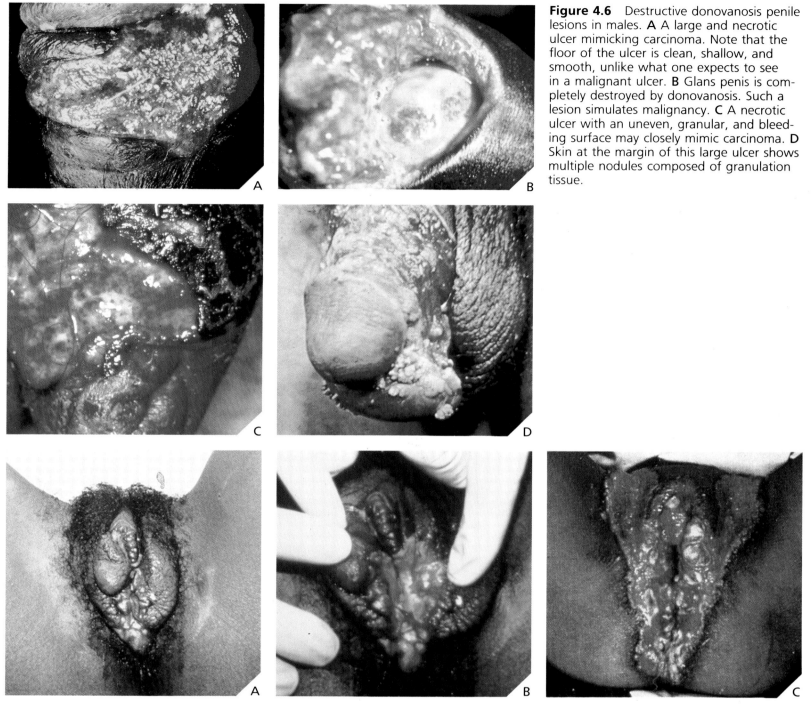

Figure 4.6 Destructive donovanosis penile lesions in males. **A** A large and necrotic ulcer mimicking carcinoma. Note that the floor of the ulcer is clean, shallow, and smooth, unlike what one expects to see in a malignant ulcer. **B** Glans penis is completely destroyed by donovanosis. Such a lesion simulates malignancy. **C** A necrotic ulcer with an uneven, granular, and bleeding surface may closely mimic carcinoma. **D** Skin at the margin of this large ulcer shows multiple nodules composed of granulation tissue.

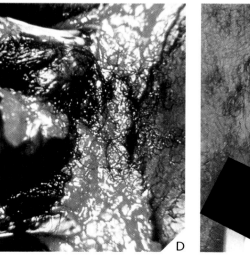
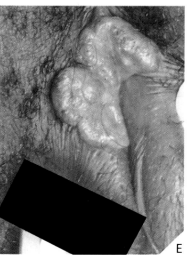

Figure 4.7 Destructive donovanosis lesions in females. **A** and **B** Pictures from the same patient showing a large, fungating ulcer obscured by edematous labia. **C** The entire vulva is destroyed by a large, fungating, necrotic ulcer. A biopsy and cytology are necessary to rule out malignancy in such cases. **D** An irregular stellate vulvar ulcer. Exuberant granulation tissue is seen in the floor of the ulcer. **E** An irregular, large vulvar ulcer with indurated, edematous, and partly everted margins mimicking carcinoma.

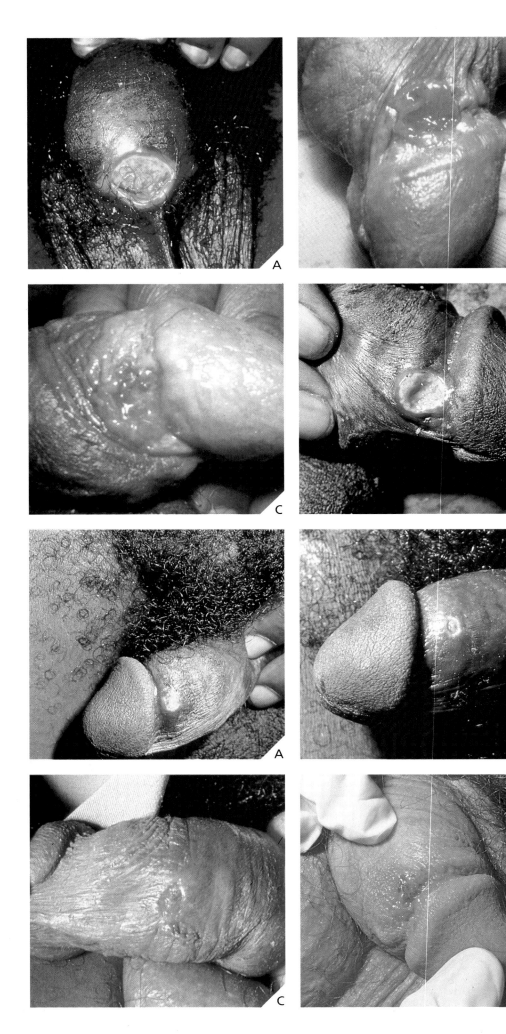

Figure 4.8 Earlier healing stages in donovanosis in males. **A** A chronic ulcer seen at the penoscrotal junction. The floor of the ulcer is grayish-white due to fibrosis, indicating attempts at healing. **B** A partially healing ulcer seen at the coronal sulcus. **C** An ulcer showing pale granulation tissue in the floor. The borders are grayish-white. These changes indicate healing. **D** This penile ulcer has a pale, grayish-white floor and thickened grayish-white margins. The ulcer cavity is partially filled by proliferating fibrous tissue indicating healing.

Figure 4.9 Later healing stages in donovanosis in males. **A** The ulcerated defect is filled by grayish-white fibrous tissue, indicating an advanced stage of healing. **B** and **C** Penile ulcers in an advanced stage of healing. **D** This lesion is almost completely healed, leaving behind a small, red area.

is necessary to rule out malignancy in these cases. Proper treatment results in healing and finally total resolution of lesions (Figs. 4.8 to 4.10). In general, the response to treatment is very satisfactory, but in long-standing cases genital deformities may occur, such as residual depigmentation of the skin (Fig. 4.11), stenosis of the urethral, vaginal, and anal orifices (Figs. 4.12 and 4.13), and massive edema (Fig. 4.14).

Extragenital lesions have been reported on the face, neck, mouth, and throat. Metastatic lesions involving the bones, joints, and viscera have been encountered. In these cases, there was an associated cervical or uterine lesion, and in some a history of a prior pregnancy or operative procedure. There is no evidence for congenital transmission of this disease.

DIFFERENTIAL DIAGNOSIS

The diagnosis of donovanosis is often overlooked because several genital infections are similar clinically, prior antibiotic therapy alters presentation, and there may be a failure to consider it as a diagnosis because of its low incidence in the United States. At present, the only conclusive method of diagnosis is to demonstrate Donovan bodies in large mononuclear cells in biopsy or cytology of the lesion.

Syphilis

The chancre of early syphilis may be confused with early lesions of donovanosis. Its exclusion is usually done by negative serology and dark field examination of the lesion for spirochetes.

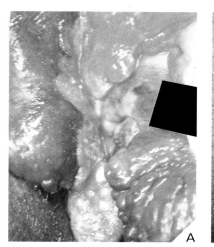
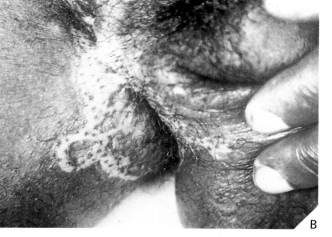
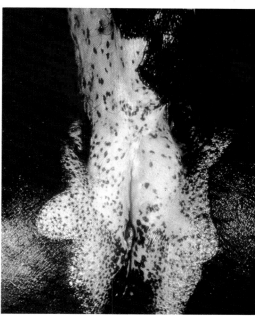

Figure 4.10 Healing stages in donovanosis in females. **A** A vulvar ulcer indicating early attempts at healing. The granulation tissue is relatively pale and avascular compared with Fig. 4.7E. **B** Fibrosis and reepithelialization of a healed lesion.

Figure 4.11 Residual depigmentation of a healed lesion.

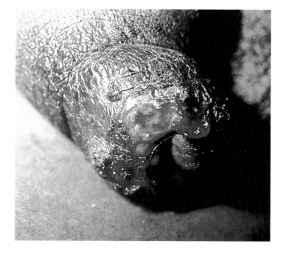
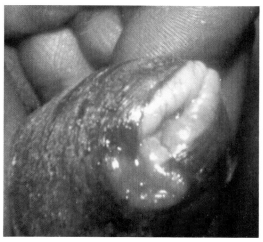
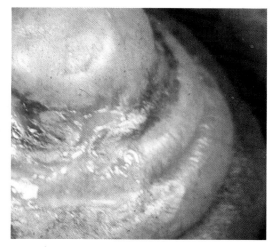

Figure 4.12 Fibrosis and edema causing a marked penile deformity. The patient had a large long-standing lesion, which healed after antibiotic therapy.

Figure 4.13 Urethral stenosis in a case of healed donovanosis.

Figure 4.14 Massive edema, phimosis, and ulceration in a case of advanced donovanosis. The ulcer shows evidence of healing by fibrosis, which can further act as a constricting band.

Lymphogranuloma Venereum

This disease is characterized by bilateral tender, inguinal nodes (buboes) that often become suppurative. Elephantiasis of the external genitalia may be seen. Exclusion is aided by serology with lymphogranuloma venereum (LGV) titers greater than 1:15.

Chancroid

Chancroid is manifested by shallow, painful, exudate-filled ulcers and tender inguinal adenopathy. The causative agent (*Hemophilus ducreyii*) can be cultured on a modified selective chocolate agar medium. Nodes will heal spontaneously.

Herpes Simplex II

This is characterized by symptomatic initial vesicles that quickly break down to form shallow, clean-based ulcers. Local edema and enlargement of inguinal lymph nodes may be present. Exclusion is by detection of intranuclear inclusions and multinucleated giant cells in smear or cultures of the herpesvirus.

Vulvar Cancer/Cervical Cancer

Both cancers are usually excluded by biopsy. Exophytic lesions or large necrotic ulcers of granuloma inguinale may closely simulate carcinoma on clinical examination. Parametrial involvement may add to this confusion.

Donovanosis can coexist with other venereal diseases. It should always be considered when genital lesions have a history of considerable duration and slow progression (weeks to months).

Laboratory Tests

BIOPSY AND CYTOLOGY

Biopsy and cytologic smears of the lesion are the most dependable tools to diagnose donovanosis. Biopsy shows that the affected skin is usually infiltrated by a dense mixed cellular infiltrate composed predominantly of mononuclear cells with occasional foci of neutrophils and histiocytes (Figs. 4.15 and 4.16). Vascular proliferation of granulation tissue is evident. Fibrosis sets in later in the process. The epithelial border of

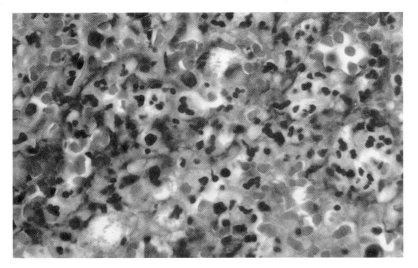

Figure 4.15 Microscopic section of the ulcer to show acute inflammation with microabscess formation and granulation tissue (hematoxylin and eosin × 50 approximately).

Figure 4.16 Donovan bodies when abundant in tissue can be seen intracellularly even by hematoxylin and eosin stain (× 120 approximately).

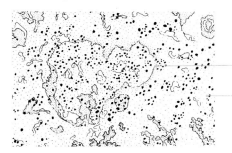

Microabscess formation

Granulation tissue

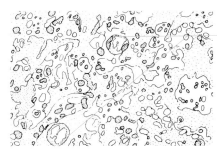

Intracellular Donovan bodies

the lesions frequently shows acanthosis, epidermal microabscesses, elongation and intercommunication of the rete pegs, and pseudoepitheliomatous hyperplasia. Caseation, suppuration, and epithelioid giant cells are not typical. Both in biopsy and cytology, there is a striking intracellular inclusion of *C. granulomatis* within histiocytes resulting in the diagnostically characteristic "pathognomonic cells." These enlarged cells (20 to 90 μm) have an eccentric nucleus and contain individual or groups of organisms in capsular or cystlike compartments of the cytoplasm. Polymorphonuclear leukocytes are rarely seen except on the surface aspects of the lesion. Pathognomonic cells are scattered in variable numbers in the upper half of the granulation tissue particularly near the margins of the ulcer. They are abundant in exuberant granulation tissue. The capsules are thought to protect the organism from degradation. The only currently effective laboratory procedure for the diagnosis of donovanosis is a properly prepared and stained tissue or smear.

Specimen Collection
An area of granulation tissue near the periphery of the lesion is carefully cleaned with several saline-soaked gauze squares and carefully dried with dry gauze. The appearance of blood does not affect specimen character. Using a punch biopsy, forceps, or small curette secure a small piece of tissue (about the size of a matchhead).

Specimen Preparation and Staining
Smear the underside of the specimen over the surface of a glass slide. Do not respread any area and cease spreading when the specimen begins to dry. The dry areas will contain rubbed, broken cells of no use as diagnostic material. The slide specimen is air dried, fixed in 95% ethanol for five minutes, and stained in a routine way. Special stains discussed below can be employed whenever possible. The tissue should be submitted for histopathologic examination. Hematoxylin and eosin stain will show marked acute and chronic inflammation with granulation tissue formation. Donovan bodies can be seen by this stain infrequently and only when present in large numbers (Fig. 4.16). For special stains, in both tissue and smear, use either Wright (Fig. 4.17), Giemsa (Fig. 4.18), Pinacyanole, or

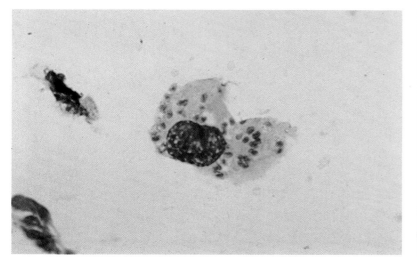

Figure 4.17 A fragmented mononuclear cell containing Donovan bodies. Bipolar staining creating a closed safety pin appearance is seen (Wright-Giemsa × 1000 approximately).

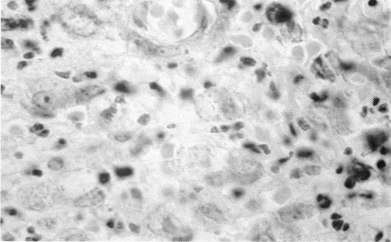

Figure 4.18 Giemsa stain of a tissue to show intracellular Donovan bodies (× 320 approximately).

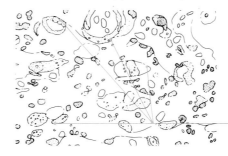

Intracellular Donovan bodies

Warthin-Starry (Fig. 4.19) stains by the usual procedures, except for the Wright stain. With the latter stain, allow the dye to remain on the preparation for 1.5 minutes before diluting with 6.4-pH phosphate buffer. A positive specimen will exhibit large mononuclear cells whose cytoplasm contains small, straight or curved dumbell-shaped (closed safety pin) rods having a blue-to-deep purple color and surrounded by pink capsules (Fig. 4.17). Broken tissue cells are not satisfactory for examination since there are many other extracellular objects of similar size and character in the specimen. The large "pathognomonic cells" can be detected with low magnification (× 45) with some experience and confirmed at a higher magnification (× 1000) (Figs. 4.20 and 4.21).

CULTURE SPECIMEN AND EXAMINATION

A specimen obtained as above is placed between two sterile glass slides and mashed between them with a twisting motion. Separate the slides and add 0.2 to 0.5 mL of sterile saline to each slide surface. Emulsify the tissue debris with a sterile toothpick or loop.

For isolation of *C. granulomatis* in chick embryos, inoculate 0.2 mL of the tissue debris into the yolk sac of a five-day-old chicken embryo and incubate at 37°C for 72 hours. Growth of *C. granulomatis* will occur in the yolk sac fluid and will demonstrate the characteristic "safety pin" morphology of this organism.

For isolation of *C. granulomatis* on "Dulaney slants," inoculate 0.2 mL of the tissue debris suspension onto the coagulated egg yolk slants, then cover 3/4 of the surface of the slant with Lockes salt solution. Close the tubes and incubate upright at 37°C for 48 to 72 hours. Slants made of egg yolks from range-fed chickens (ducks, geese, and turkeys) are effective whereas those made from egg yolks obtained from diet-fed birds are ineffective; the reasons for this are still unknown.

IMMUNOLOGY AND PATHOGENICITY

There is no serological procedure currently available either for detecting anitbodies to *C. granulomatis* in human sera or for identifying the organism as an isolate; however, antibodies have been detected in human sera by complement fixation proce-

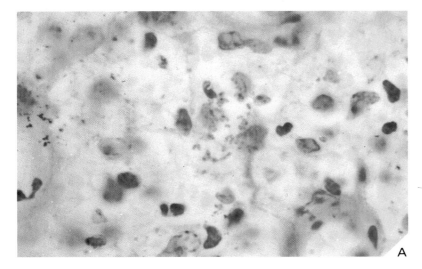
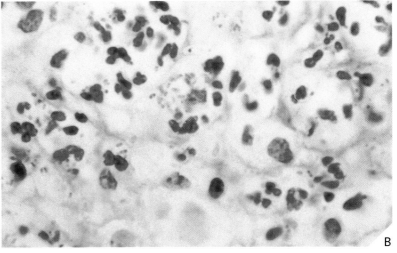

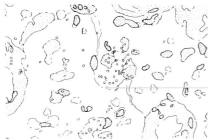
— Intracellular Donovan bodies

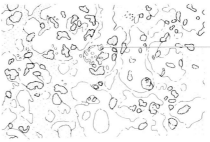
— Intracellular Donovan bodies

Figure 4.19 Warthin-Starry stain in tissue to show intracellular Dononvan bodies. **A** and **B** Same tissue, × 320 approximately. **C** × 1,000 approximately.

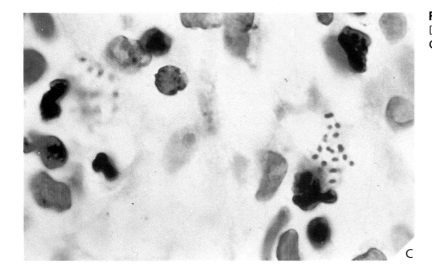

dures. Significant serum titers were found only in sera from patients in whom the duration of a lesion exceeded 3 months. The lack of protection by circulating antibodies is similar to other diseases in which the organism is found intracellularly, e.g., lepromatous leprosy, tuberculosis, and chronic mucocutaneous candidiasis. *C. granulomatis* exhibits antigenic cross-reactivity with *Klebsiella pneumoniae* and *Klebsiella rhinoscleromatis*. This observation lends some support to the proposed similarity between *K. rhinoscleromatis* and *C. granulomatis*. Other than the chick embryo, *C. granulomatis* is pathogenic only for humans.

Treatment

The treatment of choice is tetracycline or sulfasoxazole for a minimum of 2 to 3 weeks until the lesions have healed completely. The disease tends to relapse after successful treatment and healing, so prolonged follow-up is necessary. Chloramphenicol, gentamicin, streptomycin, tetracycline, and cotrimoxazole are also effective. The combination of lincomycin and erythromycin has been satisfactory for the treatment of pregnant patients. Penicillin is not efficacious and ampicillin or erythromycin alone has given inconsistent results.

PROGNOSIS
As a rule, the lesions resolve satisfactorily following proper treatment. Untreated lesions will distort, mutilate, and destroy involved tissues and spread to other areas of the body by either contiguity or systemic dissemination. Mortality is rare but its infrequent occurrence has been due to secondary causes such as pneumonia, cardiac failure, and hemorrhage.

ASSOCIATION WITH CARCINOMA
An association of donovanosis with genital carcinoma changes the treatment and therefore should be recognized early in the process. This association has been suspected for the following reasons:

1. There is a higher incidence of genital carcinoma where donovanosis is endemic
2. Carcinoma has occurred within depigmented areas of healed donovanosis
3. There has been concurrence of carcinoma and donovanosis in the same lesion

Vulvar ulcers, lesions on the cervix or vaginal vault that appear as necrotizing and proliferating masses of granulation tissue, and the thickening of the parametrial tissues seen with donovanosis are often mistaken for carcinoma.

Donovanosis is differentiated from carcinoma on the basis of dense dermal infiltration with microabscesses, plasma cells, and macrophages containing capsulated intracytoplasmic Donovan bodies. Acanthosis as well as pseudoepitheliomatous hyperplasia is present in donovanosis but nuclear hyperplasia, hyperchromasia, individual cell keratinization, and other characteristics of malignancy are absent. When a biopsy from a large, necrotic lesion clinically suspicious of carcinoma shows only inflammatory changes, a possibility of donovanosis should be considered and special stains obtained to demonstrate the diagnostic organisms. On the other hand, when the lesion remains unaltered or grows in spite of treatment, multiple biopsies should be obtained to rule out malignancy. An association between donovanosis and carcinoma, although reported, is distinctly uncommon.

Picture credits for this chapter are as follows: Figs. 4.1D and E, 4.6C, and 4.8A courtesy of American Academy of Dermatology; Figs. 4.1A, 4.2A, 4.4, 4.5B, 4.6D, 4.7D and E, 4.8B and C, 4.10A, 4.11, 4.13, and 4.14 courtesy of the Centers for Disease Control; Figs. 4.1B and C, 4.3A and B, 4.8D, 4.9, and 4.12 courtesy of Adele Moreland, MD; Fig. 4.7C courtesy of McGraw-Hill Publishing Co.; Figs. 4.5A and 4.6A courtesy of Bingham JS: Pocket Picture Guide to Sexually Transmitted Diseases. London, Gower Medical Publishing, 1984; Figs. 4.7E and 4.19 courtesy of the Journal of Reproductive Medicine.

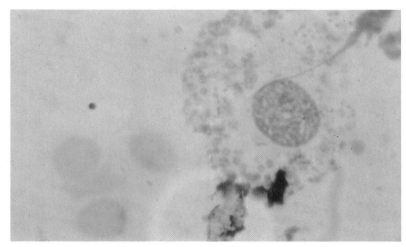

Figure 4.20 A cytologic preparation to show pathognomonic cell distended with numerous Donovan bodies (hematoxylin and eosin × 1000 approximately).

Figure 4.21 Pathognomonic intracellular Donovan bodies (methylene blue × 1500 approximately).

BIBLIOGRAPHY

Arya O: *Tropical Venerology.* New York, Churchill Livingston Press, 1980.

Bergys Manual of Systematic Bacteriology. Washington, DC, American Society of Microbiology, 1984, vol. 1, pp. 585–587.

Cannefax GR: The technic of the tissue spread method for demonstrating Donovan bodies. *J Vener Dis Info* 1948;19:201–204.

Davis C: Granuloma inguinale. *JAMA* 1970;211:632–636.

Fritz GS, Hubert WR, Dodson RE, et al.: Mutilating granuloma inguinale. *Arch Dermatol* 1975;111:1464–1465.

Goldberg J: Studies on granuloma inguinale IV. Growth requirements of *Donovania granulomatis* and its relationship to the natural habitat of the organism. *Br J Vener Dis* 1959;35:266–268.

Goldberg J: Studies on granuloma inguinale V. Isolation of a bacterium resembling *Donovania granulomatis* from the faeces of a patient with granuloma inguinale. *Br J Vener Dis* 1964;38:99–102.

Goldberg J: Studies on granuloma inguinale VII. Some epidemiological considerations of the disease. *Br J Vener Dis* 1964;40:140–145.

Goldberg J, Weaver RH, Packer H: Studies on *Granuloma Inguinale* II. The complement fixation test in the diagnosis of granuloma inguinale. *Am J Syph Gonorrhea Vener Dis* 1953;37:71–76.

Goldberg J, Annamunthodo H: Studies on granuloma inguinale VIII. Serological reactivity of sera from patients with carcinoma of the penis when tested with *Donovania* antigens. *Br J Vener Dis* 1966;42:205–209.

Greenblatt RB, Barfield WE: Newer methods in the diagnosis and treatment of granuloma inguinale. *Br J Vener Dis* 1952;28:123–128.

Janovski NA: *Diseases of the Vulva,* ed 1. Hagerstown, IN, Harper & Row, 1972.

Kalstone B, Howell JA Jr, Cline FX: Granuloma inguinale with hematogenous dissemination to the spine. *JAMA* 1961;176:152–154.

Kirkpatrick DJ: Donovanosis (granuloma inguinale): A rare cause of osteolytic bone lesions. *Clin Radiol* 1970;21:101–105.

Kuberski T: Granuloma inguinale (donovanosis). A review. *Sex Transm Dis* 1980;7:29–36.

Kuberski T, Papadimitriou JM, Phillips P: Ultrastructure of *Calymmatobacterium granulomatis* in lesions of granuloma inguinale. *J Infect Dis* 1980;142:744–749.

Lal S, Nicholas C: Epidemiological and clinical features in 165 cases of granuloma inguinale. *Br J Vener Dis* 1980;46:461–463.

Maddocks I, Anders EM, Dennis E: Donovanosis in Papua New Guinea. *Br J Vener Dis* 1976;52:190–196.

Mitchell KM, Roberts AN, Williams VM, Schneider J: *Genitourin Med* 1986;62:191–195.

Nayar M, Chandra M, Saxena HM, et al.: Donovanosis—a histopathological study. *Indian J Pathol Microbiol* 1981;24:71–76.

Pund ER, Greenblatt RB: Specific histology of granuloma inguinale. *Arch Pathol* 1937;23:224–229.

Robertson DH: *Clinical Practice in Sexually Transmissible Diseases,* ed 1. Baltimore, IN, University Park Press, 1980.

Schwartz R: Chancroid and granuloma inguinale. *Clin Obstet Gynecol* 1983;26:138–142.

Sexually Transmitted Diseases Summary. Atlanta, GA, U.S. Department of Health and Human Services, Technical Information Services, 1986.

Spagnola DV, Coburn PR, Cream JJ, Azadian BS: Extragenital granuloma inguinale (donovanosis) diagnosed in the United Kingdom: A clinical, histological, and electron microscopical study. *J Clin Pathol* 1984;37:945–949.

Stewart DB: The gynecological lesions of lymphogranuloma venereum and granuloma inguinale. *Med Clin North Am* 1964;48:773–786.

Wysoki RS, Majmudar B, Willis D: Granuloma inguinale (donovanosis) in women. *J Reprod Med* 1988;33:709–713.

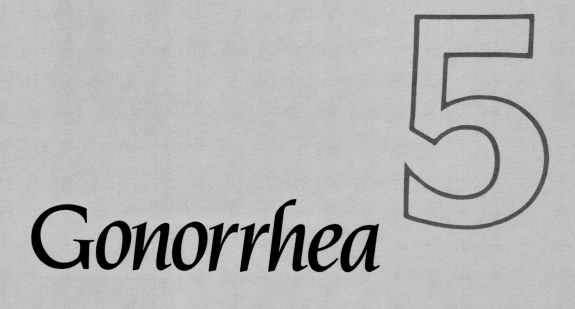

Gonorrhea

5

J.S. KNAPP, J.M. ZENILMAN, S.E. THOMPSON

Introduction

The clinical syndrome of gonorrhea was described in ancient literature, but the etiologic agent, *Neisseria gonorrhoeae* (also called the gonococcus), was not described until 1879, when Albert Neisser observed the organism in smears of purulent exudates from urethritis, cervicitis, and ophthalmia neonatorum. The genus *Neisseria* includes the pathogenic species *N. gonorrhoeae* and *N. meningitidis*, as well as species that are normal flora of the oropharynx and nasopharynx. Strains of the commensal *Neisseria* spp. may occasionally be isolated in clinical specimens from anogenital sites and observed intracellularly in polymorphonuclear leukocytes (PMNs), and are morphologically indistinguishable from the pathogenic *Neisseriae*. Thus accurate laboratory identification of the gonococcus is essential because of the social and medicolegal consequences of misidentifying strains of nonpathogenic *Neisseria* spp. as *N. gonorrhoeae*.

Because of the fastidious growth requirements of *N. gonorrhoeae*, it was difficult to culture the organism until the development of chocolatized blood agar supplemented with growth factors. In the 1960s, the development of selective media containing antimicrobial and antifungal agents (such as Martin-Lewis medium), which enhanced the isolation of the gonococcus by inhibiting not only gram-positive bacteria but also the closely related *Neisseria* spp., further simplified the laboratory diagnosis of gonorrhea. Recently, rapid biochemical and serologic tests have been developed, allowing identification of the gonococcus within a few hours of its isolation.

Although technological advances have reduced the problems involved in isolating the gonococcus, strains of some commensal *Neisseria* and related species may be isolated on gonococcal selective media and may be misidentified as *N. gonorrhoeae* in rapid tests. Thus the accurate laboratory identification of N. *gonorrhoeae* remains of paramount importance.

Epidemiology

Gonorrhea is the most frequently reported infectious disease in the U.S. Between 1977 and 1987, the number of reported cases decreased 22%, from 1 million to 781,000 cases per annum, which represents a decrease from 468/100,000 to 324/

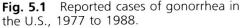

Fig. 5.1 Reported cases of gonorrhea in the U.S., 1977 to 1988.

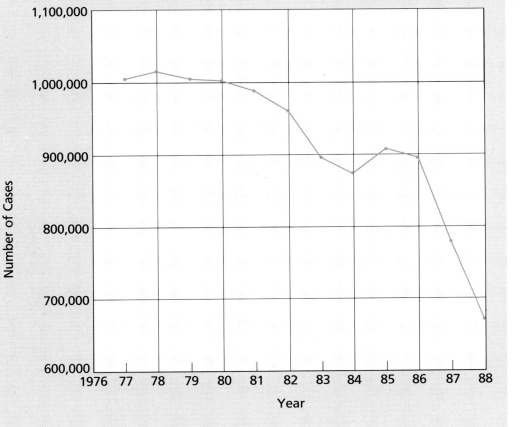

Fig. 5.2 Types of antimicrobial resistance in *N. gonorrhoeae*.

TYPES OF ANTIMICROBIAL RESISTANCE IN *NEISSERIA GONORRHOEAE*

TYPE OF RESISTANCE	ANTIMICROBIAL AGENT
Chromosomal (genes located on the chromosome)	Penicillin Tetracycline Spectinomycin Cefoxitin Ceftriaxone (decreased susceptibility)
Plasmid-mediated (genes located on plasmids)	Penicillin (β-lactam antibiotics)—PPNG Tetracycline—TRNG

100,000 population (Fig. 5.1). There are also an estimated two unreported cases for every reported case of gonorrhea.

Gonorrhea is transmitted almost exclusively by sexual contact. Persons under age 30 who have multiple sexual partners are at highest risk. Rates of gonorrhea are higher in males and in minority and inner-city populations.

Typically, gonorrhea is contracted from a sexual partner who is either asymptomatic or who has only minimal symptoms. Transmission efficiency (a measure of transmission through one sexual exposure) is estimated to be 50 to 60% from an infected man to an uninfected woman and 35% from an infected woman to an uninfected man. More than 90% of men with urethral gonorrhea will develop symptoms within five days and will seek treatment. This percentage is lower for rectal gonorrhea in men, and is less than 50% for anogenital gonorrhea in women. The rationale of public health measures such as screening and contact tracing is to identify and treat patients with asymptomatic infections, thus preventing further transmission of the disease. Additionally, because women with asymptomatic infections are at higher risk to develop disseminated gonococcal infection (DGI) and pelvic inflammatory disease (PID), early identification and treatment of asymptomatic cases in females is important.

The evolution of antimicrobial resistance in N. *gonorrhoeae* has potential negative implications for the control of gonorrhea (Fig. 5.2). Resistance to new therapeutic agents has generally developed within a few years of the agents' introduction. Strains with multiple chromosomal resistance to penicillin, tetracycline, erythromycin, and cefoxitin, as well as decreased susceptibility to ceftriaxone, have been identified in the U.S. and most of the world, especially southeast Asia. Sporadic high-level resistance to spectinomycin has also been reported.

Penicillinase-producing N. *gonorrhoeae* (PPNG) strains, which inactivate penicillins and other β-lactams, were first described in 1976. Five β-lactamase plasmids of different sizes have been identified in PPNG strains and have been used to follow the spread of PPNG geographically (Fig. 5.3). PPNG strains cause one-half of all gonococcal infections in parts of Africa and Asia, and became endemic in the U.S. in 1981. The incidence of PPNG infections has increased dramatically in the U.S. since 1984 (Fig. 5.4) and has affected nearly every major metropolitan area in the U.S.

Plasmid-mediated, high-level resistance to tetracycline was reported in N. *gonorrhoeae* (TRNG) in 1985. This plasmid has also been found in naturally occurring strains of N. *meningitidis* and

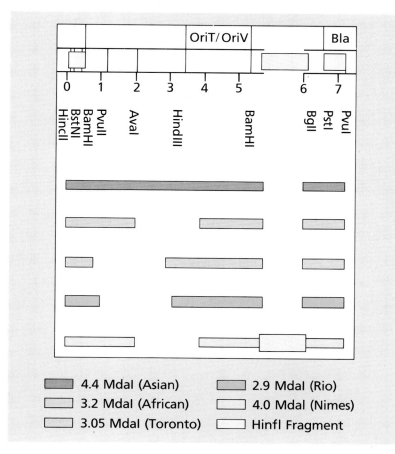

Fig. 5.3 Restriction endonuclease digestion maps of five β-lactamase plasmids described in *N. gonorrhoeae*. The 3.2-Mdal "African," 3.05-Mdal "Toronto," and 2.9-Mdal "Rio" β-lactamase plasmids appear to have been formed by deletions of segments from the 4.4-Mdal β-lactamase "Asian" plasmid. The 4.0-Mdal "Nimes" β-lactamase plasmid appears to have been formed by the insertion of a Hinfl fragment into the 3.2-Mdal plasmid. Bla is the structural gene for β-lactamase, OriT is the origin of transfer of the plasmid, and OriV is the origin of replication of the plasmid.

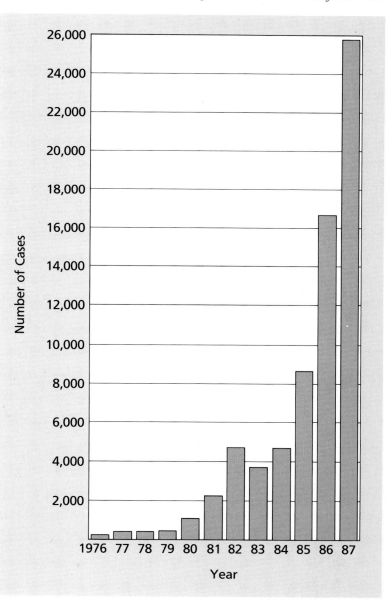

Fig. 5.4 Number of reported cases of gonorrhea caused by PPNG in the U.S., 1976 to 1987.

Kingella denitrificans. It may be transferred between gonococcal strains and strains of other *Neisseria* spp. by conjugation (Fig. 5.5) and also moblilizes β-lactamase plasmids. Isolates with plasmid-mediated tetracycline resistance have also possessed a β-lactamase plasmid.

Vancomycin-susceptible strains of N. *gonorrhoeae* occasionally occur and may not grow on selective media containing 4 μg vancomycin/mL, which was routinely used for the isolation of the gonococcus. Selective media have been modified to contain 2 or 3 μg vancomycin/mL in order to overcome this problem. Vancomycin-susceptible gonococci should be suspected in a community when false-negative cultures are obtained, as evidenced by a discrepancy between gram-stain positivity and culture positivity rates for urethral gonorrhea in men; these should agree for at least 95% of cases.

Clinical Manifestations

In the majority of cases, gonorrhea is limited to superficial mucosal surfaces. Infection occurs in areas with columnar epithelium that has contact with infected secretions. The areas most frequently involved are the cervix, urethra, rectum, pharynx, and eye. Squamous epithelium is not susceptible to infection by the gonococcus. However, the prepubertal vaginal epithelium, which has not been keratinized under the influence of estrogen, may be infected. Hence, gonorrhea in the young girl may pres-

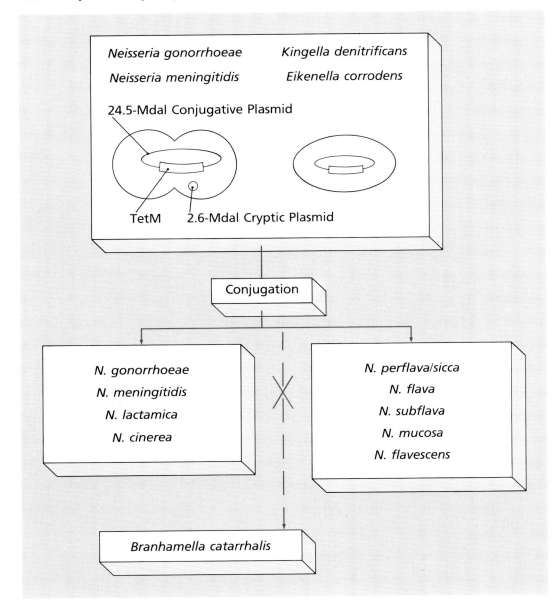

Fig. 5.5 Conjugative transfer of 25.2-Mdal TetM-containing plasmids from *N. gonorrhoeae, N. meningitidis, Kingella denitrificans,* and *Eikenella corrodens* to *Neisseria* and related spp.

ent as a vulvovaginitis. In mucosal infections, there usually is a brisk, local neutrophilic response manifested clinically as a purulent discharge (Fig. 5.6).

In women, untreated cervical infection may lead to endometritis and salpingitis, a sign–symptom complex more commonly termed PID. In approximately 0.5% of patients with mucosal infection, hematogenous spread occurs, causing DGI. In many cases of PID and DGI, the initial mucosal infection is asymptomatic. Therefore, clinical suspicion is often important in obtaining a conclusive diagnosis.

CLINICAL MANIFESTATIONS OF GONOCOCCAL INFECTIONS

SITE OF INFECTION	UNCOMPLICATED	COMPLICATED

Urethra	Symptomatic
	  Scant, clear discharge
	  Copious, purulent discharge
	Asymptomatic
		(Epididymitis)*
		
		(Penile edema)
		(Abscess of Cowper's, Tyson's glands)
		(Seminal vesiculitis)

Various		DGI
		  Bacteremia
		  Fever
		  Skin lesions: macular, erythematous, pustular, necrotic, hemorrhagic
		  Tenosynovitis
		  Joints: septic arthritis
		  Endocarditis
		  Meningitis

Cervix	Symptomatic
	  Red, friable cervical os
	  Purulent discharge from os
	  Bilateral or unilateral lower abdominal tenderness
	
	Asymptomatic
		PID
		  Endometritis
		  Salpingitis
		  Tubo-ovarian abscess
		  Pelvic peritonitis
		  Ectopic pregnancy
		  Infertility
		DGI

Rectum	Symptomatic
	  Copious, purulent discharge
	  Burning/stinging pain
	  Tenesmus
	  Blood in stools
	Asymptomatic
		DGI

Pharynx	Symptomatic
	  Mild pharyngitis
	  Mild sore throat
	  Erythema
	Asymptomatic
		DGI

Conjunctiva	Symptomatic Copius purulent discharge	Keratitis and corneal ulceration: perforation, extrusion of lens Scarring: opacification of lens Blindness

*Syndromes listed in parentheses occur infrequently.

Fig. 5.6 Clinical manifestations of gonococcal infections.

GONORRHEA

The most common symptom is a discharge that may range from a scanty, clear or cloudy fluid to one that is copious and purulent (Fig. 5.7). Dysuria usually is present. Men with asymptomatic urethritis are an important reservoir for transmission. Approximately one-half of men who are sexual partners of women with PID are asymptomatically infected. Although most men with gonorrhea develop symptoms, those who ignore their symptoms or have asymptomatic infection are at risk for developing complications (see Fig. 5.6). Endocervical infection is the most common type of uncomplicated gonorrhea in women (Figs. 5.8 and 5.9).

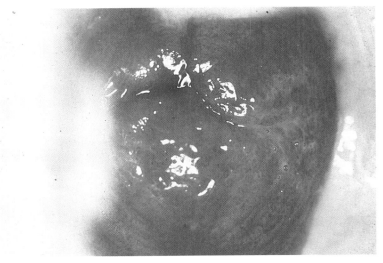

Fig. 5.7 Symptomatic gonococcal urethritis. **A** Scanty urethral discharge obtained after urethral stripping. **B** Copious spontaneous urethral discharge.

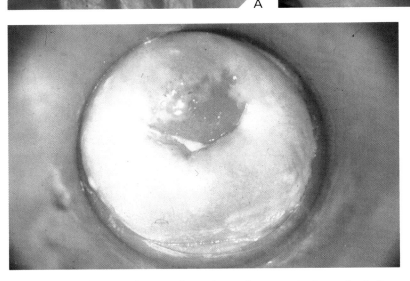

Fig. 5.8 Endocervical gonorrhea. A small amount of purulent discharge is visible in the endocervical canal.

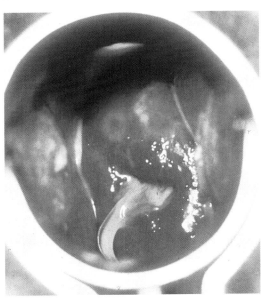

Fig. 5.9 Typical signs of endocervical gonorrhea: cervical edema and erythema as well as discharge.

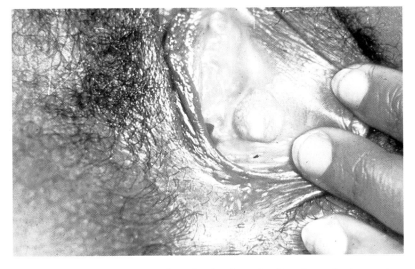

Fig. 5.10 Urethral gonorrhea in the female. Purulent discharge is visible, with involvement of Bartholin's gland.

Fig. 5.11 Gonococcal cervicitis with mucoid discharge and marked cervical erythema and edema. This is indistinguishable clinically from chlamydial cervicitis.

One-half of infected women are asymptomatic. Cervical infections usually manifest themselves by vaginal discharge and sometimes by dysuria (because of coexistent urethral involvement). Other local complications include abscesses in Bartholin's and Skene's glands (Fig. 5.10). Asymptomatic infections are found most often in women who are screened for gonorrhea in routine gynecologic examinations or who are seen as contacts of men with gonorrhea. Clinically, the cervical os may be erythematous and friable, with a purulent exudate (Figs. 5.9 and 5.11).

Rectal infections, which occur in 30% of women with cervical gonorrhea, probably represent colonization from cervical discharge and are symptomatic in less than 5% of women. Infections in homosexual men, however, result from anal intercourse and are more often symptomatic (18 to 34%). Symptoms and signs range from mild burning on defecation to itching to severe tenesmus, and from mucopurulent discharge to frank blood in the stools.

Pharyngeal "infections" are diagnosed most often in women and homosexual men with a history of fellatio. There has never been a convincing demonstration of a relationship between pharyngeal infection (or colonization, as some would put it) and the signs and symptoms of a sore throat or tonsillitis.

Ocular infections occur most commonly in newborns who are exposed to infected secretions in the birth canal of an infected mother (Fig. 5.12). Occasionally, keratoconjunctivitis is seen in adults (Fig. 5.13). Conjunctival infection, tearing, and lid edema occur early, followed rapidly by the appearance of a frankly purulent exudate. Prompt diagnosis and treatment are important because corneal scarring or perforation may result (Fig. 5.14).

DISSEMINATED GONOCOCCAL INFECTION

DGI is the result of gonococcal bacteremia. The sources of infection are primarily asymptomatic infections of the pharynx, urethra, or cervix. The most common form of DGI is the "dermatitis–arthritis" syndrome in which the patient develops fever, chills, skin lesions, and arthralgias, usually involving the hands, the feet (or, less often, ankles), and the elbows over a few days. Skin lesions, which are distributed sparsely on the extensor

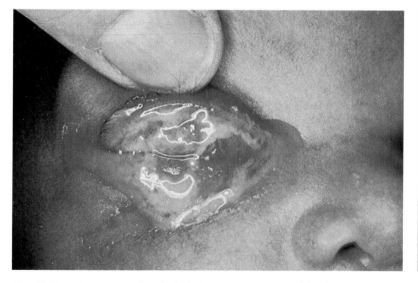

Fig. 5.12 Gonococcal ophthalmia neonatorum. Lid edema, erythema, and marked purulent discharge are seen. The Gram-stained smear was loaded with gram-negative diplococci within neutrophils.

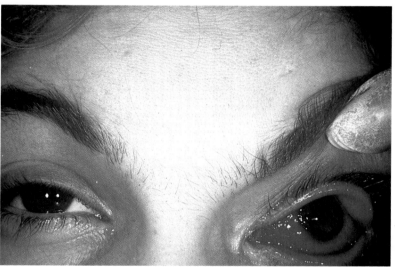

Fig. 5.13 Early gonococcal ophthalmia in an adult showing marked chemosis and tearing with no discharge.

Fig. 5.14 Corneal clouding following gonococcal ophthalmia in an adult.

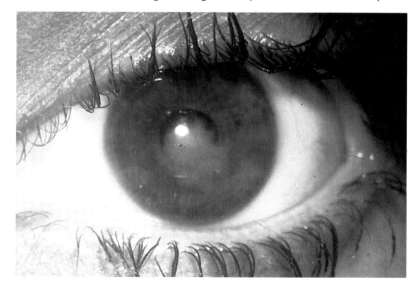

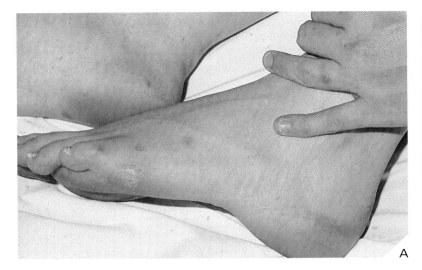

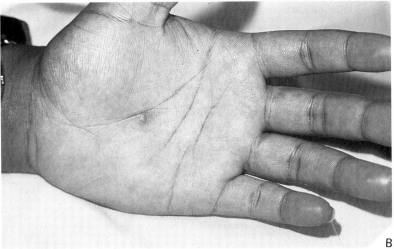

A

B

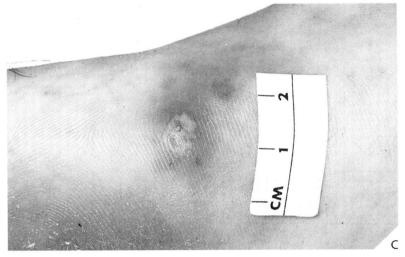

C

Fig. 5.15 Skin lesions of disseminated gonococcal infection. **A** Papular and pustular lesions on the foot. **B** Small painful midpalmar lesion on an erythematous base. **C** Classic large lesions with a necrotic, grayish central lesion on an erythematous base.

DIFFERENTIAL DIAGNOSIS OF DERMATITIS–TENOSYNOVITIS SYNDROME (POLYARTICULAR)

Meningococcemia
Staphylococcal sepsis or endocarditis
Other bacterial septicemias (rare)
HIV infection: Acute thrombocytopenia and arthritis
Hepatitis B prodrome
Acute Reiter's syndrome
Juvenile rheumatoid arthritis
Lyme disease

A

Fig. 5.16 Differential diagnosis of disseminated gonococcal infection. **A** Dermatitis–tenosynovitis syndrome. **B** Monarticular arthritis.

DIFFERENTIAL DIAGNOSIS OF MONARTICULAR ARTHRITIS

INFECTIOUS

Bacterial
  Adults
    Gonococcus*
    Staphylococcus
    Pneumococcus
    Streptococcus
  Children
    Staphylococcus
    Streptococcus
    Pneumococcus
    Haemophilus influenzae
    Gram-negative rods

Tuberculosis

Fungal

NONINFECTIOUS

Gout, pseudogout*
Rheumatoid arthritis (especially juvenile rheumatoid arthritis)
Trauma
Tumors
Hemarthrosis
Osteochondritis
Palindromic
Pigmented/villonodular syndrome

*Most common

B

surfaces of the distal extremities, may be macular, pustular, centrally necrotic, or hemorrhagic (Fig. 5.15). On careful examination, the areas of tenderness and erythema are due to periarticular inflammation of the tendon sheaths rather than true arthritis. A minority of cases develop septic joints with effusion. Gonococci may be isolated from the purulent synovial fluid in about 50% of cases, while blood cultures are positive in less than 50% of DGI cases. Occasionally, DGI may cause endocarditis or meningitis. Patients with a congenital deficiency in one of the late-acting complement components (C7, 8, 9) may experience recurrent DGI infections.

DGI must be distinguished from Reiter's syndrome, meningococcemia, acute rheumatoid arthritis, other septic arthritides, and the immune complex-mediated arthritides caused by hepatitis B virus and the human immuodeficiency virus (Fig. 5.16). A diagnosis of DGI may be based on the identification of gonococci from synovial fluid, blood, or cerebrospinal fluid. Gon-

ococci are rarely isolated from skin lesions, but a Gram-stained smear of purulent material taken from an unroofed lesion should be looked at whenever possible because diplococci occasionally may be seen with PMNs (Fig. 5.17). A direct fluorescent antibody (FA) stain of the smear is even better, if available.

In one-half of cases, gonococci cannot be isolated from blood or synovial fluid even with the best laboratory technique. A presumptive diagnosis of DGI can be made based on a combination of two of the following three criteria, provided other diagnoses have been eliminated: (1) the isolation of gonococci from a mucosal site of the patient or the patient's sexual partner (in the case of an infant, isolation from the conjunctiva or a nasogastric specimen), (2) the finding of pustular, hemorrhagic, or necrotic skin lesions on the extremities, and (3) rapid resolution of signs and symptoms on appropriate antimicrobial therapy (Fig. 5.18).

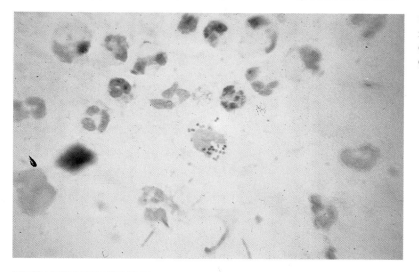

Fig. 5.17 Gram-negative diplococci visible in one neutrophil in a smear of a pustular skin lesion from a patient with disseminated gonococcal infection. Meningococci cannot be distinguished from gonococci with this method.

Fig. 5.18 Criteria supporting a clinical diagnosis of disseminated infection.

CRITERIA SUPPORTING A CLINICAL DIAGNOSIS OF DISSEMINATED GONOCOCCAL INFECTION

Gonococci are demonstrated in synovial fluid, blood, cerebrospinal fluid, or skin lesions by culture

Observation of diplococci in Gram- or methylene blue–stained smear

Clinical diagnosis of DGI may be based on two of the following three criteria:
Isolation of gonococci from urogenital, rectal, pharyngeal, or conjunctival sites of the patient or the patient's sexual partner
Infection is manifested as pustular, hemorrhagic, or necrotic skin lesions distributed on the extremities
Patient responds rapidly to appropriate antimicrobial therapy

Pelvic Inflammatory Disease (PID, Salpingitis)

The gonococcus (or chlamydia) agents may ascend from the endocervical canal through the endometrium to the fallopian tubes and ultimately to the pelvic peritoneum (Fig. 5.19), resulting in endometritis, salpingitis, and finally peritonitis. Clinically, pelvic and abdominal pain, fever, chills, and cervical motion tenderness are seen. This sign–symptom complex is termed PID. Acute pyogenic complications of PID include tubo-ovarian abscesses, pelvic peritonitis (often mimicking appendicitis), or Fitz-Hugh-Curtis syndrome, which is an inflammation of Glisson's capsule of the liver. PID may also be caused by many nonsexually transmitted bacteria that are part of the normal vaginal flora. The proportion of disease caused by N. *gonorrhoeae*, based on the recovery of the organism from laparoscopic spec-

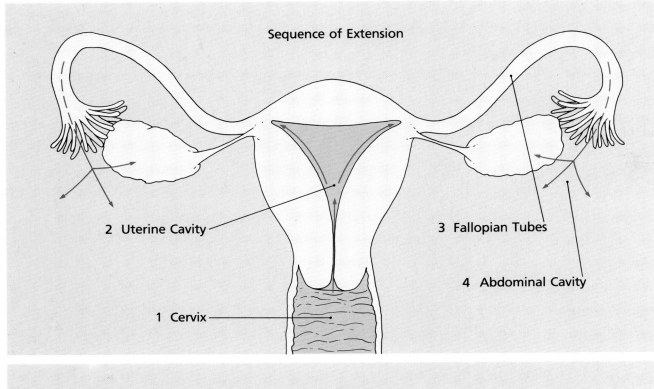

Fig. 5.19 The evolution of gonococcal pelvic inflammatory disease.

Sequence of Extension

2 Uterine Cavity
3 Fallopian Tubes
4 Abdominal Cavity
1 Cervix

Clinical Features

Peritonitis

Nausea, emesis abdominal distention, rigidity, tenderness. Pelvic or abdominal cavity abscess formation may follow.

Endosalpingitis

Constant bilateral lower quadrant abdominal pain aggravated by body motion. Tenderness in one or both adnexal areas. Abscess formation may occur.

Endocervicitis

May be asymptomatic; vaginal discharge, cervical inflammation or infection; local tenderness.

Endometritis

Menstrual irregularity

Fig. 5.20 Etiologic agents of primary and recurrent pelvic inflammatory disease.

ETIOLOGIC AGENTS OF PRIMARY AND RECURRENT PELVIC INFLAMMATORY DISEASE

Neisseria gonorrhoeae
Chlamydia trachomatis
Group B streptococci
Escherichia coli and other enterobacteria
Gardnerella vaginalis
Haemophilus influenzae

Bacteroides spp.
Peptococcus spp.
Peptostreptococcus spp.
Genital mycoplasmas (?)
Actinomyces israelii
(only with IUD-associated disease)

imens, varies from 8 to 70%. As many as 15% of women with uncomplicated cervical infections may develop PID. It is clear that PID is the most common and costly consequence of gonorrhea, and recurrent episodes of PID are common. First PID infections are more likely to be gonococcal or chlamydial, while other bacteria are isolated more frequently from recurrent episodes (Fig. 5.20). The consequences of PID include an increased probability of infertility (tubal factor infertility) and ectopic pregnancy.

The clinical diagnosis of PID is imprecise. The disease should be considered in a woman with lower abdominal pain and adnexal tenderness, or midline tenderness indicative of endometritis. Abnormally painful menses and metromenorrhagia are common. PID has been associated with the use of intrauterine contraceptive devices (IUDs). Pelvic actinomycosis, a rare cause of PID, is seen exclusively in women using IUDs. Laparoscopy

is the best method for establishing a diagnosis; however, especially in early PID, the inflammation may not have extended to the tubal surface, and the peritoneal mucosa may appear normal despite inflammation within the tubes (Fig. 5.21). Misdiagnosis is common; ectopic pregnancy and acute appendicitis may be mistaken for PID and vice versa (Fig. 5.22). In lieu of laparoscopic specimens, endocervical specimens for N. *gonorrhoeae* and *Chlamydia trachomatis* must suffice, and are essential. Empiric treatment regimens must be effective against both pathogens, especially since chlamydial disease is associated with a high incidence of tubal scarring and infertility.

Laboratory Tests

In usual practice, the laboratory diagnosis of gonorrhea is made presumptively and then confirmed, a process that involves

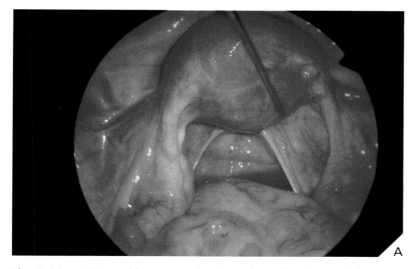

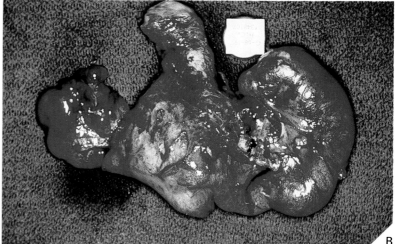

Fig. 5.21 **A** Normal laparoscopic view of the female genital tract: view from above the dome of the uterus. **B** Uterus and fallopian tubes of a patient with advanced recurrent pelvic inflammatory disease; so-called "retort" tubes.

ABDOMINAL PAIN SYNDROMES ERRONEOUSLY DIAGNOSED AS OTHER THAN SALPINGITIS

VISUAL FINDINGS (PREOPERATIVE DIAGNOSIS)

Ovarian tumor	20
Acute appendicitis	18
Ectopic pregnancy	16
Chronic PID	10
Acute peritonitis	6
Pelvic endometriosis	5
Uterine myoma	5
Uncharacteristic pelvic pain	5
Miscellaneous	6
	91

Modified from Jacobson and Westrom.

A

ABDOMINAL PAIN SYNDROMES ERRONEOUSLY DIAGNOSED AS SALPINGITIS

VISUAL FINDINGS

Acute appendicitis	24
Pelvic endometriosis	16
Corpus luteum hematoma	12
Ectopic pregnancy	11
Ovarian tumor	7
Chronic PID	6
Mesenteric lymphadenitis	6
Miscellaneous	16
	98

Modified from Jacobson and Westrom.

B

Fig. 5.22 **A** Abdominal pain syndromes erroneously clinically diagnosed as other than salpingitis. **B** Abdominal pain syndromes erroneously clinically diagnosed as salpingitis. The correct diagnoses in **A** and **B** were confirmed by laparoscopy.

Fig. 5.23 Characteristics of human *Neisseria* and related spp. that grow on routine laboratory media selective for the gonococcus. **A** Growth on selective and simple media, requirement for supplemental CO_2. **B** Differential biochemical reactions.

SPECIES	EXTRA CO_2 NEEDED[a]	GROWTH ON MTM, ML, OR NYC MEDIUM	GROWTH ON CHOCOLATE OR BLOOD AGAR AT 22°C	NUTRIENT AGAR AT 35°C
N. gonorrhoeae	VI	+[b]	−	−
N. meningitidis	I	+	−	+
N. lactamica	D	+	−	+
N. cinerea	D	−[c]	−	+
N. polysaccharea	D	+	−	+
N. flavescens	I	+	−	+
N. sicca	No	−	+	+
N. subflava biovar *perflava*	No	−[d]	+	+
B. catarrhalis	No	D	+	+
K. denitrificans	I	+	−	−

MTM = modified Thayer-Martin medium; ML = Martin-Lewis medium; NYC = New York City medium; + = Most strains (≥ 90%) positive; − = Most strains (≥ 90%) negative; D = Some strains positive, some strains negative.
[a]Extra CO_2: VI, very important for growth; I, important for growth; No, not needed for growth; D, some strains require extra CO_2.
[b]≥ 90% of vancomycin-susceptible strains of *N. gonorrhoeae* may not grow on TM or MTM media.
[c]Some strains of *N. cinerea* have been isolated on gonococcal selective medium but are colistin-susceptible and will not grow when subcultured on selective media.
[d]Some strains of *N. subflava* biovar *perflava* grow on gonococcal selective media in primary culture, are colistin-resistant, and grow on selective media on subculture.

A

DIFFERENTIAL BIOCHEMICAL REACTIONS

SPECIES	PIGMENT[a]	SUPEROXOL[b]	ACID PRODUCED FROM GLUCOSE	MALTOSE	FRUCTOSE	SUCROSE	LACTOSE (ONPG)	POLYSACCHARIDE[c] FROM 1% SUCROSE	NO$_3$	NO$_2$[d]	DNase
N. gonorrhoeae	−	+	+	−	−	−	−	−	−	−	−
N. meningitidis	−	−	+	+	−	−	−	−	−	D	−
N. lactamica	−	−	+	+	−	−	+	−	−	D	−
N. cinerea	−	−	−[e]	−	−	−	−	−	−	+	−
N. polysaccharea	−	−	+	+	−	−	−	+	−	D	−
N. flavescens	+	−	−	−	−	−	−	+	−	−	−
N. sicca	−	−	+	+	+	+	−	+	−	+	−
N. subflava biovar *perflava*	+	−	+	+	+	+	−	+	−	+	−
B. catarrhalis	−	−	−	−	−	−	−	−	+	−	+
K. denitrificans	−	−	+	−	−	−	−	−	+	−	−

ONPG = o-nitrophenyl-β-D-galactopyranoside; DNase = deoxyribonuclease; − = Most strains (≥ 90%) negative; + = Most strains (≥ 90%) positive; D = Some strains positive, some strains negative.
[a]Pigment observed in colonies on nutrient agar. Strains of *N. cinerea* and *N. lactamica* are yellow-brown and yellow pigmented when growth is harvested on a cotton applicator or smeared on filter paper.
[b]All *Neisseria* spp. and *B. catarrhalis* give a positive catalase test using 3% H_2O_2; *N. gonorrhoeae* strains give strong reactions with 30% H_2O_2 (superoxol) on chocolatized blood media, whereas other species are usually negative. This test should be used only in conjunction with other tests.
[c]Some strains may be inhibited by 5% sucrose; reactions may be obtained on a starch-free medium containing 1% sucrose. Strains of *N. gonorrhoeae* and *N. meningitidis* do not grow on this medium.
[d]Results for tests in 0.1% (w/v) potassium nitrite; *N. gonorrhoeae* strains and strains of some other species that are negative in 0.1% nitrite can reduce 0.01% (w/v) nitrite.
[e]Some strains of *N. cinerea* may give a weak reaction in glucose in some rapid tests for the detection of acid from carbohydrates.

B

identifying characteristics that distinguish N. *gonorrhoeae* from other *Neisseria* spp. that may be present in the specimen (Fig. 5.23). Nonpathogenic *Neisseria* and related spp. are normal flora of the oropharynx and nasopharynx and occasionally are isolated from other sites infected by the gonococcus—for example, the urethra, cervix, and rectum.

PRESUMPTIVE LABORATORY DIAGNOSIS
A provisional diagnosis of gonorrhea may be made from urethral, cervical, and rectal specimens (Fig. 5.24) if gram-negative diplococci are observed intracellularly in PMNs (Fig. 5.25). Gram stain diagnosis is ≥95% sensitive in men with symptomatic urethritis. This criterion is less sensitive in cervical specimens (50%) and may be even less in rectal specimens. A presumptive diagnosis of gonorrhea can be made in cervical and rectal specimens if oxidase-positive, gram-negative diplococci grow on medium selective for the isolation of N. *gonorrhoeae*. Presumptive diagnoses cannot be made from pharyngeal specimens because the oropharynx is the normal habitat of *Neisseria* and related spp. Strains isolated from pharyngeal specimens must be confirmed to distinguish the gonococcus from *Neisseria* and related spp. that may grow on selective media.

SPECIMEN COLLECTION AND TRANSPORTATION
Specimens for the laboratory diagnosis of gonorrhea should always be collected before the patient is treated. N. *gonorrhoeae* is most successfully isolated when the specimen is inoculated onto media and incubated at 35 to 36.5°C in a CO_2-enriched atmosphere immediately after collection. It is more important to incubate inoculated plates immediately in a CO_2-enriched atmosphere than to place the specimens at 35°C. This can best be done by immediately placing streaked plates in a CO_2 candle-extinction jar held at room temperature until they can be transported to the laboratory incubator. Specimens may be kept at room temperature for up to five hours without loss of viability. A candle-extinction jar is easily made from a wide-mouthed screw-cap jar such as a commercial-sized (1 gallon) mayonnaise or relish jar. A damp paper towel is placed on the

---

PRESUMPTIVE LABORATORY DIAGNOSIS OF *NEISSERIA GONORRHOEAE*

Fig. 5.24 Presumptive laboratory diagnosis of N. *gonorrhoeae*.

Gram-negative diplococci observed intracellularly in PMNs (≥ 95% sensitive in men with symptomatic urethritis)

Gram-negative, oxidase-positive diplococci are isolated on selective media

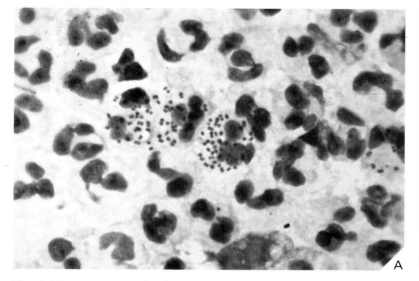 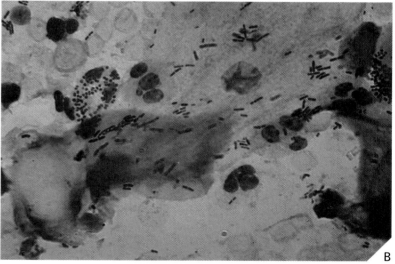

Fig. 5.25 **A** Gram-stained smear of urethral exudate from a male showing a sheet of neutrophils (PMN) and many gram-negative diplococci within PMN. This is sufficient for a presumptive diagnosis of gonorrhea in the male. **B** Gram-stained smear of endocervical exudate showing scattered neutrophils and squamous epithelial cells. Gram-negative diplococci are present in one neutrophil. This is sufficient to make a presumptive diagnosis of gonorrhea in the female, but should be confirmed by culture.

bottom, and a plain wax candle is lit and placed on the floor of the jar and relit each time a new plate is added to the stack. The cover is then screwed on firmly. This will produce a humid, 3 to 4% CO_2 atmosphere (Fig. 5.26).

Specimens for the laboratory diagnosis of uncomplicated gonorrhea may be collected from the urethra, cervix, rectum, and pharynx (Fig. 5.27). The precise choice of anatomic sites from which to collect specimens is made on the basis of the patient's potential for sexual exposure (Fig. 5.28). Specimens are collected with cotton, polyester, or calcium alginate swabs. Normally, only urethral specimens are collected from heterosexual men, while urethral, rectal, and pharyngeal specimens are collected from homosexual men. For urethral specimens, calcium alginate swabs are preferred because they can be inserted into the urethra in patients with no discharge. Cervical and rectal specimens are routinely collected from women;

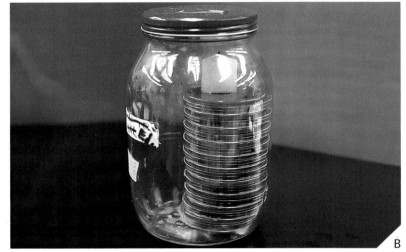

Fig. 5.26 **A** Homemade candle-extinction jar properly filled with candle on the floor of the jar and cover screwed on tightly. **B** Homemade candle-extinction jar improperly filled. The candle is too close to the lid and will be extinguished before generating the required amount of carbon dioxide.

Fig. 5.27 Specimen collection for laboratory diagnosis of gonorrhea.

SPECIMEN COLLECTION FOR LABORATORY DIAGNOSIS OF GONORRHEA

SPECIMEN	METHOD OF COLLECTION
Urethral, men	**Symptomatic:** Express urethral exudate. **Asymptomatic:** Compress meatus vertically to open the distal urethra, and insert and withdraw a calcium alginate swab to 2 cm with a rotary motion.
Urethral, women	**Symptomatic:** Massage urethra gently against pubic symphysis. **Asymptomatic:** Insert and withraw a calcium alginate swab to 2 cm with a rotary motion.
Endocervical	Insert speculum moistened with warm water (NOT surgical lubricant) into the vagina. Insert a swab 2 to 3 cm into the cervical canal and move in and out with a rotary motion over 10 sec to allow absorption of exudate.
Vaginal	Insert speculum. Rub sterile cotton swab against the posterior vaginal wall and allow swab to absorb specimen. (A swab of the vaginal orifice can be taken if hymen is intact.)
Rectal	Ask patient to spread buttocks and bear down slightly. Insert sterile cotton swab approximately 3 cm into anal canal and rotate to sample crypts just inside the anal ring; allow swab to absorb specimen for 10 sec.
Oropharyngeal	Rub two or three sterile swabs together over the posterior pharynx and tonsillar crypts carefully for 10 sec.

specimens may also be collected from the urethra and from Bartholin's and Skene's glands when appropriate. In men, N. gonorrhoeae may also be isolated from sediment obtained from centrifuged urine. Blood cultures should be collected from patients with suspected disseminated infection. In patients with septic arthritis, synovial fluid should be cultured.

If swab specimens must be transported to a laboratory, they should be inoculated onto an isolation medium, ideally Jembec or Transgrow, and incubated overnight before being shipped. The transport medium should be shipped by courier or an express mail service to ensure delivery of the inoculated medium within 24 to 48 hours. The transport of specimens in Amies' or Stuart's medium is not advised.

Urethral, cervical, and pharyngeal specimens are inoculated onto selective media such as Thayer-Martin (TM) medium, Martin-Lewis (ML) medium, New York City (NYC) medium, or GC-Lect (GC-L) medium, which are composed of GC base or equivalent media supplemented with growth factors and antimicrobial and anti-fungal agents; some media contain hemo-globin. Rectal specimens are inoculated onto modified TM (MTM) containing trimethoprim lactate, which inhibits the growth and swarming of *Proteus* spp. If the specimen is obtained from a site that is normally sterile (e.g., blood, synovial fluid, conjunctiva), it may be inoculated on nonselective media such as chocolate agar. It should be remembered that other *Neisseria* spp. may grow on nonselective media and therefore confirmation procedures should be scrupulously followed.

The specimen is inoculated over the entire surface of the plate in a "Z" pattern, followed by streak inoculation of the plate (Fig. 5.29). This inoculation technique yields isolated colonies that can be more easily processed, particularly in pharyngeal specimens from which strains of N. *meningitidis*, N. *lactamica*, and K. *denitrificans* may also be isolated.

Inoculated plates are immediately incubated at 35 to 36.5°C in a CO_2-enriched, humid atmosphere. Gonococci require CO_2 for primary isolation; the supplemental CO_2 can be provided in a CO_2 incubator, a container with a CO_2-generating tablet, or a candle-extinction jar with white, unscented, nontoxic candles.

Fig. 5.28 Sites for usual collection of specimens for the laboratory diagnosis of uncomplicated gonorrhea.

SPECIMEN COLLECTION SITES

PATIENT	SITES
Heterosexual men	Urethra
	Oropharynx
Homosexual men	Urethra
	Rectum
	Oropharynx
Women	Cervix
	Rectum
	Oropharynx

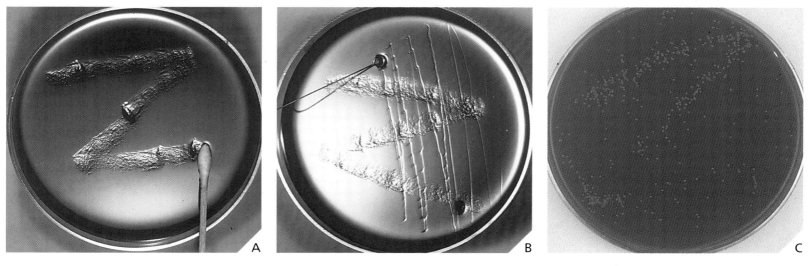

Fig. 5.29 A "Z" streak method of inoculation to obtain isolated colonies for the identification of *Neisseria*. **B** Cross-streaking of "Z" inoculated plate to ensure separation of colonies. **C** Inoculated plate after 24 hours of incubation.

GRAM STAIN

A thin smear prepared from the specimen or suspect colonies on the isolation medium is Gram stained and examined under an oil-immersion objective (×100) for intracellular gram-negative diplococci in PMNs. Cells of Neisseria spp. occur as diplococci composed of kidney-shaped cells (0.8 μm × 0.6 μm) with adjacent sides flattened (see Fig. 5.25A). A confirmed identification of N. gonorrhoeae also can be made from Gram-stained smears prepared from colonies on primary isolation plates or smears; confirmation of the gonococcus can be made in cultures with a monoclonal FA stain (Fig. 5.30). This reagent has shown no cross-reaction with nongonococcal species, but occasionally has not reacted with gonococcal strains. FA confirmation with polyvalent antibodies is not recommended because the reagent may react with other Neisseria spp. (false-positive) and occasionally has not reacted with some PPNG strains (false-negative).

GROWTH CHARACTERISTICS

Plates are examined for growth after incubation for 24 hours; those that show no growth at this time are reincubated for 24 hours before being discarded and before a report of negative for N. gonorrhoeae is issued. Translucent, nonpigmented-to-brownish colonies measuring 0.5 to 1.0 mm in diameter on isolation media should be characterized. Representative colonies are Gram stained and examined for oxidase production. Oxidase is detected either by placing a drop of oxidase reagent (tetramethyl-paraphenylenediamine-dihydrochloride) on a few representative colonies or by rubbing representative colonies on filter paper moistened with oxidase reagent with a platinum loop; nichrome loops may react with the oxidase regent, giving a false-positive reaction. In a positive test, the growth will turn purple within 10 seconds (Fig. 5.31). The oxidase reagent should not be placed on all suspect colonies. If few suspect colonies are available, they must be subcultured to chocolate agar immediately after the application of the oxidase reagent because it is toxic for the cells. Thin smears of suspect colonies are Gram stained as described above. If the suspect colonies are oxidase-positive, gram-negative diplococci, a report of presumptive N. gonorrhoeae may be made for cervical, urethral, or rectal specimens. Ideally, all isolates should be confirmed as N. gonorrhoeae. Certainly, pharyngeal isolates must be confirmed because other Neisseria and related spp. frequently may be isolated on gonococcal selective media (Fig. 5.32).

PRESERVATION

Isolates of N. gonorrhoeae must be subcultured every 24 to 48 hours or suspended in a solution of trypticase soy broth containing 15% glycerol and frozen at −70°C. Strains cannot be stored at −20°C for long periods but can be stored at this temperature for a short time (approximately 2 months).

IDENTIFICATION OF ISOLATES

Traditionally, Neisseria and related spp. have been identified by a series of biochemical tests, including acid production from glucose, maltose, sucrose, and lactose; reduction of nitrate; and production of polysaccharide. Traditional biochemical tests must be incubated for 24 to 48 hours before results can be

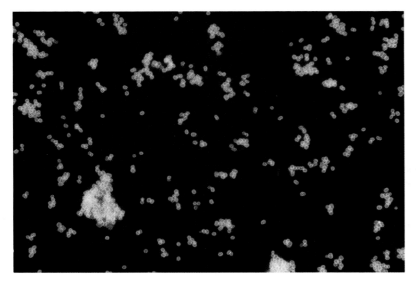

Fig. 5.30 Monoclonal FA stain.

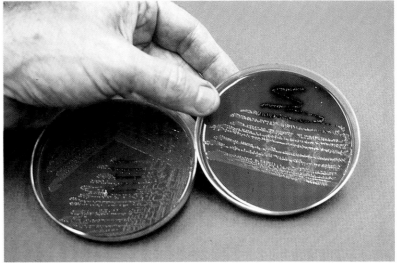

Fig. 5.31 Positive oxidase reaction on culture of N. gonorrhoeae.

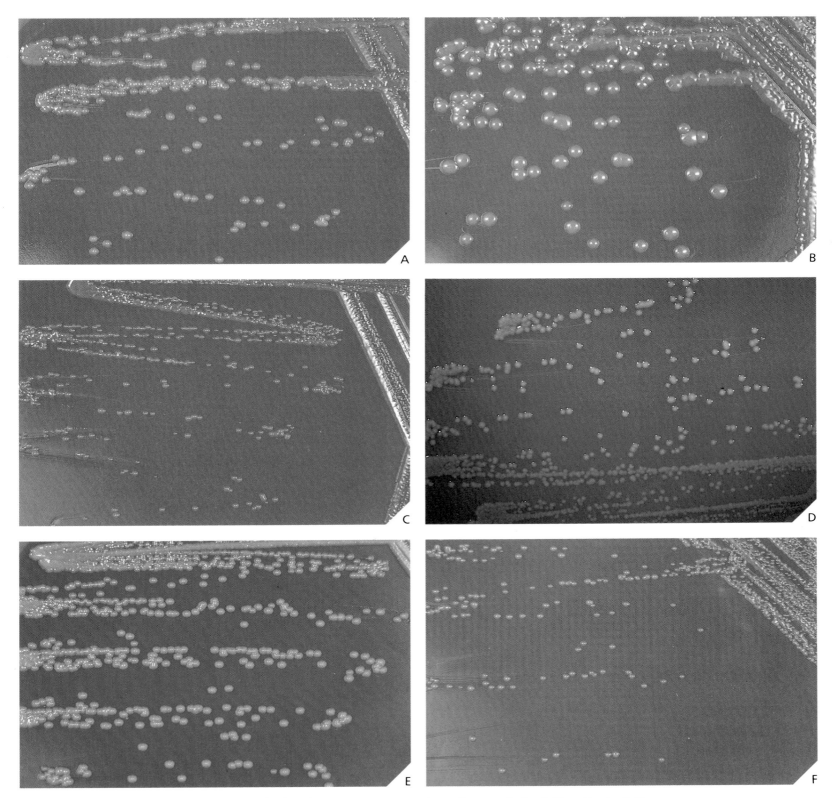

Fig. 5.32 Typical colonies of *Neisseria* and related spp. **A** *N. gonorrhoeae.* **B** *N. meningitidis.* **C** *N. lactamica.* **D** *N. cinerea.* **E** *Bran-hamella catarrhalis.* **F** *Kingella denitrificans.*

interpreted (Fig. 5.33). Acid production tests should be incubated at 35 to 36.5°C without CO_2, which will produce an acid reaction in the media. Rapid tests have been developed that permit identification of strains from the primary isolation plate or within several hours of the isolation of a pure subculture. The rapid confirmation tests may be divided into four categories: rapid carbohydrate, enzyme substrate, serologic, and DNA probe tests.

Rapid Carbohydrate Tests

Rapid carbohydrate tests permit detection of acid production from glucose, maltose, lactose, and sucrose. Strains of N. *gonorrhoeae* are distinguished by their ability to produce acid only from glucose; most other N*eisseria* spp. produce acid from maltose and thus are easily differentiated from N. *gonorrhoeae*. However, because strains of other N*eisseria* and related spp. may also give strong or weak acid reactions from glucose, additional tests may be required to differentiate between them (Fig. 5.34). Strains of several species (maltose-negative N. *meningitidis*, N. *cinerea*, Bran-hamella catarrhalis, and K. *denitrificans*) may be misidentified as N. *gonorrhoeae*. In addition, some strains of N. *gonorrhoeae* produce very weak reactions in glucose tests and may appear to be glucose-negative. Supplemental tests that can be used to distinguish N. *gonorrhoeae* from these species are listed in Figure 5.23.

Enzyme Substrate Tests

Strains of N*eisseria* spp. produce enzymes that may be used to differentiate between them (Fig. 5.35). N. *gonorrhoeae* strains pro-duce hydroxyprolyl aminopeptidase, N. *meningitidis* strains pro-duce γ-glutamyl aminopeptidase, and N. *lactamica* strains pro-duce β-galactosidase; strains of B. *catarrhalis* produce none of these enzymes. The use of enzyme substrate tests is limited to the identification of strains isolated on gonococcal selective media because strains of the commensal N*eisseria* spp. may pro-duce hydroxyprolylaminopeptidase and would be identified as N. *gonorrhoeae* without supplemental tests. In addition, strains of K. *denitrificans* and some strains of N. *subflava* biovar *perflava* and N. *cinerea* have also been isolated on gonococcal selective media and will be misidentified as N. *gonorrhoeae* without additional char-acterization. Thus using a combination of enzyme substrate and other biochemical tests, strains isolated on selective media can be identified by a process of elimination (see Fig. 5.23).

Products that combine acid production, enzyme substrate, and other biochemical tests are also commercially available. These tests provide a more detailed characterization of isolates that will permit the laboratorian to distinguish N. *gonorrhoeae* from related species. Pure cultures of clinical isolates are re-quired to inoculate all rapid biochemical tests.

Serologic Tests

There are currently no tests that permit the laboratory diagnosis of N. *gonorrhoeae* in patient's serum. There are also no tests that can permit confirmed identification of the gonococcus in specimens.

Serologic tests for the identification of N. *gonorrhoeae* in pri-mary cultures are commercially available as FA tests (discussed above) or as coagglutination tests. Coagglutination tests consist

Fig. 5.33 Acid production from carbohydrates in Cystine Trypti-case Soy (CTA) medium. Tubes from left to right are CTA base me-dium containing no carbohydrate, CTA medium containing 1% glu-cose and CTA medium containing 1% maltose. **A** N. *gonorrhoeae*. **B** N. *meningitidis*.

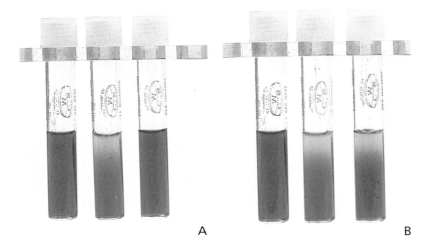

A   B

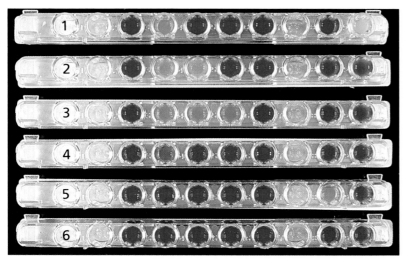

Fig. 5.34 Reactions of N*eisseria* and related spp. in the API Quad-ferm + rapid carbohydrate test. Tests, from left to right, are con-trol (no carbohydrate), glucose, maltose, lactose, sucrose, DNase, and β-lactamase. 1. N. *gonorrhoeae* (β-lactamase-positive). 2. N. *meningitidis*. 3. N. *lactamica*. 4. K. *denitrificans*. 5. B. *catarrhalis*. 6. N. *cinerea*.

of cocktails of monoclonal antibodies directed toward gonococcal protein I which have been adsorbed to protein A-producing *Staphylococcus aureus* cells. Suspect colonies are suspended in buffer or saline and heated in a boiling water bath. A drop of the cooled suspension is mixed with a drop each of the antigonococcal and a negative control reagent. After rotation for one to two minutes, the reactions are interpreted. If a suspension gives a positive reaction with the antigonococcal and a negative reaction with the control reagent, the isolate is identified as N. *gonorrhoeae* (Fig. 5.36). Cross-reactions between nongonococcal N*eisseria* and related spp. and the coagglutination reagents have been reported, and some gonococcal strains have not reacted with the reagents.

DNA Probes

Recently, tests that use DNA probes to detect DNA or RNA sequences in strains of N. *gonorrhoeae* have been developed. Initial reports suggest that these tests are highly specific and sensitive for the confirmed identification of N. *gonorrhoeae*.

Antimicrobial Susceptibility Testing

Surveillance for antimicrobial resistance in N. *gonorrhoeae* should be an integral part of a routine STD laboratory program. If resources permit, all isolates of N. *gonorrhoeae* should be tested for their susceptibility to clinically important antimicrobial agents. If resources are limited, clinically and epidemiologically important isolates (e.g., isolates from patients with positive test-of-cure culture) should be tested. Clusters of treatment failures may indicate an outbreak of a resistant strain. When an outbreak is suspected, a consecutive sample of 50 isolates should be evaluated to determine the prevalence of a resistant strain.

β-LACTAMASE TESTS

All gonococcal isolates should be tested for β-lactamase, which can be detected in colonies on primary or subculture. Several tests for β-lactamase are available commercially; these include chromogenic cephalosporin, acidometric, and iodometric tests

Fig. 5.35 Reactions of *Neisseria* and related spp. to the enzyme substrate test, Gonochek II. From left to right N. *gonorrhoeae*, N. *meningitidis*, N. *lactamica*, B. *catarrhalis*, N. *cinerea*, and K. *denitrificans*. The production of γ-glutamylaminopeptidase and β-galactosidase by N. *meningitidis* and N. *lactamica*, respectively, is determined directly without removing the clear inner cap. The ability of strains to produce hydroxyprolylaminopeptidase is determined by exposing the organism suspension to the substrate contained in the red cap. Note that N. *gonorrhoeae*, N. *cinerea*, and K. *denitrificans* give identical reactions in this test—that is, they produce hydroxyprolylaminopeptidase. Strains of B. *catarrhalis* do not produce any of these enzymes; suspensions will be yellow or colorless after exposure to the substrate contained in the red cap.

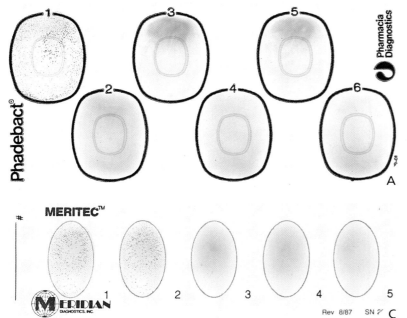

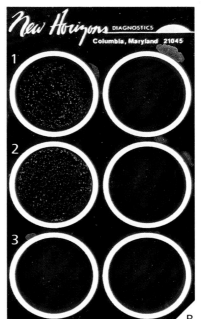

Fig. 5.36 Reactions of N. *gonorrhoeae*, N. *meningitidis*, and related spp. in coagglutination tests. **A** Phadebact: 1. N. *gonorrhoeae*. 2. Negative control. 3. N. *meningitidis*. 4. N. *cinerea*. 5. N. *lactamica*. 6. Negative control. **B** GonoGen: From top to bottom, left to right: 1. Positive control and its control (negative) reaction. 2. N. *gonorrhoeae* and its control (negative) reaction. 3. N. *meningitidis* and its control (negative) reaction. **C** Meritec: 1. Positive control. 2. N. *gonorrhoeae*. 3. Negative control. 4. N. *meningitidis*. 5. Negative control.

(Fig. 5.37). The chromogenic cephalosporin (nitrocefin, PADAC) tests are preferred because the substrates are stable and the reactions are specific and highly sensitive for β-lactamase. The specificity and sensitivity of the acidometric and iodometric tests may be affected by several factors, including improper storage of the product, which may result in nonspecific hydrolysis of the substrate. β-lactamase-positive and β-lactamase-negative strains should be included as controls with each batch of clinical isolates.

DETERMINATION OF ANTIMICROBIAL SUSCEPTIBILITY

With the exception of specific β-lactamase tests, resistance in N. *gonorrhoeae* must be detected by measuring the level of susceptibility of strains to an antimicrobial agent. Two methods, the agar-dilution and disk-diffusion procedures, may be used to measure the susceptibilities of isolates.

Agar-Dilution Susceptibility Testing

Agar-dilution susceptibility testing is the reference method for measuring antimicrobial susceptibilities of strains of N. *gonorrhoeae* because it is the most accurate and reproducible procedure. Resistance to antimicrobial agents is measured as the minimal inhibitory concentration (MIC) of the agent that inhibits growth of an isolate. Measurement of resistance to penicillin, tetracycline, spectinomycin, cefoxitin, and ceftriaxone is recommended. Susceptibility testing is performed on GC agar base medium containing 1% (vol/vol) IsoVitaleX or an equivalent supplement; antimicrobial agents are incorporated into the base medium in serial twofold dilutions. Isolates to be tested are grown overnight on chocolate agar and suspended in Mueller-Hinton broth to an optical density equivalent to a 0.5 McFarland standard to contain approximately 10^8 colony-forming units (CFU)/mL. The suspensions are diluted 1:10 in Mueller-Hinton broth, and 10^4 CFU/mL are inoculated onto the surface of the antibiotic-containing media and an antibiotic-free control medium with a Steer's replicator or a calibrated loop. Plates are incubated at 35 to 36°C in a CO_2-enriched atmosphere for 24 hours and then examined for growth. The MIC of the antimicrobial agent for an isolate is the lowest concentration that inhibits its growth.

Disk-Diffusion Susceptibility Testing

Agar-dilution susceptibility testing of N. *gonorrhoeae* isolates is not routinely performed in clinical microbiology laboratories. Instead, disk-diffusion susceptibility testing is most frequently used to measure the antimicrobial resistance of isolates of N. *gonorrhoeae*. The results of disk-diffusion susceptibility testing can be correlated with treatment outcome (Fig. 5.38).

ANTIBIOTIC-CONTAINING MEDIA

Medium containing 1.5 μg penicillin/mL has been used to screen for resistant isolates in primary culture. Penicillin-containing media have not been extensively evaluated but have been useful in some geographic areas. The major concern about this method is that it is not standardized. The number of organisms inoculated onto the medium will vary according to their numbers in specimens; urethral specimens from symptomatic men may contain many more organisms than those from women or asymptomatic men. As with the agar-dilution procedure, the result is inoculum dependent—that is, the resistance level may be higher if a larger inoculum is used. Whereas a clinical specimen containing many resistant diplococci may yield a positive culture on the penicillin-containing medium, a specimen containing few resistant diplococci may fail to grow on the same medium.

INTERPRETATION OF ANTIMICROBIAL SUSCEPTIBILITY TEST RESULTS

An antimicrobial susceptibility result determined in the laboratory is only a measure of the in vitro susceptibility of an isolate. A patient may have a positive test-of-cure culture for

Fig. 5.37 Reactions of β-lactamase-positive (left) and negative (right) strains of N. *gonorrhoeae* in a nitrocefin test.

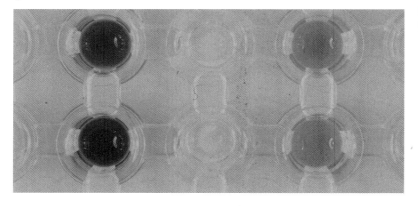

Fig. 5.38 Correlates of disk-diffusion susceptibility results with clinical outcome.

CORRELATES OF DISK-DIFFUSION SUSCEPTIBILITY RESULTS WITH CLINICAL OUTCOME

Susceptible	Less than 5% likelihood of treatment failure
Intermediate	Predictable failure rates of 5 to 15% if the patient is treated with the tested antibiotic in the standard dosage (in most cases of intermediate susceptibility, a higher dose or prolonged therapy results in greater than 95% cure rates)
Resistant	May be associated with treatment failure rates of greater than 15%

a variety of reasons: (1) failure of therapy because of infection with a resistant isolate, (2) failure of therapy even when the patient is infected with a strain that is susceptible by in vitro measurements, or (3) reinfection. Thus, antimicrobial susceptibilities must be used as an adjunct to, but cannot be substituted for, clinical findings.

Antimicrobial Therapy

In response to the continued emergence of PPNG and other resistant strains in the U.S., the 1989 Centers for Disease Control STD Treatment Guidelines recommend treatment of all gono-coccal infections presumptively with antibiotic regimens effective against resistant strains (Fig. 5.39). Ceftriaxone 250 mg, intramuscularly as a single dose, is recommended therapy in most cases. For patients with a strong history of allergy to β-lactam drugs, spectinomycin 2 g, intramuscularly, is recommended. The penicillins are not recommended as therapy unless either the patient was infected in a geographic area that is nonendemic for PPNG or the organism is known to be penicillin-sensitive. The 1989 STD Treatment Guidelines, to be published by the CDC in the fall of 1989, will include detailed discussions of antimicrobial therapy and treatment recommendations for complicated gonococcal disease such as PID and DGI (Fig. 5.40).

Fig. 5.39 Recommended antimicrobial therapy for uncomplicated gonorrhea according to the prevalence of infections caused by PPNG.

RECOMMENDED THERAPY FOR UNCOMPLICATED GONORRHEA

RECOMMENDED THERAPY

Ceftriaxone: 250 mg IM
or
Spectinomycin: 2.0 g IM
or
Ciprofloxacin: 500 mg, PO

Plus
Doxycycline: 100 mg, by mouth, twice a day for 7 days
or
Tetracycline HCl: 500 mg, by mouth, four times a day for 7 days
or
Erythromycin* base or stearate, 500 mg, by mouth, four times a day for 7 days
or
Erythromycin ethylsuccinate,* 800 mg, by mouth, four times a day for 7 days
or
Other erythromycin* preparations in appropriate doses

*For patients in whom tetracycline is contraindicated (e.g., pregnant women and children).

RECOMMENDED THERAPY FOR PATIENTS WITH COMPLICATED GONOCOCCAL INFECTIONS

Fig. 5.40 Recommended therapy for patients with complicated gonococcal infections.

SYNDROME	RECOMMENDED THERAPY*
Disseminated gonococcal infection	Ceftriaxone[†]: 1g, IV, once a day for 7 days.
Meningitidis/endocarditis	Consult with an expert. In general, high-dose third-generation cephalosporin recommended. Patients with meningitis should be treated for 10 to 14 days; those with endocarditis should be treated for at least 1 month.

Ophthalmia
  Neonatal
  Adult
	
	Ceftriaxone[†]: 25 to 50 mg/kg body weight/day, IM or IV, for 7 days.[‡]
	Ceftriaxone[†]: 1g, IM or IV, 1 dose.

*Recommendations are for PPNG-endemic and PPNG-hyperendemic areas.
[†]Equivalent third-generation cephalosporin may be used in appropriate doses in lieu of ceftriaxone.
[‡]In some cases with nonsepticemic ophthalmia, single-dose therapy may be effective.

BIBLIOGRAPHY

Centers for Disease Control: Policy guidelines for the detection, management, and control of antibiotic-resistant strains of *Neisseria gonorrhoeae*. MMWR 36:5S, 1987.

Dallabetta G, Hook EW: Gonococcal infections. *Infect Dis Clin North Am* 1:25, 1987.

Ehret JM, Judson FN, Biddle JW: Gonorrhea, in Wentworth BB,Judson FN (eds): *Laboratory Methods for the Diagnosis of Sexually Transmitted Diseases*. Washington, DC, American Public Health Association, 1984, pp 43–79.

Morello JA, Janda WM, Bohnhoff M: *Neisseria* and *Branhamella*, in Lennette EH, Balows A, Hausler WJ Jr, Shadomy HJ (eds): *Manual of Clinical Microbiology*, ed 4. Washington, DC, American Society for Microbiology, 1985, pp 176–192.

Morse SA, Holmes KK: Gonococcal infections, in Hoeprich PD (ed): *Infectious Diseases*, ed 4. New York, Harper & Row, 1989 (in press).

Morse SA, Knapp JS: Neisserial infections, in Wentworth BB (ed): *Diagnostic Procedures for Bacterial Infections*, ed 7. Washington, DC, American Public Health Association, 1987, pp 407–432.

Weisner PJ, Thompson SE: Gonococcal infections, in Evans AS, Feldman HA (eds): *Bacterial Infections of Humans*. New York, Plenum Medical Book Company, 1982, pp 235–237.

Infections Caused by Chlamydia trachomatis

6

R. C. BARNES

Introduction

Chlamydia trachomatis is a bacterium with incomplete metabolic capability that restricts its growth to within the intracellular environment of parasitized host cells. The organism is distributed worldwide and apparently is restricted to human hosts, unlike the distantly related *Chlamydia psittaci*, which has a broad host range among non-human vertebrates. The first recognition that chlamydial organisms were responsible for STDs occurred in the 1930s, when the association with lymphogranuloma venereum (LGV) was noted. Sexually acquired LGV is rare in the U.S. (Fig. 6.1) but occurs frequently in the tropics. The pathogenic role of *C. trachomatis* in STDs other than LGV has been widely recognized only within the past two decades. *C. psittaci* is responsible for the zoonotic disease *ornithosis* (formerly "psit-

tacosis"), which is characterized by respiratory disease in humans who become accidental hosts for avian strains of the organism. Recently, respiratory illness in humans has been associated with another organism that is morphologically similar to the chlamydiae: the so-called "TWAR" organism. The distribution and clinical epidemiology of this organism is poorly understood.

C. trachomatis has been successfully propagated only within embryonated hens' eggs or in cell or tissue culture. This has impeded study of both the biology and clinical manifestations of infection. Until the recent recognition of the high prevalence of sexually transmitted chlamydial infections within developed countries, cell culture methods for isolation and identification of chlamydia were limited to research laboratories.

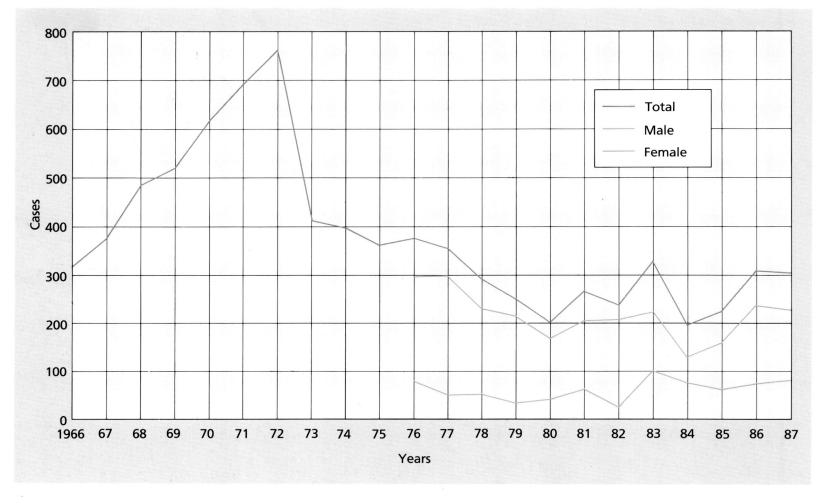

Figure 6.1   Reported cases of LGV by year in the U.S. The accuracy of such reporting is unknown.

DISTINGUISHING FEATURES OF CHLAMYDIAE

Obligate intracellular parasites

Deficient in endogenous ATP production

Contain DNA, RNA, and typical procaryotic ribosomes

Have outer membrane similar to other gram-negative bacteria

Have a dimorphic developmental cycle, which takes place in an intracellular cytoplasmic inclusion

Have small genome sizes (ca. ⅛ of *Escherichia coli*)

Extremely diverse in DNA homology

Figure 6.2   Distinguishing features of chlamydiae.

Because of their small size and the difficulty encountered in propagation, chlamydia were considered viruses from their original description until the 1960s. However, they possess a characteristic bacterial cell wall, ribosomes, both DNA and RNA, and metabolic functions that confirm their bacterial nature (Fig. 6.2).

Knowledge of the distinctive intracellular development cycle of the chlamydial organism is important in understanding parasite–host interaction (Fig. 6.3). Much of what is known has been obtained through studies of chlamydiae grown in mammalian cell culture. The organism is dimorphic. The infectious form, the elementary body (EB), is a condensed, sporelike spheroid with a diameter of 200 to 400 nm. (Fig. 6.4A and B) It is metabolically inactive, and contains a tightly compressed nucleoid and an outer membrane composed primarily of lipopolysaccharide and proteins that are highly disulfide-linked. Upon contact with a suitable host cell, the EB appears to induce its own entry by a process of "induced phagocytosis." The ingested EB resides within a membrane-limited phagosome that is able to avoid fusion and destruction by the primary lysosomes of the parasitized cell by an unknown mechanism.

Several hours following invasion of the host cell, the EB undergoes conversion to the vegetative form, the reticulate body (RB). The RB is metabolically active, and competes with

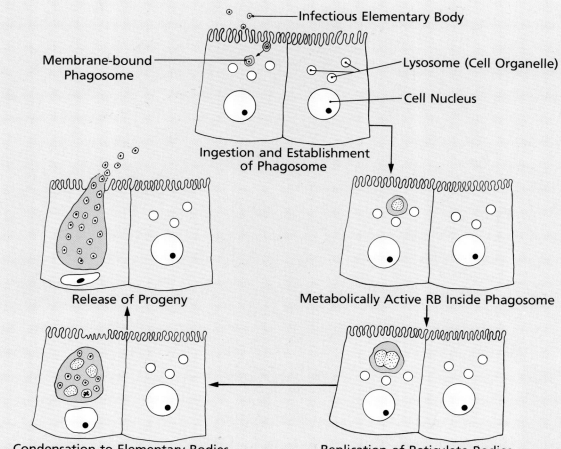

Figure 6.3 Chlamydial development cycle. The infectious elementary body (EB) attaches to the host cell and is ingested by a process that is poorly understood. The EB resides within a membrane-bound endosome. The normal process of fusion with lysosomes is aborted, and transformation to the metabolically active reticulate body (RB) begins. Synthesis of chlamydial constituents and replication of the RBs through binary fission occurs next. A chlamydial inclusion body containing numerous replicative forms can be seen 24 to 48 hours following infection. At 48 to 72 hours following infection, RBs condense to the sporelike EBs. The inclusion body contains several hundred infectious particles at the peak of its maturation. The infectious progeny EBs are released from the infected host cell by extrusion of the inclusion body and/or by lysis of the host cell.

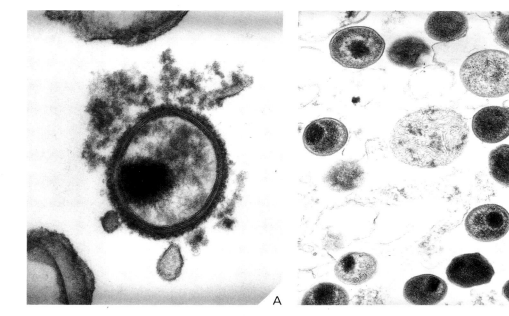

Figure 6.4 Transmission electron micrographs of *C. trachomatis* EBs. **A** Single EB (×120,000). **B** EBs outside host cell. A single, electron-lucent RB and a mitochondrion are also seen (×67,500).

the host cell for metabolic precursors. It is less electron-dense, suggesting relaxation of the condensed DNA, and has a diameter of 500 to 900 nm (Fig. 6.5).

Approximately 12 hours following invasion of the host cell, the RB begins to replicate by binary fission. By 24 hours, the RBs appear to form visible "inclusions" within the membrane-limited phagosome (Fig. 6.6), each inclusion containing up to several hundred organisms. During the next 24 to 36 hours the RBs condense into EBs, such that by 60 to 72 hours the inclusion contains primarily EBs.

Between 48 and 60 hours of development, polysaccharide components within the inclusion may be seen following iodine staining. This staining distinguishes C. *trachomatis* from C. *psittaci*, which does not produce large quantities of glycogen or glycogenlike deposits and does not stain with iodine. Other biologic properties that distinguish these species are illustrated in Figure 6.7. The processes by which EBs egress from the host cell are unclear, and may include both lysis of the host cell and extrusion of intact inclusions without the immediate death of the host cell. Most serotypes of C. *trachomatis* are unable to establish multiple cycles of infection in vitro in mature cell monolayers, greatly limiting their ability to propagate to high concentrations.

The infectious EB possesses a distinct outer membrane with protein and lipopolysaccharide (LPS) components. A single major outer membrane protein (MOMP) comprises the bulk of outer membrane protein. The MOMP has an approximate subunit mass of 40,000 daltons, although the mass appears to differ among the various serotypes of C. *trachomatis*. The MOMP has genus, species, subspecies, and serotype-specific epitopes, and appears to be antigenic in humans. Other prominent antigens in human infections appear with apparent molecular masses

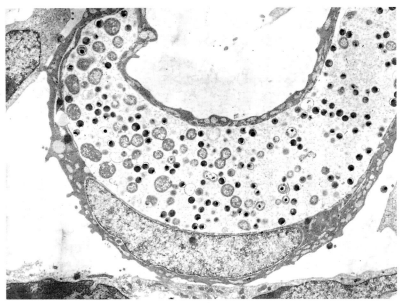

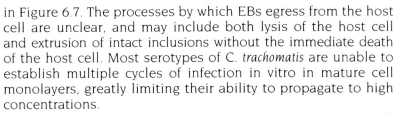

Figure 6.5 A mature C. *trachomatis* inclusion displaces the host cell nucleus and includes various chlamydial developmental forms.

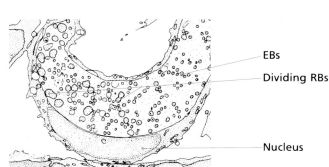

EBs
Dividing RBs
Nucleus

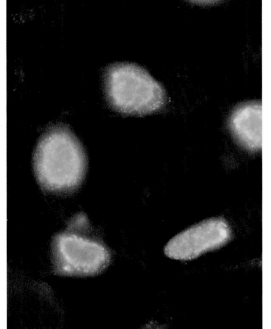

Figure 6.6 Chlamydial inclusions in cell monolayer stained with fluorescein-labeled monoclonal antibody specific for C. *trachomatis*.

DISTINGUISHING CHARACTERISTICS OF C. TRACHOMATIS AND C. PSITTACI

	C. TRACHOMATIS	C. PSITTACI
HOST RANGE	Humans, mice	Non-human vertebrates
INCLUSION MORPHOLOGY	Granular, vacuolar	Lucent, dense
INCLUSION STAINING	Iodine +	Iodine −
FOLATE ANTAGONISTS	Sensitive	Resistant

Figure 6.7 Distinguishing characteristics of C. *trachomatis* and C. *psittaci*.

of 62, 60, 28, and less than 12 kD. The most prominent genus-specific antigen is the chlamydial LPS that resembles the rough LPS of Re ("deep rough") mutants of *Salmonella minnesota*.

C. *trachomatis* strains can be classified by antiserum or monoclonal antibodies into 15 readily distinguished serotypes. Endemic trachoma is usually associated with infection by serotypes A, B, Ba, and C, while nontrachomatous oculogenital infection is usually caused by serotypes B and D–K. Lymphogranuloma venereum (LGV) infections (discussed under Clinical Manifestations) are caused by the invasive LGV biovar strains of serotypes L1–L3 (Fig. 6.8). Chlamydial genital infection by multiple serotypes has been reported, and can be observed in vitro (Fig. 6.9).

C. *trachomatis* EBs contain a plasmid that exhibits considerable similarity among the serotypes (Fig. 6.10). This plasmid is approximately 7,500 base pairs in size, and has several open reading frames capable of encoding polypeptide products. The ubiquitous nature of this cryptic plasmid suggests that it may be important in the survival of the organism; however, no clear functions have been ascribed to it.

DISEASES COMMONLY ASSOCIATED WITH SEROTYPES OF C. TRACHOMATIS	
SEROTYPE	**DISEASE**
A, B, Ba, C	Endemic trachoma
B, D–K	Genitourinary disease
L1, L2, L3	LGV

Figure 6.8 Diseases commonly associated with serotypes of C. trachomatis.

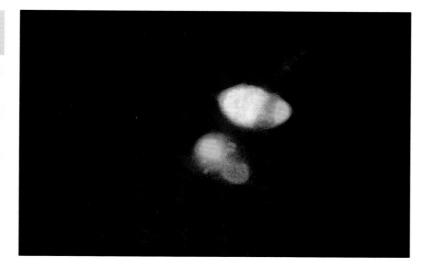

Figure 6.9 HeLa cells infected simultaneously with two serotypes of C. trachomatis and stained with two type-specific monoclonal antibodies, each labeled with a different fluorochrome. The upper cell shows two inclusions, one containing both serotypes, illustrating that multiple serotypes can coexist within the same host cell. Clinical examples of chlamydial infection by two serotypes have been reported.

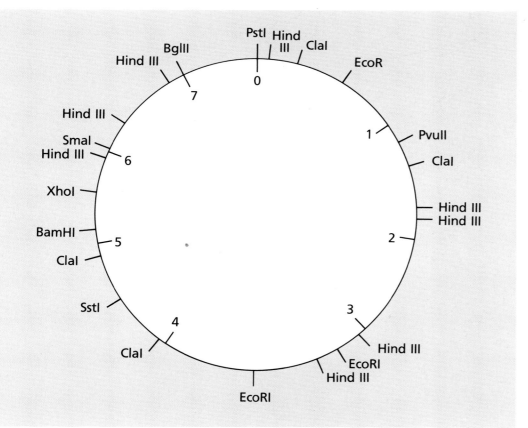

Figure 6.10 Restriction endonuclease map of the 7.5-kB cryptic plasmid from C. trachomatis serotype L2. The same or a similar plasmid has been found in all serotypes investigated.

Epidemiology

Chlamydial infections are the most frequently occurring sexually transmitted diseases (STDs) in the U.S. (Fig. 6.11), and probably in most developed countries. As they are not uniformly reported in the U.S., only crude estimates of incidence of these infections, based on extrapolation of data from particular clinics, are available. The U.S. Public Health Service estimates that between 3 and 5 million cases occur each year (Fig. 6.12). Data from private health care reports suggest that although cases of urethritis due to Neisseria gonorrhoeae have been decreasing in the past decade, office visits by men with nongonococcal urethritis—due in large part to C. trachomatis infection—have been increasing (Fig. 6.13). Risk factors for chlamydial genitourinary infection are shown in Figure 6.14.

The classic venereal disease caused by chlamydia is lymphoganuloma venereum, or LGV. This disease is rare in the U.S. but common in developing countries, especially in central Africa. Figure 6.1 illustrates the number of cases of LGV reported to the Centers for Disease Control between 1966 and 1987.

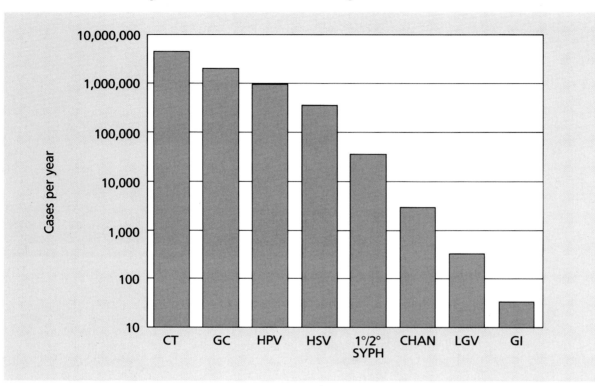

Figure 6.11 Estimated incidence of non-HIV STDs in the U.S. Note the logarithmic scale.

ESTIMATED ANNUAL INCIDENCE OF *C. TRACHOMATIS* INFECTIONS IN THE U.S.

Figure 6.12 Estimated annual incidence of *C. trachomatis* infections in the U.S.

INFECTION	INCIDENCE
MALE	
Nongonococcal urethritis	1,550,000
Epididymitis	250,000
FEMALE	
Asymptomatic cervical infection	700,000
Symptomatic cervical infection	300,000
Pelvic inflammatory disease	300,000
NEONATAL	
Total infections	247,000
Conjunctivitis	74,000
Pneumonia	37,000

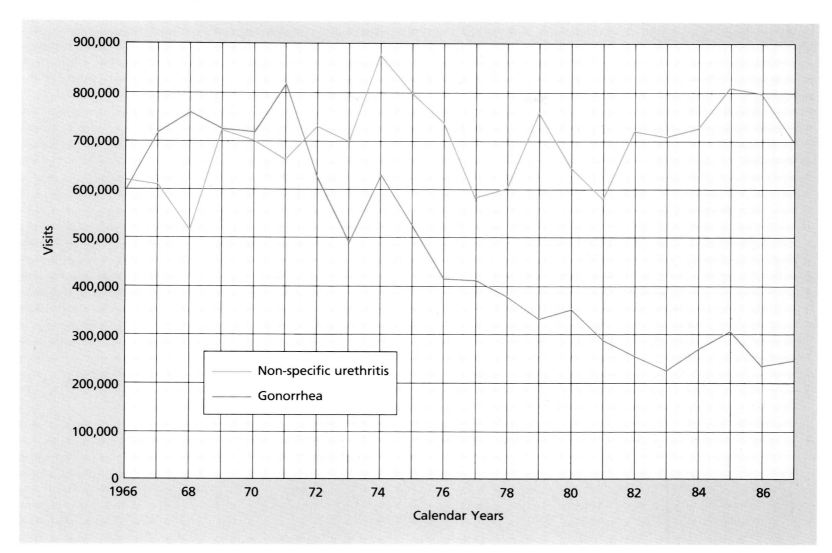

Figure 6.13 Number of physician's office visits for urethritis in the U.S., 1966 to 1987. Although visits by men with urethritis due to *Neisseria gonorrhoeae* have decreased, there has been a substantial increase in number of visits for nongonococcal urethritis. These data suggest that chlamydial genitourinary infection may be increasing.

Figure 6.14 Patient groups at high risk for chlamydial STDs.

PATIENT GROUPS AT HIGH RISK FOR CHLAMYDIAL STDs

Patients with multiple sexual partners

Younger patients

Patients with other STDs

Patients with chlamydia-associated syndromes

Sexual partners of patients with gonorrhea or chlamydia-associated syndromes

Neonates born to infected mothers

Genital infection in adults occurs through sexual intercourse. In recent years, the U.S. has witnessed substantial increases in ectopic pregnancy (Fig. 6.15) and involuntary infertility, particularly among populations at high risk for prior chlamydial infection. Studies of antibody prevalence to chlamydia have shown that chlamydial exposure is more common among infertile women in the U.S. than in control populations, suggesting a role of C. trachomatis in tubal infertility. Ocular infection may accompany genital infection, suggesting that transmission of infection from the genitals to the eye may occur. In neonates, infection most commonly occurs through exposure to organisms in the birth canal. Although infection of the genitals and conjunctivae are common, the mucosal surfaces of the pharynx, urethra, and rectum also are sites of chlamydial colonization. C. trachomatis may reside for months within the genital tracts of infected patients who have not been treated with antimicrobials. Some infants born to infected mothers may have a clinically inapparent infection for many months following birth.

As the causative agent of endemic trachoma, C. trachomatis is one of the most frequent infections leading to blindness in the developing world.

Clinical Manifestations

Infection by C. trachomatis can occur at several anatomic locations and cause a variety of distinct disease syndromes. Several animal models of C. trachomatis genital infection have been used to explore the pathophysiology of chlamydial infection. Models of immunity have been explored using a mammalian C. psittaci, the Guinea Pig Inclusion Conjunctivitis (GPIC) agent, in both

mice and guinea pigs. Several models of pneumonitis have been developed in the mouse. Models of upper genital tract infection have been developed using mice, guinea pigs, and non-human primates (Fig. 6.16). The latter have also been used as animal models for C. trachomatis rectal infections.

LYMPHOGRANULOMA VENEREUM
After genital inoculation there is apparently systemic spread of the organism until localization in the genital or rectal lymph node tissues occurs. This infection of the lymphatics becomes locally invasive, and is characterized by induration, multifocal suppuration, and fistula formation. Involvement of both femoral and inguinal lymph node groups, more frequent among infected men than women, can produce swelling on both sides of the inguinal ligament. The resulting "groove sign" (Fig. 6.17) has been said to be pathognomonic of LGV, but occurs in only 10 to 15% of infected patients. LGV can produce chronic scarring and lymphedema, particularly if the rectum is infected. Cicatricial scarring in the lower rectum can produce long fibrotic narrowings of the colonic lumen.

URETHRITIS AND PROCTITIS IN MEN
Chlamydia causes about half of the infections in men presenting to STD clinics with urethral inflammation from which Neisseria gonorrhoeae cannot be identified. The majority of men with chlamydial infection of the urethra have symptoms of urethral discharge, dysuria, or pruritus of the urethra. Up to 25% of men found upon culture screening to have urethral infection by C. trachomatis are asymptomatic. Infrequently, chlamydia may cause acute epididymitis (Fig. 6.18), apparently due to infection

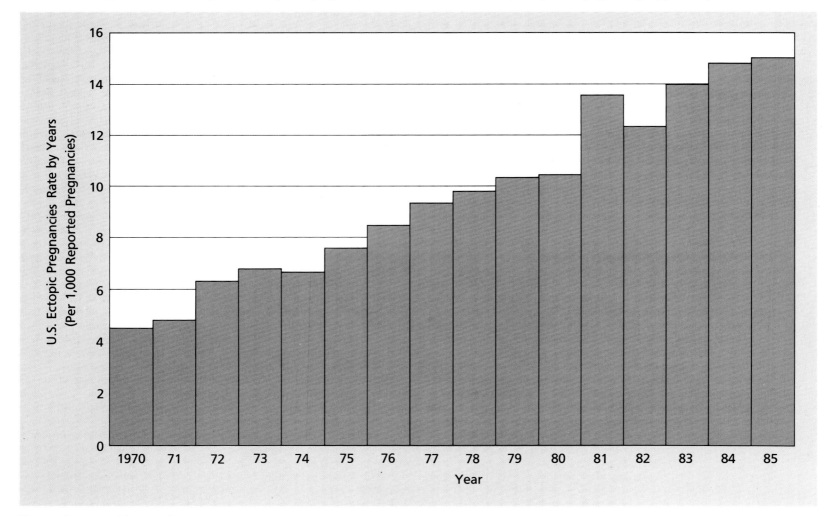

Figure 6.15 Incidence of ectopic pregnancy in the U.S., 1970 to 1985.

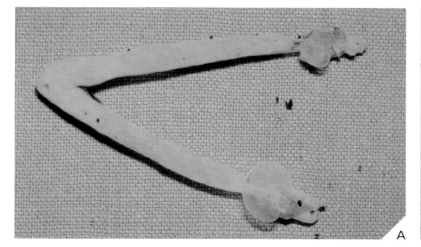

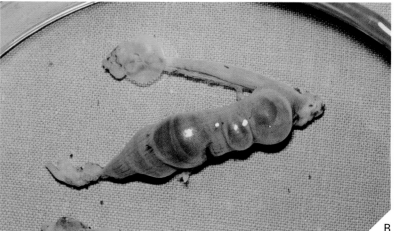

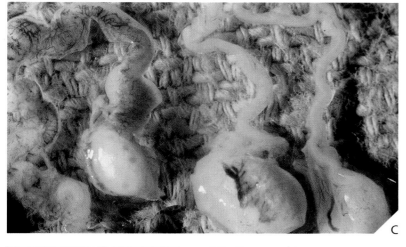

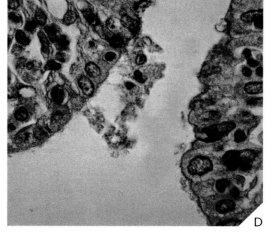

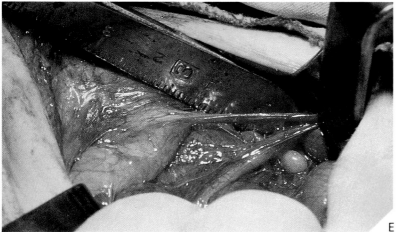

Figure 6.16 Salpingitis in animal models. **A** Resected reproductive tract from a mouse experimentally infected with *C. trachomatis*. Bilateral hydrosalpinx is seen at the distal extremities of both uterine horns. **B** Specimen from a mouse impregnated following unilateral hydrosalpinx development. Embryos are implanted in the normal horn, while the hydrosalpinx side is unimplanted. **C** Resected fallopian tubes from guinea pigs, showing tubes inflamed and swollen with acute salpingitis due to chlamydial infection (left) compared with the uninfected control (right). **D** Immunoperoxidase stain of *C. trachomatis* inclusions (dark black) in a segment of monkey fallopian tube transplanted subcutaneously and stained five days following infection. **E** Adhesions seen at laparotomy in a monkey following experimentally induced *C. trachomatis* salpingitis. Such experimental animal models provide knowledge regarding mechanisms of scarring following salpingitis.

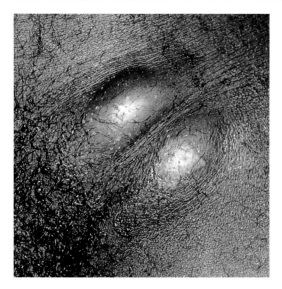

Figure 6.17 "Groove sign" in a man with LGV. Although frequently said to be pathognomonic for LGV, this sign is seen infrequently in LGV patients and may be produced by other conditions.

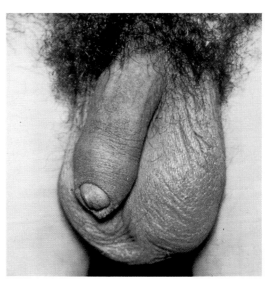

Figure 6.18 Red, swollen scrotum of a man with chlamydial epididymitis.

ascending from the urethra. Chlamydia causes most cases of epididymitis in young heterosexual men without anatomic anomalies of the genitourinary system.

In homosexual men, infection of the rectal mucosa by C. *trachomatis* can result in a severe proctocolitis (Fig. 6.19). Although infection is usually asymptomatic, infection by organisms of the more virulent LGV strains can produce a severe and symptomatic form.

CERVICITIS AND URETHRITIS IN WOMEN

In women, chlamydia have been isolated from the cervix, the urethra, Bartholin's duct, the fallopian tubes, the uterus, and the rectal mucosa. However, up to 70% of genital infections in women are asymptomatic. When symptoms of cervicitis and urethritis are described in association with proven infection of the cervix, they are nonspecific, and may include dysuria, vaginal discharge, or vaginal pruritus, although several studies have failed to associate specific symptoms with endocervical chlamydia infection. Upon examination of the infected patient, a mucopurulent cervical discharge and/or friability of the cervix (Figs. 6.20 to 6.25) may be noted, although these signs also are neither sensitive nor specific for chlamydial infection. Sampling from the endocervical canal can produce gross evidence of purulent

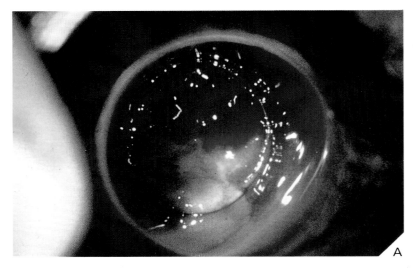

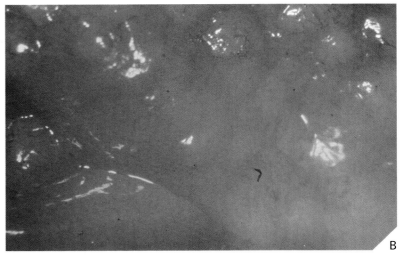

Figure 6.19 **A** Anoscopic view of rectal mucosa with area of focal purulence in a man with chlamydial proctitis. **B** Lymphoid follicular proctitis seen in a case of *C. trachomatis* rectal infection.

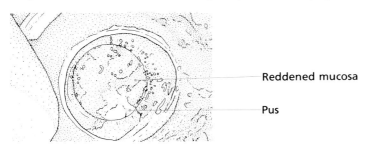

Reddened mucosa

Pus

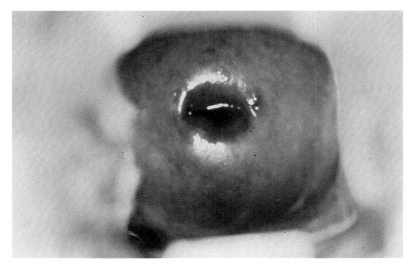

Figure 6.20 Normal nulliparous cervix of a postmenarchal female, showing no cervical ectopy.

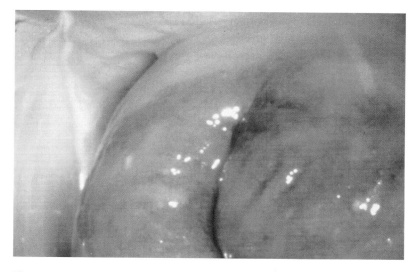

Figure 6.21 Colposcopic view of early metaplastic changes in the cervical epithelium). This is a normal finding with sexual maturity.

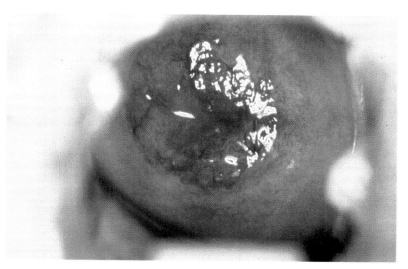

Figure 6.22 Cervix showing effacement of the transitional zone (squamocolumnar junction) as might be observed in a young patient or in an oral contraceptive user.

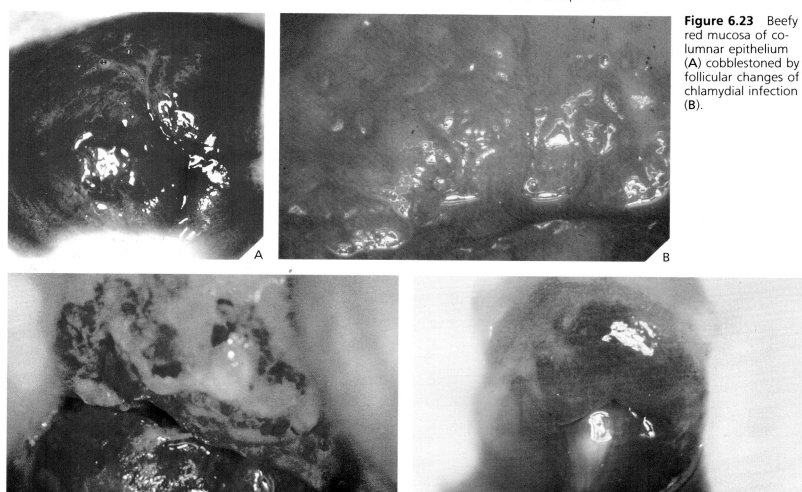

Figure 6.23 Beefy red mucosa of columnar epithelium (**A**) cobblestoned by follicular changes of chlamydial infection (**B**).

A

B

Figure 6.24 Cervicitis showing purulent discharge from the os. Focal bleeding at areas previously touched during external cleansing of the cervix is evidence of friability.

Figure 6.25 Mucopurulent discharge seen coming from the cervical os following removal of ectocervical mucus. Endocervical swab from this patient was culture-positive for *C. trachomatis*.

inflammation (Figs. 6.26 and 6.27). C. *trachomatis* has been isolated from the urethra and urinary bladder of women presenting with dysuria; it is also responsible for a large proportion of abacteriuric pyuria in sexually active women—the "acute urethral syndrome."

SALPINGITIS AND PERIHEPATITIS
The most serious complication of chlamydia genital infection in women is acute salpingitis, presumably caused by ascent of the organism from the lower genital tract to the endometrium and fallopian tubes (Fig. 6.28). The clinical manifestations of upper reproductive tract infection by C. *trachomatis* are nonspecific but can be severe, with fever, lower abdominal pain, prostration, and tenderness of the uterus and adnexae. A severe inflammatory response can be observed on laparoscopy to involve the fallopian tubes and peritoneum (Fig. 6.29) Peritoneal inflammation can result in hepatic capsular adhesions, which may produce the Fitz-Hugh-Curtis syndrome: pain, tenderness in the right upper quadrant, and occasionally a hepatic friction rub on auscultation (Fig. 6.30).

In addition to the acute morbidity of pelvic inflammatory disease, scarring of the tubal transport system following chlamydial salpingitis may lead to infertility and/or ectopic pregnancy (Fig. 6.31).

PERINATAL INFECTIONS
Exposure to C. *trachomatis* during passage through an infected birth canal can cause infection in newborns. The most common

Figure 6.26 Swab from the endocervical canal of a chlamydia-infected woman (left) compared with fresh swab. The yellow-green exudate may reflect infection of the endocervix or endometrium.

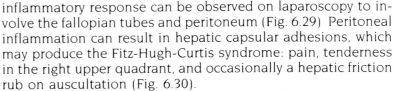

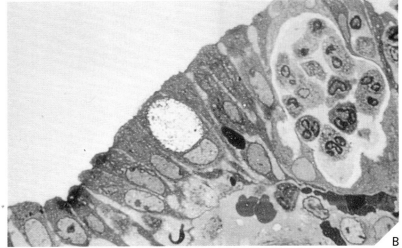

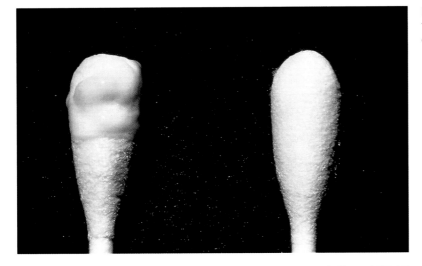

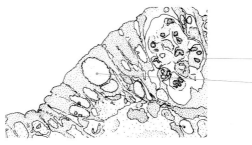

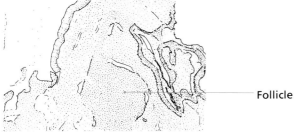

Figure 6.27 Histologic (**A**) and transmission electron micrographic (**B**) images of chlamydia-infected human cervix on biopsy. An intense follicular inflammatory infiltrate is seen on low power, while both a chlamydial inclusion and microabscess are observed in the electron micrograph.

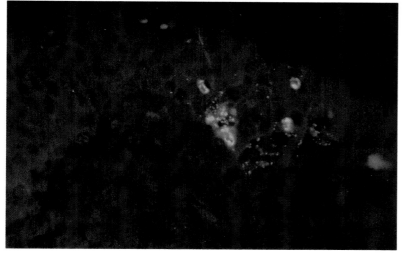

Figure 6.28 Fluorescence micrograph showing chlamydial inclusions developing in experimentally infected monkey fallopian tube. Chlamydial infection may ascend from the endocervix to infect the endometrium and fallopian tube epithelium.

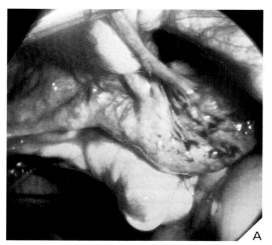

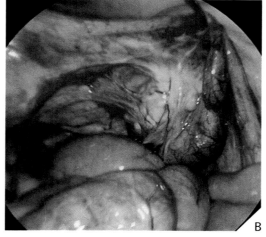

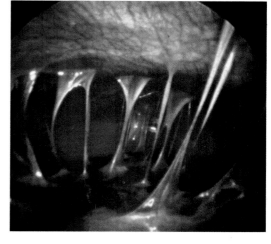

Figure 6.29 **A** Acute salpingitis. The fallopian tube is congested and swollen. A dense adhesion has formed between the ampulla of the tube and the pelvic side

wall. **B** Hydrosalpinx with adhesions. Dye has been instilled into the grossly swollen fallopian tube on the right. Dense adhesions obscure the ovary.

Figure 6.30 Laparoscopic view of "violin-string" adhesions in a patient with perihepatitis (Fitz-Hugh-Curtis syndrome).

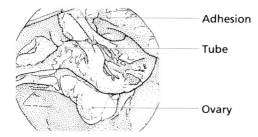

Adhesion

Tube

Ovary

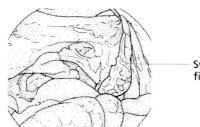

Swollen dye-filled tube

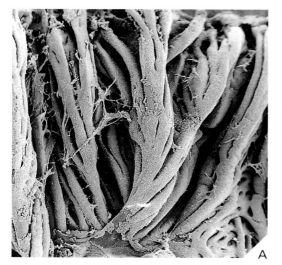

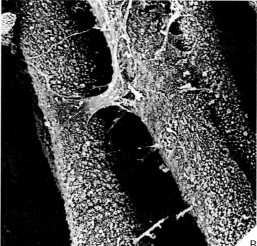

Figure 6.31 **A** and **B** Scanning electron micrographs of a monkey fallopian tube ampulla following experimental infection with *C. trachomatis*. Adhesions such as seen on both the low power and magnified images are presumably responsible for the development of tubal obstruction with infertility and/or ectopic pregnancy.

symptomatic illness of these children is a self-limited purulent conjunctivitis (Fig. 6.32), which usually occurs within several weeks following birth. Ten to thirty percent of children born to infected mothers develop this infection. In fewer than 10% of children exposed, a distinctive pneumonitis develops. This infection is characterized by occurring several weeks to several months following delivery, by a notable lack of fever, and by a hacking, nonproductive cough. The radiographic picture is not distinctive, but frequently shows hyperaeration and generalized interstitial changes (Fig. 6.33). C. *trachomatis* is the most commonly identified cause of infant pneumonitis in the first 6 months of life.

OTHER CHLAMYDIAL INFECTIONS IN ADULTS
Ocular infection by C. *trachomatis* is not limited to perinatally acquired infection. Although not primarily an STD, endemic trachoma is one of the most common causes of visual impairment in the developing world, causing millions of cases of

blindness (Fig. 6.34). Similarly, ocular infection in sexually active adults can occur frequently, probably as a consequence of genital–ocular autoinoculation. This infection is usually self-limited and without severe sequellae, although a distinctive follicular conjunctivitis can result (Fig. 6.35).

Genital infection by C. *trachomatis* has been associated in serologic studies with the development of reactive arthropathy in Reiter's syndrome, which consists of conjunctivitis (see Fig. 8.75), urethritis, and arthritis (Fig. 6.36). Recently, chlamydial particles have been seen in joint aspirates from patients with this postinfectious arthropathy, suggesting that direct infection of the joint space may produce this complication. Reiter's syndrome is a chronic, fluctuating disease that may have striking rheumatologic and dermatologic presentations (Figs. 6.37 and 6.38).

In humans, uncomplicated genital infection by C. *trachomatis* produces few diagnostic symptoms and signs. Similarly, a number of organisms can be responsible for pelvic inflam-

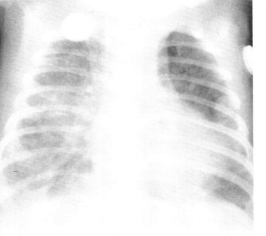

Figure 6.33
Chlamydial pneumonitis. x-ray of a neonate showing the generalized patchy infiltrates.

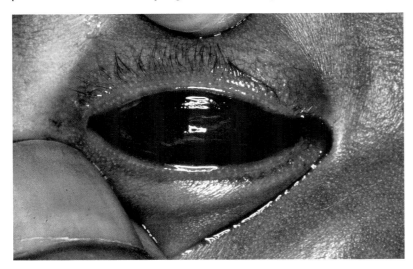

Figure 6.32 Chlamydial ophthalmia. Erythematous conjunctiva is seen in this infant.

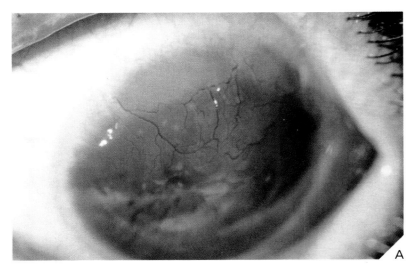
A

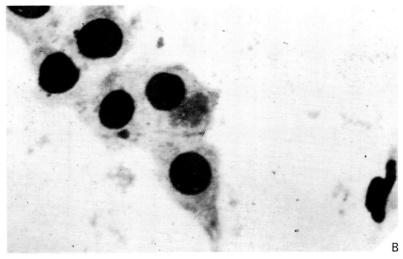
B

Figure 6.34 A Scarring of cornea (pannus) resulting from long-standing ocular trachoma. Similar destructive lesions are infrequently observed in ocular infection by genital strains of C. *trachomatis*

(paratrachoma). B Giemsa stain of an ocular scraping from a patient with trachoma, showing a C. *trachomatis* intracellular inclusion.

matory disease. The lack of specific clinical criteria in the diagnosis of chlamydial infection mandates laboratory diagnosis in almost all cases of infection.

Laboratory Tests

The diagnosis of endemic trachoma can usually be made by an experienced clinician on the basis of patient history and physical examination. The diagnosis of C. *trachomatis* genital infection, however, is dependent upon specific laboratory identification. Infection is asymptomatic in the majority of infected women and a substantial proportion of infected men. In addition, the symptoms and signs of infection are highly variable when present, and may be caused by other infectious agents or by noninfectious processes. The medical history and physical examination, while necessary in every instance, are neither sensitive nor specific enough to identify infected patients.

Isolation of chlamydia in cell culture or eggs was, until recently, the only practical method for detection of infection. The recent development of monoclonal antibodies directed against the organism and increased knowledge about the components of the EB have resulted in new tests capable of detecting the presence of chlamydial antigen in clinical specimens. Since 1982, there has been a dramatic increase in the use of the antigen detection tests in clinical laboratories. Future improvements in the performance and costs of rapid diagnostic methods are likely.

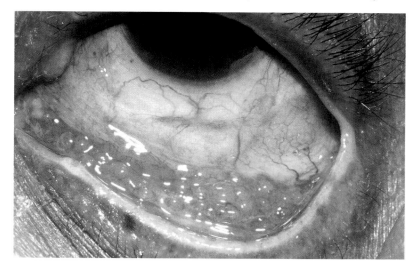

Figure 6.35 Follicular conjunctivitis. Infection of the palpebral conjunctiva with lymphocytic follicle formation by C. *trachomatis.*

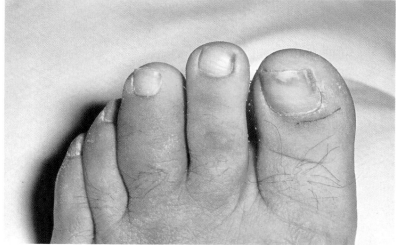

Figure 6.36 A red and swollen third toe is seen in this photograph of the foot of a man presenting with Reiter's syndrome arthritis.

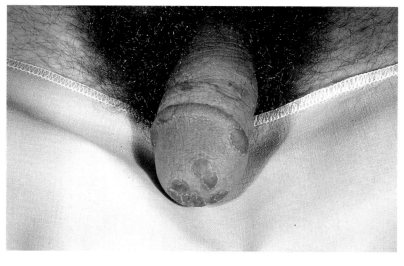

Figure 6.37 Scaling erythematous plaques on the penis. Circinate balanitis of Reiter's syndrome. This is one of the infrequent but distinctive cutaneous findings associated with this syndrome.

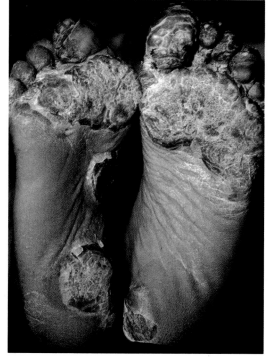

Figure 6.38 Keratodermia blennorrhagica in Reiter's syndrome. Note the thick scales and crusts on the feet of this patient.

PATHOLOGY

Gram Stains

The diagnosis of nongonococcal urethritis, or NGU, in men is usually based on the clinical presentation of scanty urethral discharge (Fig. 6.39) and a Gram stain of urethral exudate. The Gram stain is sensitive and specific for the diagnosis of gonorrhea (Fig. 6.40A), but as many men with gonococcal urethritis also have chlamydial infection, it is not useful in specific chlamydial diagnosis in the presence of N. *gonorrhoeae*. Thus only the absence of intracellular gram-negative diplococci (Fig. 6.40B) is useful in microscopically distinguishing NGU from gonorrhea.

Histopathology

Histopathologic characteristics of chlamydial infection include chronic inflammation and fibrotic changes with granulation. Left untreated, these processes lead to morbid complications regardless of location of the infection. In LGV, there is local acute and granulomatous inflammation in involved lymph nodes, often with gross formation of stellate abcesses (Fig. 6.41).

SPECIMEN COLLECTION

Isolation of C. *trachomatis* in cell culture remains the preferred method for identifying an infected patient. Proper collection of a specimen for culture is essential for successful results. A fiber-tipped swab is the most commonly used instrument for collection of a clinical specimen. Swab shafts should be made of inert material, preferably plastic or metal. Aluminum shafts and soluble components eluting from wooden shafts may be cytotoxic in chlamydial culture systems. Swab tips made of cotton or dacron appear to be less inhibitory to propagation than tips of nylon or alginate; however, individual lots of swabs should be tested to assure lack of toxicity to the cell monolayer and lack of growth inhibition. Recently, collection devices resembling biopsy brushes have been developed to improve the sensitivity of sample collection from the endocervix. Typical sample collection instruments are shown in Figure 6.42.

Transport media for chlamydia may contain buffered salt solution, sucrose, and antibiotics that do not inhibit chlamydia such as vancomycin, gentamicin, and nystatin. Many laboratories add fetal bovine serum to the media to enhance specimen recovery.

Figure 6.39 Chlamydial urethritis. Mucoid, penile discharge with meatal erythema. C. *trachomatis* was isolated whereas N. *gonorrhoeae* was not.

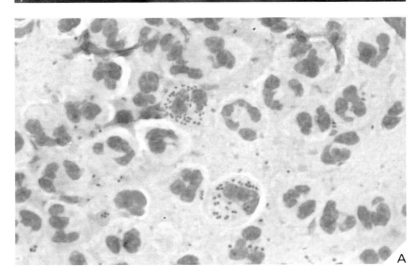

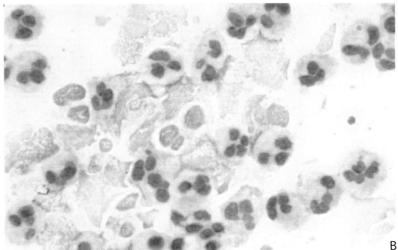

Figure 6.40 **A** Gonorrhea. **B** Nongonoccal urethritis. Gram stains of penile urethral exudate show inflammatory cells (**A**) containing gonococci and (**B**) without visible gonococci.

The organism may be difficult to isolate from specimens containing excess mucus or inflammatory cells, such as from bubo aspirates in patients with LGV. Likewise, components in semen are toxic to cell culture systems (Fig. 6.43). C. trachomatis can exhibit direct cytotoxicity to cell monolayers when inoculated at high multiplicities of infection. Cytopathic effects seen in clinical specimens are unlikely to be due to chlamydia, as the number of organisms in clinical samples is probably never sufficient to produce this effect. Cytotoxicity due to collection or transport system components or due to semen components, inflammatory cells, or genital microorganisms other than chlamydia may interfere with cell culture identification of chlamydia in up to 5% of specimens from STD clinics. Dilution of such specimens prior to attempting cell culture has improved organism recovery.

C. trachomatis in clinical specimens has limited viability at temperatures above −70°C. Once collected, specimens should be refrigerated on ice or at 4°C and inoculated into cell culture within 24 hours. If specimens must be stored for longer periods prior to culture, they should be frozen at temperatures below −70°C.

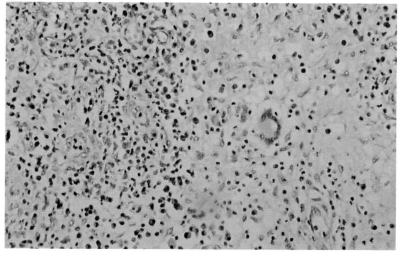

Figure 6.41 Biopsy specimen of a lymph node in LGV showing acute and chronic inflammation with occasional multinucleate giant cells.

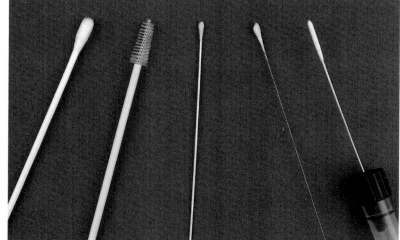

Figure 6.42 Various instruments available for sampling for chlamydia from the genitourinary tract. Left to right: The large-diameter cotton or dacron swab on a nontoxic plastic shaft or the brushlike device are satisfactory for endocervical sampling, though the latter is more traumatic. Urethral specimens may be obtained with the rigid aluminum-shafted swab or a flexible, steel, cotton-tipped device. An example of a swab for urethral enzyme immunoassay is seen on the far right.

Figure 6.43 Cytotoxicity in cell culture. Cells exhibit a round morphology and have sloughed from the coverslip, resulting in a diffuse cytopathic effect.

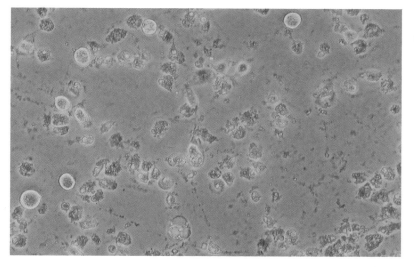

CELL CULTURE

The typical procedure for isolation of C. *trachomatis* by cell culture is seen in Figure 6.44. If frozen, specimens to be cultured are thawed at 37°C and mixed. The specimen is inoculated onto the surface of confluent monolayers of susceptible cells. Commonly used cells include McCoy, HeLa 229, and BHK lines. The inoculated cell monolayers are centrifuged at 30 to 35°C at 2,000 to 3,000 ×g to improve the sensitivity of the culture. Following

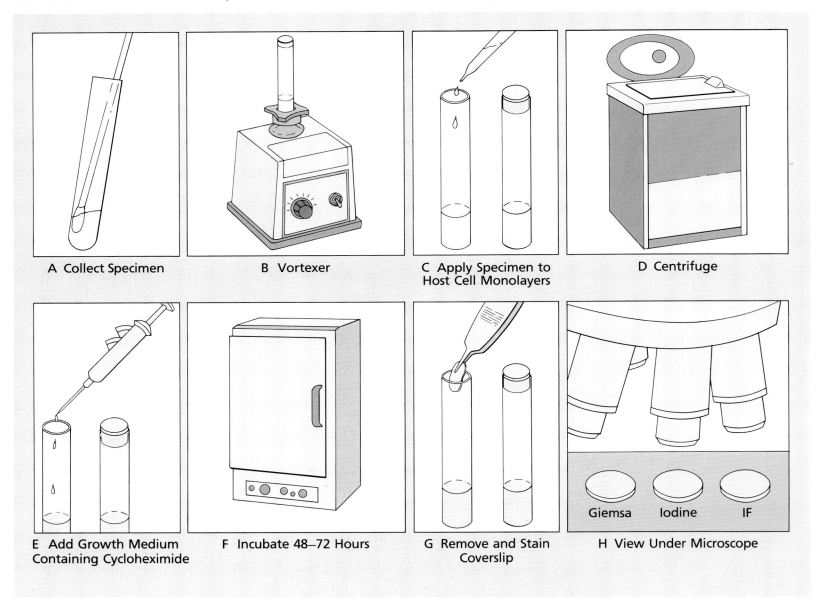

A Collect Specimen

B Vortexer

C Apply Specimen to Host Cell Monolayers

D Centrifuge

E Add Growth Medium Containing Cycloheximide

F Incubate 48–72 Hours

G Remove and Stain Coverslip

H View Under Microscope

Giemsa   Iodine   IF

A Collection of the specimen and transport to the laboratory on ice.

B Processing of the specimen by mixing or sonication.

C Inoculation of specimen onto fresh cell culture monolayers, usually following treatment of the monolayers with DEAE-dextran to improve chlamydial infectivity.

D Centrifugation of inoculated monolayers to enhance ingestion of chlamydia.

E Addition of cell growth medium containing cycloheximide to inhibit most cell metabolism.

F Incubation of infected cell monolayers.

G Staining for the presence of chlamydial inclusions.

H Microscopic examination of stained cell monolayers.

Figure 6.44 Culture method of chlamydia isolation. Although recognized as the standard method for sensitive and specific laboratory identification of C. *trachomatis* organisms, the required skill and laboratory resources, coupled with the 2-to-7-day turnaround for results, has made less demanding techniques generally more acceptable for routine clinical diagnosis.

inoculation and centrifugation, the monolayer is overlaid with growth medium. Cycloheximide is included at a predetermined concentration to increase the number and size of chlamydial inclusions by inhibiting host cell protein synthesis.

After incubation of the inoculated cell monolayer for 48 to 72 hours, characteristic inclusions may be observed. The inclusion of C. *trachomatis* is surrounded by a distinct membrane and is visible under direct microscopic examination, particularly using phase microscopy. The inclusions may be visualized by staining with iodine, Giemsa, acridine orange, fluorescein-conjugated monoclonal or polyclonal antibody preparations, or with immunochemical stains using enzyme-conjugated antichlamydial monoclonal antibodies (Figs. 6.45 to 6.49). The most common stains used are iodine and fluorescein-labeled anti-

Figure 6.45 Cell monolayer infected with C. *trachomatis*. Dark red inclusions are positive in this specimen stained with Jones' iodine.

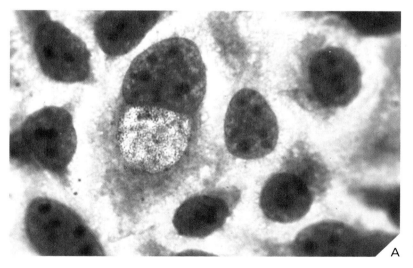

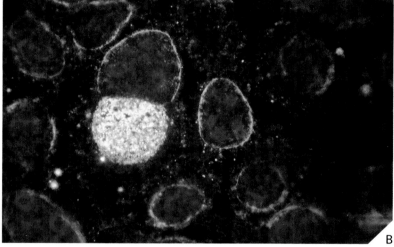

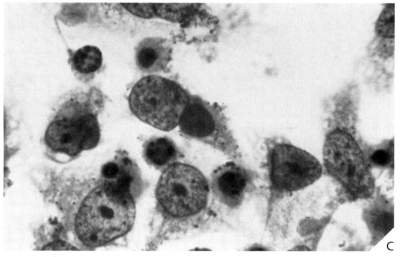

Figure 6.46 Giemsa-stained inclusions. **A** (Bright-field) and **B** (dark-field) show open, granular nature of an intracellular inclusion of C. *trachomatis* in contrast to the dense inclusion seen in "TWAR" (**C**) and C. *psittaci* inclusions following staining.

bodies. Staining with fluoresceinated monoclonal antibodies to the MOMP of C. *trachomatis* is more sensitive and specific than iodine staining. Iodine stains intracellular glycogen, which is maximal at 40 to 60 hours following infection. Though inexpensive and easily performed, iodine stains are more subject to artifact due to staining of nonchlamydial material.

Several studies have indicated that isolation of chlamydia in cell culture is relatively insensitive. Studies using multiple sampling in the same patient or repeated passage of inoculated host cells have suggested that a single endocervical swab may detect infection in only 70% of infected women. Additional sampling of women using a urethral swab has been shown to improve the sensitivity substantially.

DIRECT FLUORESCENT ANTIBODY DETECTION

Detection of C. *trachomatis* infection by nonculture methods (antigen detection) became feasible with the recent development of immunologic reagents specific for chlamydial outer

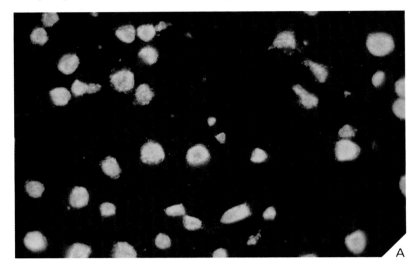

Figure 6.47 Chlamydial inclusions in cycloheximide-treated Mc-Coy cell monolayers stained with a fluorescein-labeled genus-specific monoclonal antibody. C. *trachomatis* inclusions (**A**) occur individually, while C. *psittaci* or "TWAR" (**B**) may produce multiple or multilobed inclusions within a single infected cell.

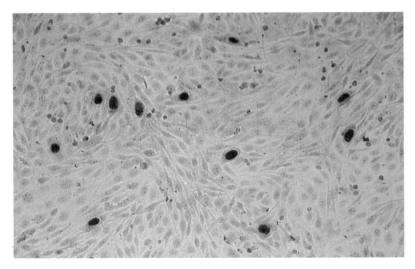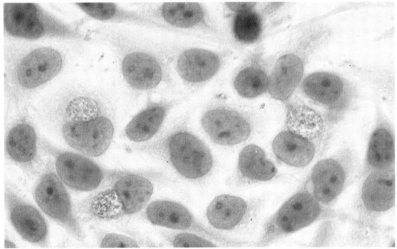

Figure 6.48 Distinct red chlamydial inclusions detected using an alkaline-phosphatase monoclonal antibody method with naphthol-AS chromogenic substrate (original magnification ×250).

Figure 6.49 Black, granular C. *trachomatis* inclusion produced using peroxidase-labeled monoclonal antibody and 1-chloro-4-naphthol chromogenic substrate (original magnification ×400).

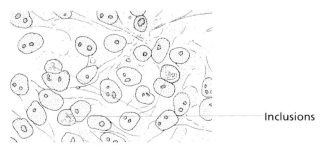

Inclusions

membrane components. Direct fluorescent antibody (DFA) detection uses one or more monoclonal antibodies (MAbs) conjugated to fluorescent molecules as shown in Figure 6.50. Monoclonal antibodies directed against species-, subspecies-, and genus-(LPS) specific antigens have been developed for this method. Data to date suggest that monoclonal antibodies reacting to the chlamydial MOMP produce superior staining and characteristic morphology compared with anti-LPS antibodies. As with chlamydia culture, proper technique in the collection of the clinical specimen is necessary to ensure adequate test performance. Upon addition to a specimen smear, these reagents bind to chlamydial EBs, producing brightly fluorescent

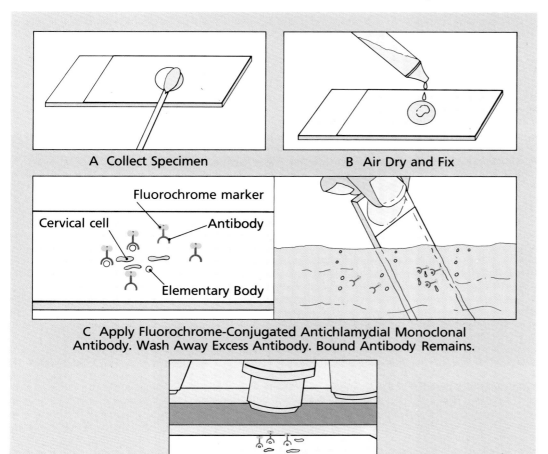

A Collect Specimen

B Air Dry and Fix

Fluorochrome marker

Cervical cell   Antibody

Elementary Body

C Apply Fluorochrome-Conjugated Antichlamydial Monoclonal Antibody. Wash Away Excess Antibody. Bound Antibody Remains.

D View under fluorescence microscope

Figure 6.50 Direct fluorescent antibody detection of *C. trachomatis.*

A Ectocervical exudate is removed. A swab or brush is then used to collect endocervical epithelial cells, which are smeared onto a slide.

B The specimen is then air dried fixed.

C Specimen is stained with fluorescein-labeled monoclonal antibody. Unbound antibody is removed by washings.

D Chlamydial EBs labeled with fluoresceinated antibody are visualized by fluorescence microscopy.

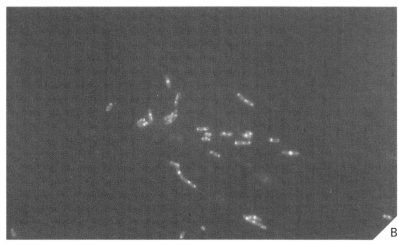

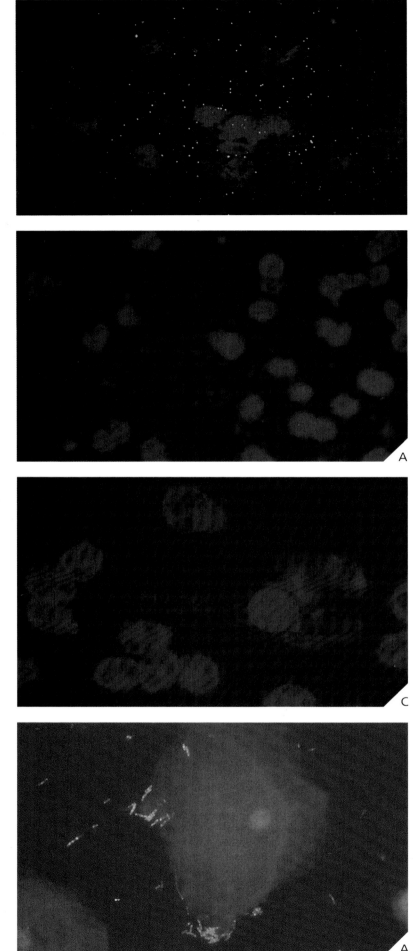

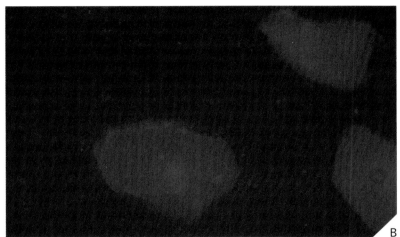

Figure 6.51 Direct fluorescent antibody stain of chlamydia EBs from a smear of cervical exudate.

Figure 6.52 **A** Normal endocervical epithelial cells stained with a commercial chlamydial DFA reagent. The presence of such cells indicates to the microscopist the satisfactory quality of the sample collection. **B** An abundance of squamous cells is seen in this genital specimen from a women. This indicates that specimen collection has been unsatisfactory. **C** Inflammatory cells stained as above (all original magnification ×630).

Figure 6.53 **A** and **B** Examples of cross-reacting microorganisms seen in clinical specimens stained with a chlamydia MOMP-specific monoclonal antibody. Such artifacts are infrequent and are not confusing to an experienced microscopist.

and morphologically distinctive dots. Several to several hundred organisms may be seen in any smear (Fig. 6.51). The sensitivity of the DFA method in comparison with cell culture has varied in published studies, but averages 80 to 90% in women and symptomatic men. When a cutoff value for positive test results of 10 EBs is used, the test specificity exceeds 95%.

A significant advantage of DFA is the lack of necessity for rapid transporting of specimens to the laboratory and storage of specimens in cold, since slides can be fixed and mailed to a central area for staining and interpretation. In addition, the cellular background observed on the smear allows the microscopist to reject slides without sufficient cellular material from the endocervix (Fig. 6.52). Some studies have shown that up to 10% of all specimens are inadequate for DFA, suggesting that inadequate specimen collection contributes significantly

to the insensitive nature of all chlamydia detection methods. Disadvantages of the DFA method include the need for a trained microscopist, who must devote several minutes to the interpretation of each specimen, and the need for a fluorescence microscope. Some artifacts have been noted to occur due to cross-reactivity of reagents with nonchlamydial organisms (Fig. 6.53), but an experienced microscopist is rarely confused by these.

ENZYME IMMUNOASSAY

Other methods for rapid detection of chlamydial components use chlamydia-specific or second antibodies labeled with an enzyme. Following incubation of a specimen with the antibody preparation, an enzyme substrate is added to generate a colored product, which can be detected visually or photometrically (Fig. 6.54). These enzyme immunoassay (EIA) tests can be designed

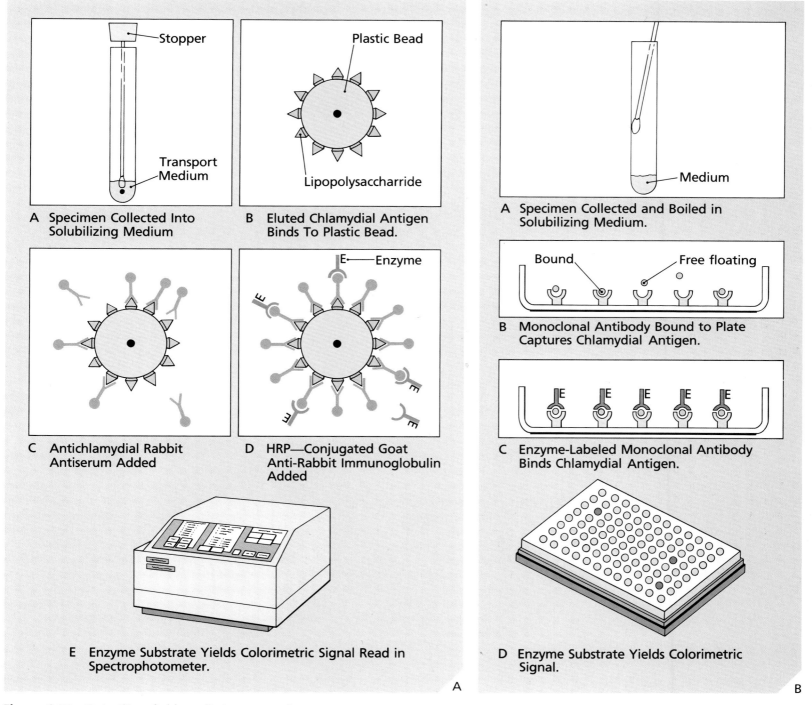

A Specimen Collected Into Solubilizing Medium

B Eluted Chlamydial Antigen Binds To Plastic Bead.

C Antichlamydial Rabbit Antiserum Added

D HRP—Conjugated Goat Anti-Rabbit Immunoglobulin Added

E Enzyme Substrate Yields Colorimetric Signal Read in Spectrophotometer.

A

A Specimen Collected and Boiled in Solubilizing Medium.

B Monoclonal Antibody Bound to Plate Captures Chlamydial Antigen.

C Enzyme-Labeled Monoclonal Antibody Binds Chlamydial Antigen.

D Enzyme Substrate Yields Colorimetric Signal.

B

Figure 6.54 Detection of chlamydia by enzyme immunoassay (EIA). **A** Direct Antigen Capture technique. **B** MAb Sandwich Antigen Capture technique.

to allow testing of numerous specimens for chlamydial antigen. EIA tests, like DFA, are reported to be less sensitive than culture methods; they are also somewhat less specific than DFA. The advantages of EIA include the high throughput capability for screening large numbers of patients, and, due to the objective nature of the test results, the lack of requirement for highly skilled personnel to interpret the information. The reagents for EIA are expensive, costing $3 to $7 per test. Tests based upon reactivity of polyvalent antisera with the chlamydial LPS may cross-react with bacteria of the gastrointestinal tract that share common LPS antigenic determinants. For this reason, these tests are limited to those sites not potentially contaminated by gastrointestinal flora. EIA tests to date appear to be less specific than are necessary for acceptable predictive values of a positive test result in populations with prevalences below 15%. Relative advantages of cell culture and antigen detection (DFA, EIA) methods are shown in Fig. 6.55A. Advantages of DFA and EIA are compared in 6.55B.

SEROLOGY
Although not occurring in every case of uncomplicated genital infection, antibody to C. trachomatis usually occurs following infection and persists for years. IgM responses can be seen in first episodes of infection. These antibody responses have been used for decades to diagnose chlamydial infection.

Complement Fixation
With the availability of high-quality antigen in the 1940s, the chlamydial group complement fixation (CF) test was developed. The CF test uses the chlamydial "group" antigen to detect serum antibody to any of the members of this genus. This test is still used in the diagnosis of LGV, in which a negative single-serum test rules out the disease, and in ornithosis, in which a change in titer between acute and convalescent sera can be diagnostic.

MICROIMMUNOFLUORESCENCE
The limited sensitivity and genus specificity of the CF test limits its use in seroepidemiologic studies. The development of the microimmunofluorescence (MIF) test in the 1970s allowed studies of the clinical epidemiology of chlamydial infection. The MIF uses fixed, purified chlamydial antigens, which are dotted onto a glass slide and reacted with the patient serum (Figs. 6.56 and 6.57). The test is sensitive, and, in most cases, provides information regarding the infecting serotype in C. trachomatis infections. It is also capable of determining IgM responses, characteristic of acute infection, and is of particular use in the diagnosis of infant chlamydial pneumonia. However, the technique is laborious and technically demanding, and interpretation requires extensive experience. Less demanding ELISA tests or inclusion–indirect immunofluorescent tests using a single serovar have been described or are available commercially, but have not been critically examined in large clinical trials. Several studies have indicated the association of local antibody in acute chlamydial disease, and serum IgA has been suggested to predict infection; however, these tests have not been sufficiently researched to be recommended. Due primarily to the background prevalance of chlamydial infections, serologic diagnosis of C. trachomatis infection has limited utility (Fig. 6.58).

PAPANICOLAOU SMEAR
Another method used in the laboratory diagnosis of chlamydial infection is examination of Papanicolaou-stained cervical smears (Pap smear). The detection of intact chlamydial inclusions in the PAP smear is insensitive, as most EBs are extra-

RELATIVE ADVANTAGES OF CELL CULTURE AND ANTIGEN DETECTION METHODS FOR IDENTIFICATION OF C. TRACHOMATIS

CELL CULTURE	ANTIGEN DETECTION
Superior sensitivity	Transport ease
Absolute specificity	Decreased laboratory hazard
Allows strain characterization	Technologically easier
Suitable for specimens from any anatomic site	Cost may decrease with technical improvements

A

RELATIVE ADVANTAGES OF DIRECT FLUORESCENT ANTIBODY AND ENZYME IMMUNOASSAY TESTS FOR C. TRACHOMATIS DETECTION

DIRECT FLUORESCENT ANTIBODY	ENZYME IMMUNOASSAY
Sample quality verifiable	Objective test signal
Individual tests rapid	Batch processing
Reagent cost low	Automatible
Suitable for gastrointestinal specimens	

B

Figure 6.55 **A** Relative advantages of cell culture and antigen detection methods for identification of C. trachomatis. **B** Relative advantages of direct fluorescent antibody and enzyme immunoassay tests for C. trachomatis detection.

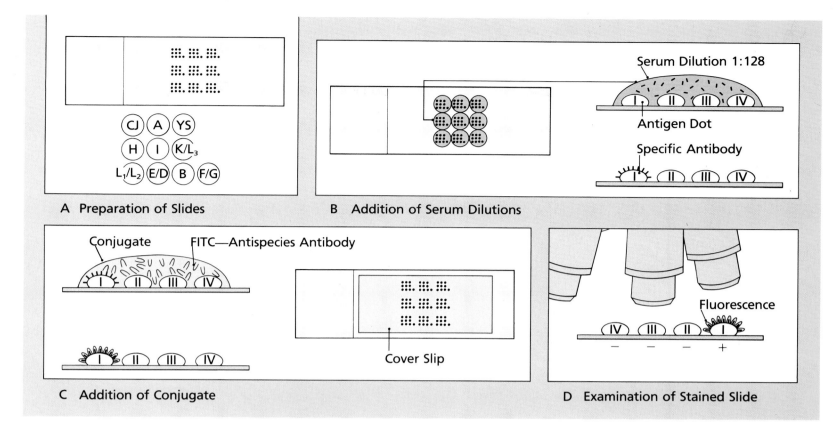

A   Preparation of Slides

B   Addition of Serum Dilutions

Serum Dilution 1:128

Antigen Dot

Specific Antibody

C   Addition of Conjugate

Conjugate   FITC—Antispecies Antibody

Cover Slip

D   Examination of Stained Slide

Fluorescence

Figure 6.56   Microimmunofluorescence assay.

Figure 6.57   Fluorescein chlamydial EBs suspended in egg yolk sac material viewed with the microimmunofluorescence method. The laborious nature of this test and the degree of skill required for proper interpretation have limited its acceptance outside research laboratories.

Figure 6.58   Uses of serology in chlamydial diagnosis.

USES OF SEROLOGY IN CHLAMYDIAL DIAGNOSIS

TEST	DIAGNOSTIC USE	PERFORMANCE
Complement fixation	LGV Ornithosis	Sensitive but not specific. Can rule out LGV if negative.
Microimmunofluorescence	Trachoma Genital infection Infant pneumonia	Sensitive and specific. Type responses in majority of infections.
ELISA	Unknown	Sensitivity and specificity undefined. Various methods not standardized.

cellular in endocervical scrapings. In addition, the cytologic changes that accompany C. trachomatis cervical infection are nonspecific. For these reasons, Pap smear alone cannot be used to diagnose chlamydial endocervical infection; however, the finding of inflammatory cells may indicate the need for specific chlamydial testing.

NUCLEIC ACID PROBES

Several published studies have examined the use of DNA probes, usually using the common C. trachomatis plasmid as a probe. These have shown far less sensitivity than culture methods, and are at the present time research tools only. Nucleic acid probes based on ribosomal RNA are currently under study, and one such product is commercially available. The performance parameters of these products will be determined by currently ongoing comparative trials. New techniques of nucleic acid detection such as sandwich amplification and polymerase chain reaction have not yet been applied to detection of C. trachomatis, but may improve the sensitivity of chlamydial detection dramatically.

Figure 6.59 Representative values of C. trachomatis MICs.

REPRESENTATIVE VALUES OF C. TRACHOMATIS MICs

ANTIMICROBIAL	MIC (μg/mL)
Tetracycline	0.03–0.50
Doxycycline	0.02–0.03
Erythromycin	0.50–2.0
Clindamycin	2.0–16
Rifampicin	0.005–0.25
Sulfamethoxazole	0.50–4

Variability of strains and methods used in the determination of chlamydial susceptibilities limits the clinical utility of these in vitro data.

TREATMENT REGIMENS FOR CHLAMYDIAL INFECTIONS AND CHLAMYDIA-ASSOCIATED CONDITIONS

PATIENT	CONDITION	THERAPY	COMMENTS
Adults	NGU, MPC, gonorrhea, or sexual partners in past 30 days to persons with these conditions	Doxycycline 100 mg PO BID for 7 days or Tetracycline HCl 500 mg PO QID for 7 days	Alternatives: Erythromycin base 500 mg PO QID for 7 days. or Sulfamethoxazole 1 g PO BID for 10 days.
Pregnant women	Urogenital infection	Erythromycin base 500 mg PO QID for 7 days	If 2 g daily dose not tolerated, decrease to 250 mg PO QID for 14 days.
Neonates or infants	Conjunctivitis or pneumonitis	Erythromycin syrup 12.5 mg/kg PO QID for 14 days	Concurrent gonococcal conjunctival infection must be ruled out in conjunctivitis. Topical therapy not beneficial. Repeat therapy for relapses.
Young men	Epididymitis (in presence of urethritis and absence of bacteriuria)	Doxycycline 100 mg PO BID for 10 days or Tetracycline HCl 500 mg PO QID for 10 days	Given in conjunction with effective antigonococcal therapy.
Women	PID (regimen varies depending on clinical severity)	Doxycycline 100 mg PO BID for 14 days	For ambulatory patients only. Given in conjunction with immediate therapy effective for gonorrhea and anaerobes.
Adults	LGV	Doxycycline 100 mg PO BID for 21 days or Tetracycline HCl 500 mg PO QID for 21 days	Efficacy not established in clinical trials.

Figure 6.60 Treatment regimens for chlamydial infections and chlamydia-associated conditions.

Treatment

Treatment of chlamydial infection in the acute stages of disease is straightforward; chlamydiae are susceptible to many antibiotics, and acquired resistance to antimicrobials has not yet been recognized (Fig. 6.59). Because the cell wall differs from that of many bacteria, beta-lactam antibiotics such as penicillin lack bactericidal activity against these organisms. The tetracyclines and macrolides of the erythromycin class are the currently recommended choices for proven or suspected chlamydial infection. Sulfonamides have activity against C. trachomatis, as does rifampin and its derivatives. Quinolones have variable activity against C. trachomatis in vitro, but sufficient clinical trials have not yet been performed to evaluate their efficacy. Similarly, long-acting cogeners of erythromycin are now being tested for use against infection in short-term therapeutic regimens. The currently recommended therapy is presented in Figure 6.60.

BIBLIOGRAPHY

Barnes RC: Laboratory diagnosis of human chlamydial infections. Clin Microbiol Rev 1989;2 (April).

Bird BR, Forrester F: Laboratory diagnosis of Chlamydia trachomatis infections. HHS:PHS:CDC. U.S. Government Printing Office, 1981.

Centers for Disease Control: C. trachomatis infections. Policy guidelines for prevention and control. MMWR 1985;34 |suppl|:53S–74S.

Grayston JT, Wang S-P: New knowledge of chlamydiae and the diseases they cause. J Infect Dis 1975;132:87–105.

Schachter J: Chlamydial infections. N Engl J Med 1978;298:428–435, 490–495, 540–549.

Schachter J: Biology of C. trachomatis. In: Holmes KK, Mårdh P-A, Sparling PF, Weisner PJ, eds. Sexually Transmitted Diseases. New York, McGraw Hill Book Company, 1984, pp 243–257.

Schachter J, Dawson CR: Human Chlamydial Infections. Littleton, MA, Publishing Sciences Group, 1978.

Stamm WE: Diagnosis of C. trachomatis genitourinary infections. Ann Intern Med 1988;108:710–717.

Thompson SE, Washington AE: Epidemiology of sexually transmitted C. trachomatis infections. Epidemiol Rev 1983;5:96–123.

Genital Mycoplasmas

G.H. CASSELL, K.B. WAITES, D. TAYLOR-ROBINSON

Introduction

Mycoplasmas are the smallest known free-living microorganisms, intermediate in size between bacteria and viruses (Fig. 7.1). They are unique among prokaryotes, differing by one or more characteristics from all other major groups of human pathogens and viruses (Fig. 7.2). The absence of a cell wall (Fig. 7.3) is the single most distinguishing feature of mycoplasmas as a group and is responsible for their inclusion as a separate class, the Mollicutes. Many of the biological properties of mycoplasmas are due to the absence of a rigid cell wall, including resistance to all beta-lactam antibiotics and marked pleomorphism among individual cells. In contrast to L-phase variants of bacteria, mycoplasmas are unable to synthesize cell wall precursors under any conditions. The mycoplasmal cell membrane contains phospholipids, glycolipids, cholesterol, and various proteins. The extremely small size of the mycoplasmal genome (approximately one-sixth the size of that of *Escherichia coli*) severely limits their biosynthetic capabilities, helps to explain their complex nutritional requirements for cultivation, and necessitates a parasitic or saprophytic existence for most species.

Mycoplasmas usually reside on mucosal surfaces of the respiratory and urogenital tracts. Unlike chlamydiae, they are strictly extracellular pathogens. They are generally limited

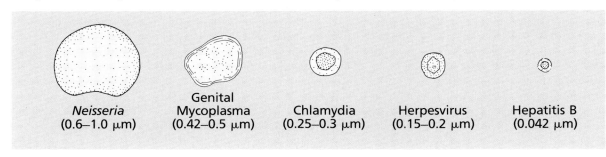

Neisseria (0.6–1.0 μm)	Genital Mycoplasma (0.42–0.5 μm)	Chlamydia (0.25–0.3 μm)	Herpesvirus (0.15–0.2 μm)	Hepatitis B (0.042 μm)

Fig. 7.1 Relative size of mycoplasmas in comparison with other sexually transmitted microorganisms. An individual mycoplasmal cell may be as small as 300 nm in diameter.

Fig. 7.2 Comparison of mycoplasmas with other microbial agents.

COMPARISON OF MYCOPLASMAS WITH OTHER MICROBIAL AGENTS

CHARACTERISTIC	MYCOPLASMAS	BACTERIA	CHLAMYDIAE	RICKETTSIAE	VIRUSES
Growth on cell-free media	+	+	−	−	−
Generation of metabolic energy	+	+	−	+	−
Independent protein synthesis	+	+	+	+	−
Contain both DNA and RNA	+	+	+	+	−
Reproduce by fission	+	+	+	+	−
Contain cell wall	−	+	+	+	−
Require sterol for growth	+ *	−	−	−	−

*Except for the genus *Acholeplasma*.

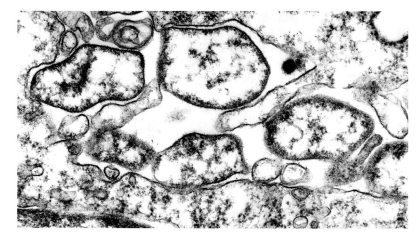

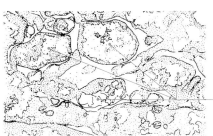

Mycoplasmas

Fig. 7.3 Transmission electron micrograph showing mycoplasmas between two epithelial cells. Unlike other bacteria, mycoplasmas lack a cell wall.

to the epithelial surface and rarely penetrate the submucosa (Fig. 7.4).

Of the eight species of mycoplasmas isolated from the urogenital tract of humans (Fig. 7.5), *Ureaplasma urealyticum* and *Mycoplasma hominis* are found most commonly and are the only two known to cause disease. *Mycoplasma genitalium* is a newly identified species first isolated from males with urethritis (Fig. 7.6).

There are only a few reported isolations of this organism, which is very slow growing and difficult to isolate. Epidemiologic surveys using a DNA probe suggest that M. *genitalium* may be a cause of nongonococcal urethritis. Serologic studies of women with pelvic inflammatory disease and experimental inoculation of primates also suggest that this organism may be pathogenic for humans, but its prevalence is unknown.

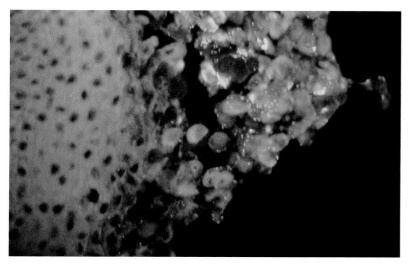

Fig. 7.4 Mycoplasmas attach to epithelial cell surfaces but rarely penetrate the submucosa. Unlike chlamydiae, they are extracellular. They are seen in this immunofluorescence micrograph showing mycoplasmas attached to the surface of inflammatory cells in the cervix. Note that neither *U. urealyticum* nor *M. hominis* have been shown to be a cause of cervicitis.

MYCOPLASMAS ISOLATED FROM THE GENITOURINARY TRACT OF HUMANS

| | | | | ANATOMIC SITE | | | | |
MYCOPLASMA	KIDNEY	BLADDER URINE	VOIDED URINE	URETHRAL SWAB	SEMINAL FLUID	FALLOPIAN TUBE	CERVIX/ VAGINA	AMNIOTIC FLUID
Mycoplasma hominis	+	+	+	+	+	+	+	+
Ureaplasma urealyticum	+	+	+	+	+	+	+	+
Mycoplasma fermentans			+	+			+	
Mycoplasma primatum				+				
Mycoplasma salivarium	+						+	
Mycoplasma genitalium				+				
Acholeplasma laidlawii							+	
Acholeplasma oculi								+

Fig. 7.5 Mycoplasmas isolated from the genitourinary tract of humans.

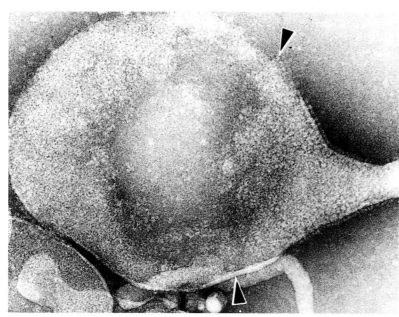

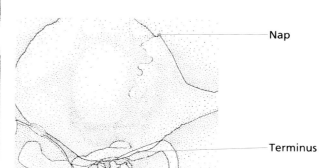

Nap

Terminus

Fig. 7.6 Transmission electron micrograph of *M. genitalium*. Negative staining of an intact mycoplasma cell with ammonium molybdate. The terminus is covered with a nap extending peripherally to the tip. (Courtesy of A.M. Collier, University of North Carolina, Chapel Hill.)

EPIDEMIOLOGY OF *UREAPLASMA UREALYTICUM* AND *MYCOPLASMA HOMINIS*

POPULATION	ISOLATION RATES	
	U. UREALYTICUM	*M. HOMINIS*
Sexually mature, asymptomatic females (cervix or vagina)	40–80%	21–53%
Babies born to infected mothers	ca. 40%	ca. 40%
Older children	<10%	<10%
Sexually inexperienced adults	<10%	<10%
Normal males	34%	22–54%

Fig. 7.7 Epidemiology of *U. urealyticum* and *M. hominis.*

RELATIONSHIP OF *UREAPLASMA UREALYTICUM* AND *MYCOPLASMA HOMINIS* TO DISEASES OF THE GENITOURINARY TRACT OF HUMANS

DISEASE	CAUSATIVE AGENT	
	U. UREALYTICUM	*M. HOMINIS*
Urethritis of males	+*	–*
Urethroprostatitis	±	–
Female urethral syndrome	±	–
Pyelonephritis	±*	+
Urinary calculi	±	–
Vaginitis	–	–
Cervicitis	–	–
Pelvic inflammatory disease	±	+
Infertility	±	–
Chorioamnionitis	+	±
Spontaneous abortion	±	±
Prematurity/low birth weight	±	–
Intrauterine growth retardation	±	–
Postpartum fever	±	+
Congenital pneumonia	+	+
Pneumonia in newborns	+	+
Meningitis in newborns	+	+
Abscesses in newborns	–	+
Extragenital disease in adults (including septic arthritis)	+	+

*– = No association or causal role demonstrated; + = causal role; ± = significant association and/or strong suggestive evidence but causal role not proven.

Fig. 7.8 Relationship of *U. urealyticum* and *M. hominis* to diseases of the genitourinary tract of humans.

Epidemiology

Isolation rates of U. *urealyticum* and M. *hominis* in various populations are given in Figure 7.7. U. *urealyticum* can be found in the cervix or vagina of 40 to 80% of sexually mature, asymptomatic women, and M. *hominis* in 20 to 50%. The incidence of each is somewhat lower in the urethra of normal males. In women, colonization is linked to younger age, lower socioeconomic status, sexual activity with multiple partners, black ethnicity, and oral contraceptive use. U. *urealyticum* and M. *hominis* may be transmitted to about 40% of babies born to infected mothers. Colonization of most infants appears to be transient, with a sharp decline in the rate of isolation after 3 months of age. Less than 10% of older children and sexually inexperienced adults are colonized. Colonization after puberty increases with sexual activity.

Clinical Manifestations

Neither U. *urealyticum* nor M. *hominis* has been shown to cause disease in the lower genital tract of the female. In fact, these organisms are probably commensals in this site. Genitourinary diseases for which they have been suspected to play an etiologic role are listed in Figure 7.8. All are either diseases of the upper genitourinary tract of females or diseases of the male. The difficulty with accepting these organisms as the cause of disease in each usually has arisen from the fact that either cultural samples cannot be easily obtained from the affected site or the organisms can be recovered from the affected site in asymptomatic individuals.

Even in diseases in which Koch's postulates have been fulfilled [i.e., M. *hominis* and pelvic inflammatory disease (PID)], attempts to link inflammatory lesions of the upper tract with cultural isolation from the lower tract have delayed recognition of the etiologic significance of these organisms. Recent carefully controlled clinical studies and experimental infection of laboratory animals have confirmed the disease-producing potential of both U. *urealyticum* and M. *hominis*. A major principle amply illustrated in these studies is that only in a subpopulation of individuals infected in the lower genitourinary tract do the organisms reach the upper tract, and only in some of these individuals does disease ensue. In no instance have the factors that predispose to upper tract colonization or development of disease been delineated. In many of the diseases considered, these factors may be of more importance for the development of lesions than the organism involved. While U. *urealyticum* or M. *hominis* may be responsible for directly inducing lesions in some instances, they primarily appear to be opportunists. In fact, U. *urealyticum* and M. *hominis* are increasingly being recognized as common causes of extragenital disease in immunocompromised patients and in newborn infants, particularly in those infants born preterm.

URINARY TRACT

Two conditions of the urinary tract definitively proven to be due to the genital mycoplasmas are urethritis in males due to U. *urealyticum* and pyelonephritis caused by M. *hominis*. It is possible that some urinary calculi are due to U. *urealyticum* infection.

Urethritis in Men

Human and animal inoculation studies and the occurrence of urethritis in immunodeficient patients provide indisputable evidence of a causal role for U. *urealyticum* in nonchlamydial, nongonococcal urethritis, although the proportion of cases for which the organism is responsible has not been established with certainty (Fig. 7.9). Carefully controlled antibiotic and serologic studies are also supportive of a causal role. The common occurrence of ureaplasmas in the urethra of asymptomatic men suggests either that only certain serotypes of ureaplasmas are pathogenic or that predisposing factors, such as a lack of mucosal immunity, must exist in those individuals who do develop disease. There is no evidence supporting a role for M. *hominis* as a cause for urethritis.

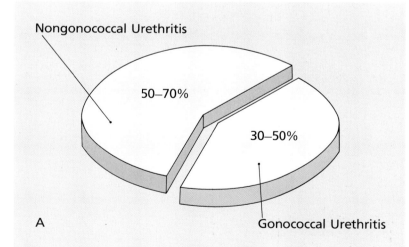

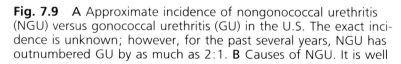

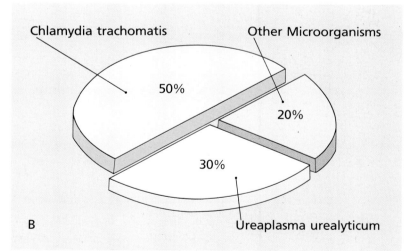

Fig. 7.9 **A** Approximate incidence of nongonococcal urethritis (NGU) versus gonococcal urethritis (GU) in the U.S. The exact incidence is unknown; however, for the past several years, NGU has outnumbered GU by as much as 2:1. **B** Causes of NGU. It is well established that approximately one-half of NGU cases are due to C. *trachomatis*, with the remainder caused by either U. *urealyticum* or other microorganisms whose precise contributions have yet to be identified.

Urinary Calculi

Urinary calculi composed of magnesium ammonium phosphate (struvite) and carbonate-apatite account for 20% of all urinary tract stones (Fig. 7.10), and may be the most deleterious variety in terms of urologic complications. These so-called "infection stones" are induced by the enzymatic breakdown of urea by bacterial urease (Fig. 7.11). *Proteus* and to a lesser extent *Klebsiella, Pseudomonas, Providencia, Staphylococcus,* and other bacterial species are the usual causes in humans. However, U. *urealyticum* also produces urease and has been demonstrated to induce crystallization of struvite and calcium phosphates in artificial urine in vitro and to produce calculi in animal models. However, the evidence that it does so under natural conditions in humans in the absence of other urease-producing organisms is scanty. The major remaining questions concerning the possible role of this organism in production of urinary calculi are the frequency with which it reaches the kidney, the predisposing factors that allow this to occur, and the relative frequency of renal calculi that seem to be induced by this organism compared with those induced by other organisms.

Pyelonephritis

Despite the high incidence of M. *hominis* in the lower urogenital tract, this organism has been isolated from the upper urinary tract only in patients with symptoms of acute infection, and often with development of a significant antibody response. Overall, M. *hominis* is thought to be involved in 5% of cases of acute pyelonephritis in humans. Predisposing factors, including obstruction or instrumentation of the urinary tract, occur in about 50% of cases in which M. *hominis* is thought to be the etiologic cause.

REPRODUCTIVE TRACT
Pelvic Inflammatory Disease

Pelvic inflammatory disease (PID) is an increasingly common disease of multifactorial etiology. It can be caused iatrogenically or can occur naturally from infections with various bacteria, the most common of which are *Chlamydia trachomatis* and, to a lesser extent, *Neisseria gonorrhoeae.* M. *hominis,* but probably not U. *urealyticum,* is also a likely cause of PID, although the exact proportion of cases attributable to it is unknown. The organism

Fig. 7.10 Staghorn renal calculus typically associated with urinary tract infections due to urease-producing bacteria.

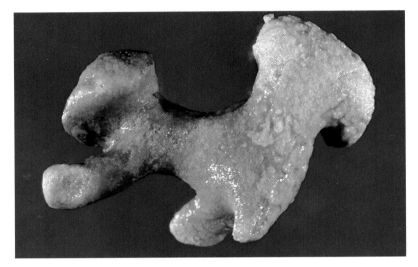

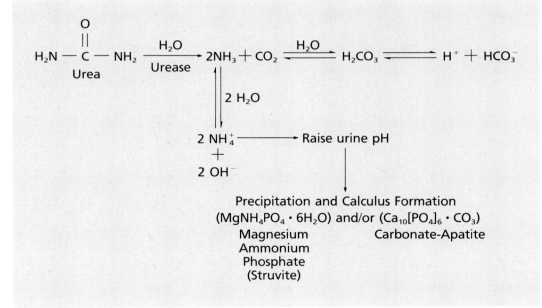

Fig. 7.11 Biochemical reactions leading to the formation of urinary calculi by urease-producing bacteria such as *U. urealyticum.*

has been isolated in pure cultures from the fallopian tubes of approximately 8% of women with salpingitis diagnosed by laparoscopy, compared with 0% of women without lesions. The organism can also be isolated from the endometrium. In addition, a role for M. *hominis* in cases of PID not associated with either C. *trachomatis* or N. *gonorrhoeae* is supported by significant increases in specific antibody. PID due to M. *hominis* is clinically indistinguishable from similar conditions caused by other organisms, so that antimicrobial coverage for M. *hominis* should always be included in the therapy.

While U. *urealyticum* has been isolated directly from affected fallopian tubes, it is found usually in the presence of other known pathogens. Furthermore, the results of serologic studies in humans and those involving animal inoculation and inoculation of fallopian tube organ cultures do not support a causal role.

Prostatitis

A number of studies suggest that the prostate can be infected during the course of an acute ureaplasmal infection of the urethra. Ureaplasmas are isolated more frequently and in greater numbers from patients with acute prostatitis than from controls. Men with more than 10^4 organisms respond to tetracycline therapy, while those with fewer organisms do not. U. *urealyticum* has not been found in prostatic biopsies from patients with chronic abacterial prostatitis, and M. *hominis* has not been associated with prostatitis of any kind in most studies.

DISORDERS OF REPRODUCTION

Given that M. *hominis* is a cause of salpingitis, it is reasonable to assume that severe tubal infection with this organism may lead to occlusion and infertility. However, this has not been proven. Although the possibility that ureaplasmas may play a role in involuntary infertility in humans was first raised over 20 years ago, the association remains speculative. Prospective studies based on isolation of U. *urealyticum* and M. *hominis* from the endometrium or placenta, but not studies based only on vaginal–cervical isolation, consistently show an association with spontaneous abortion. Individual case reports indicate that in some patients the infection is probably causal.

CHORIOAMNIONITIS AND PREGNANCY OUTCOME

In a subpopulation of women colonized in the lower genital tract, both M. *hominis* and U. *urealyticum* can colonize the endometria (Fig. 7.12), with or without evidence of inflammation. Attachment of the organisms to sperm (Fig. 7.13) has been suggested as one mechanism whereby the organisms are introduced into the upper tract. Both organisms can invade the amniotic sac in the first 16 to 20 weeks of gestation in the presence of intact fetal membranes and in the absence of other microorganisms. Mycoplasmas can be isolated from the endometrium of 20% of unselected individuals with intact fetal membranes at the time of cesarean section and from the placentas of about 10% of unselected individuals with intact membranes and no labor who are undergoing cesarean section. Isolation from fetal membranes increases with onset of labor, rupture of membranes, and number of vaginal examinations.

Isolation of M. *hominis* from amniotic fluid is virtually always associated with clinical symptoms (maternal fever, uterine tenderness, foul vaginal discharge) and a specific serologic response. U. *urealyticum*, on the other hand, can persist in amniotic fluid for as long as two months in the presence of an intense inflammatory response without discernible clinical signs or symptoms of amnionitis. The demonstration of inflammatory cells and ureaplasmas in amniotic fluid over a two-month period in the absence of other demonstrable microorganisms, as well as demonstration of ureaplasmas alone directly in inflam-

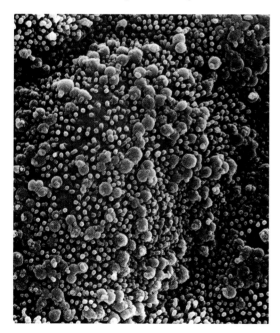

Fig. 7.12 Scanning electron micrograph showing U. *urealyticum* attached to the endometrium. Both U. *urealyticum* and M. *hominis* can be isolated from the endometrium with or without evidence of inflammation. The presence of this organism was demonstrated also by culture of the endometrium and by immunofluorescence.

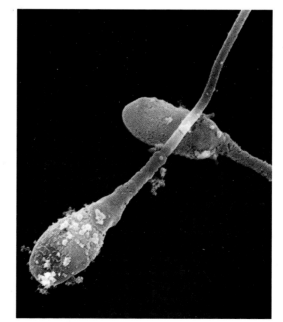

Fig. 7.13 U. *urealyticum* attached to human sperm. These organisms were shown to be ureaplasmas by immunofluorescence and culture.

matory infiltrates in the fetal membranes (Figs. 7.14 to 7.17) at the time of premature delivery, provide a convincing argument that these organisms alone can actually produce chorioamnionitis.

Isolation of U. *urealyticum* from the placenta is significantly associated with histologic chorioamnionitis and funisitis, stillbirth, and perinatal morbidity and mortality. Individual case reports indicate that, at least in some instances, the infection is causal. Isolation of ureaplasmas from the placenta is inversely related to gestational age and birth weight.

PERIPARTUM INFECTIONS

M. *hominis* is a proven cause of postpartum endometritis and is the single most common cause of postpartum fever. M. *hominis* and U. *urealyticum* are both known to cause postabortal fever. These infections are often self-limited and do not require treatment. However, M. *hominis* septicemia results in a longer hospital stay and in some cases results in suppurative septic arthritis and postcesarean wound infections.

M. *hominis* has been isolated from the joints of women with acute, suppurative arthritis following childbirth, the onset of arthritis occurring from six hours to three weeks after delivery. In most cases the organism was isolated not only from affected joints but also from blood. A tetracycline was given to those patients for whom therapy was prescribed, and recovery appeared to be rapid. One patient was found to have narrowing of the joint space at nine months' follow-up, but in the other reports the long-term outcome was not described.

DISEASES OF THE NEWBORN
Respiratory Disease

U. *urealyticum* and M. *hominis* are causes of congenital pneumonia and respiratory disease in the newborn (Fig. 7.18). U. *urealyticum*, in particular, is a significant cause of respiratory disease in very-low-birth-weight infants. Infants whose birth weights are less than 1000 g and who have ureaplasmas isolated from the lower respiratory tract within 24 hours of birth are twice as likely to develop chronic lung disease and also twice

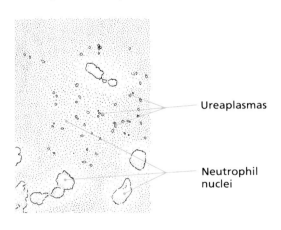

Fig. 7.15 DNA-fluorochrome-stained cytocentrifuged preparation of amniotic fluid collected at 20 weeks' gestation showing large numbers of U. *urealyticum* (identified by culture) and large numbers of polymorphonuclear leukocytes (×750). The fluid was culturally negative for other bacteria, viruses, and chlamydiae.

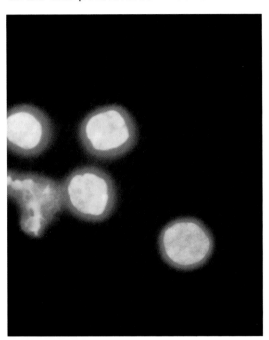

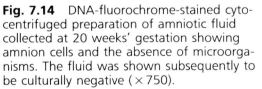

Fig. 7.14 DNA-fluorochrome-stained cytocentrifuged preparation of amniotic fluid collected at 20 weeks' gestation showing amnion cells and the absence of microorganisms. The fluid was shown subsequently to be culturally negative (×750).

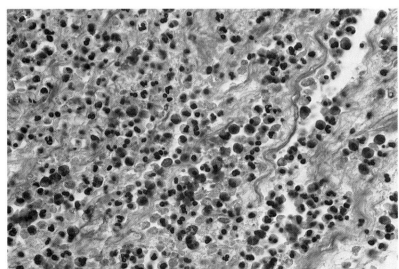

Fig. 7.16 Placenta at 26 weeks' gestation (hematoxylin and eosin, ×25). U. *urealyticum* was isolated in pure culture from amniotic fluid six weeks prior to delivery. Note the extensive inflammation in the amnion and chorion.

as likely to die as are infants of similar birth weights who are uninfected or infants weighing more than 1000 g. Pneumonia and sepsis due to U. urealyticum can be associated with persistent pulmonary hypertension of the newborn. Evidence indicates that many ureaplasmal and M. hominis respiratory infections are acquired in utero.

U. urealyticum and M. hominis isolated from tracheal aspirates are likely to represent true infection of the lower respiratory tract since most strains are isolated in pure culture and often are concomitantly isolated from blood. That the tracheal isolates are not merely a reflection of contamination from the nasopharynx is supported by the discrepancy in isolation rates between the two sites. U. urealyticum has been isolated more frequently from endotracheal aspirates than from nasopharyngeal swabs. Furthermore, M. hominis has been isolated from as many as 11% of endotracheal aspirates from infants weighing less than 2500 g who have respiratory disease, but rarely from the nasopharynx of these infants. Further evidence that tracheal

isolates represent true infection of the lower respiratory tract includes initial isolation from tracheal aspirates in numbers exceeding 10^3, and in some cases more than 10^6 colony-forming units, and repeated isolations of the organisms from tracheal aspirates over a period of months. Cerebrospinal fluid (CSF) of infants with respiratory disease is found often to be positive for U. urealyticum and M. hominis, again indicating the invasive nature of these organisms in preterm infants.

Central Nervous System and Other Systemic Infections

Both U. urealyticum and M. hominis cause meningitis in the newborn. Although their overall prevalence as central nervous system pathogens has not been thoroughly evaluated, recent evidence suggests that they may be among the most common causes of CSF infections in premature infants within the first few days of life. Congenital infection has been documented in some cases (Fig. 7.19).

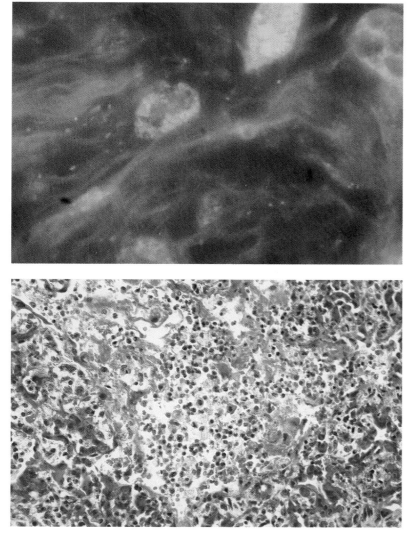

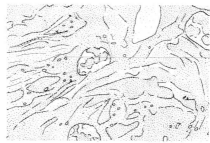

Fig. 7.17 Adjacent section of placenta shown in Fig. 7.16 (×750) stained with rabbit anti-U. urealyticum serovar 1 serum and reacted with affinity-purified, fluorescein-labeled, goat anti-rabbit IgG. Ureaplasmas present in the most intense areas of inflammation are indicated. Adjacent sections reacted with normal rabbit serum and conjugate were negative. Brown- and Bren-stained adjacent sections of placenta were negative for other bacteria.

Ureaplasmas

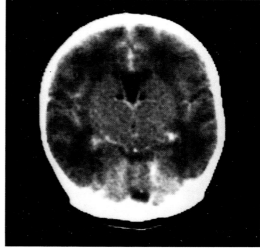

Fig. 7.18 Lung tissue (hematoxylin and eosin, ×100) collected at autopsy from a 1-week-old term infant. U. urealyticum was isolated in pure culture from blood, tracheal aspirate, and pleural fluid prior to death, and from lung and brain tissue at post mortem. There is a mixed mononuclear and polymorphonuclear cell infiltrate with abundant macrophages, fibrin deposition, and early interstitial fibrosis.

Fig. 7.19 Cranial computerized axial tomogram of an infant nine days after birth. M. hominis was isolated from CSF six days after birth. There is decreased attenuation, predominantly involving the supratentorial white matter symmetrically, with a few punctate lesions of increased attenuation suggestive of small focal hemorrhage or early calcification. These findings are compatible with diffuse intrauterine infection or a degenerative process.

U. *urealyticum* in the CSF is significantly associated with severe intraventricular hemorrhage and is found often in the presence of hydrocephalus. Chronic CSF infection of greater than one month's duration has been observed with both M. *hominis* and U. *urealyticum*. Changes in the CSF may be similar to those seen in bacterial meningitis, namely low glucose, elevated protein, and mononuclear or polymorphonuclear pleocytosis, or there may be no abnormalities detected whatsoever. The range of infection varies, from a mild subclinical course with no sequelae to more severe neurologic damage with permanent handicaps.

M. *hominis* is also a cause of pericardial effusion, adenitis, and subcutaneous abscesses associated with breaks in the skin due to fetal monitoring electrodes or forceps wounds.

SEPTICEMIA AND OTHER EXTRAGENITAL INFECTIONS

There are numerous individual reports of both M. *hominis* and U. *urealyticum* gaining access to the bloodstream. In the case of U. *urealyticum*, this has been reported in cases of postabortal and postpartum septicemia, as well as in newborn infants with respiratory distress and/or pneumonia. Septicemia due to M. *hominis* has been demonstrated in a variety of conditions following renal transplantation, trauma, and genitourinary manipulations. Wound infections, brain abscesses, and osteomyelitis also have been reported.

The true incidence of extragenital infections due to either ureaplasmas or M. *hominis* is not known since these organisms are not sought routinely. Most of the reported cases have been discovered by "accident" due to the occasional growth of M. *hominis* on blood agar and in routine blood cultures, or after specific mycoplasmal cultures were obtained following exclusion of other possible infectious causes.

ARTHRITIS AND OTHER EXTRAGENITAL DISEASES IN IMMUNOCOMPROMISED HOSTS

Approximately 8% of individuals with agammaglobulinemia develop "septic" joint inflammation. There is evidence to suggest that mycoplasmas may be responsible for the majority of these, since these organisms can be isolated repeatedly from the joints in the absence of any other microbial agent.

In many reported cases the arthritis has been persistent, lasting from several months to over a year. Aggressive, erosive arthritis that progresses in the face of antiinflammatory therapy and gamma-globulin replacement can occur. In some of the cases involving U. *urealyticum*, the arthritis is associated with subcutaneous abscesses, persistent urethritis, and chronic urethrocystitis/cystitis. Most cases have required aggressive antibiotic therapy, but some of the strains involved are or have become resistant to multiple antibiotics.

Septic arthritis, surgical wound infections, septicemia, and peritonitis due to M. *hominis* appear to occur rather frequently in patients following organ transplantation and in other types of patients undergoing immunosuppressive therapy. Sternal wound infections due to M. *hominis* in heart–lung transplant patients seem to be particularly common. Polyarthritis with recovery of both U. *urealyticum* and M. *hominis* has been seen in a kidney allograft patient on an immunosuppressive regimen. However, further evidence that ureaplasmas cause a problem in immunosuppressed patients or in those with AIDS is lacking.

Laboratory Tests

Many infections caused by mycoplasmas are discovered accidentally, either by observing the presence of M. *hominis* growing on blood agar or because of treatment failure with antibiotics directed at common bacterial pathogens but ineffective against mycoplasmas. Unfortunately, a mycoplasmal etiology is often considered only as a last resort.

A mycoplasmal etiology should be sought in diseases in which these organisms have been shown to play a role and when common bacteria have neither been revealed by Gram stain nor isolated. For conditions in which a mycoplasmal etiology has not been proven, it is difficult to justify either examination for the organisms or treatment. In particular, isolation of either M. *hominis* or U. *urealyticum* from the lower female genital tract or urine (other than that collected by catheter or suprapubic aspiration) is not meaningful.

Mycoplasmas are very demanding in terms of laboratory cultivation requirements. Diagnosis of mycoplasmal infections in general bacteriology laboratories is hampered because the organisms are not visible on Gram stain, reliable culture media specifically designed to support mycoplasmal growth has not been available commercially, and the organisms grow poorly or not at all in conventional bacteriological media. M. *hominis* can be recovered occasionally from blood cultures or other clinical material without special techniques, but this approach is unreliable. Ureaplasmas and M. *genitalium* are more fastidious than M. *hominis* and would not be recovered from clinical material unless specific techniques and media are used. If a mycoplasmal infection is suspected, care should be taken to collect a suitable specimen, to ensure that it is transported or stored under conditions known to maintain mycoplasmal viability, and to see that its examination is performed by a laboratory experienced in isolation and identification of mycoplasmas. Reliable information will be obtained only if these conditions are met.

SPECIMENS FOR CULTURE: ANATOMIC SITES

Liquid specimens, including blood, synovial fluid, cerebrospinal fluid, urine, prostatic secretions, sputum, pleural fluid, or tracheal secretions, are acceptable for mycoplasmal culture depending on the nature of the clinical condition. Other suitable specimens include placenta or any tissue collected from a biopsy or at autopsy if there is reason to suspect the presence of mycoplasmas.

SPECIMEN COLLECTION AND TRANSPORT

Only calcium alginate-, dacron-, or polyester-tipped swabs should be used, and the swab must always be extracted from the specimen. Blood should be collected free of anticoagulants.

Unlike many bacteria, mycoplasmas, due to their lack of a cell wall, are extremely susceptible to adverse environmental conditions, especially drying, osmotic changes, and toxic metabolites. Particular care must be taken to ensure that specimens are not subjected to extreme environmental fluctuations. No specific transport medium is necessary for tissue or fluid specimens if they can be inoculated directly into mycoplasmal medium within a reasonable period of time (i.e., no more than one hour after collection). However, if specimens are allowed to remain at room temperature and are not inoculated into appropriate transport media, significant loss of mycoplasmal viability or overgrowth of bacterial contaminants is to be expected. When possible, specific mycoplasmal medium such as Shepard's 10 B broth should be provided for direct inoculation of clinical specimens at the time they are collected. If specimens are collected in a facility that does not have immediate access to mycoplasmal broth for transport, satisfactory alternatives include 2SP medium (0.2 M sucrose in 0.02 M phosphate buffer, pH 7.2), trypticase soy broth with 0.5% bovine serum albumin, and commercially available Stuart's medium. Body fluids should be inoculated in an approximately 1:10 ratio (usually 0.1 mL fluid per 0.9 mL broth/transport medium). Ideally, some uninoculated material should also be sent to the laboratory. Specimens should be kept refrigerated at 4°C and protected from drying in a sealed container until they can be transported to the laboratory. If transport is not possible within a maximum of 24 hours after collection, the specimen should be stored at −70°C and transported frozen on dry ice. Mycoplasmas are stable for indefinite periods if kept frozen at −70°C in a stable protein-containing supporting medium such as 10 B broth. Storage at −20°C is less reliable and is subject to a significant gradual loss in titer.

CULTIVATION

Although by definition mycoplasmas are free-living (capable of growth on cell-free media), they are fastidious and demanding in their requirements for special media. A variety of media is available. Those sold commercially have yet to be evaluated thoroughly in a clinical setting. In using any medium, but in particular one obtained commercially, it is important to rule out mycoplasmal contamination. Fetal calf serum and horse serum used in most media are occasionally contaminated with mycoplasmas of animal origin.

Mycoplasmas are very sensitive to inhibitors present in some batches of horse serum, yeast extract, and even mycoplasma media base, and it is common for the standard medium in a laboratory to be temporarily insufficient for cultivation of mycoplasmas. Without proof of adequacy, negative cultures have little meaning. Rigorous quality control procedures using recent clinical isolates and stock strains (including multiple serotypes, especially with ureaplasmas) are critical. A reference mycoplasma laboratory should be consulted prior to obtaining any specimen if a reliable experienced laboratory is not locally available.

Clinical specimens for mycoplasmal culture should always be diluted serially in broth to at least 10^{-3} and each dilution inoculated onto agar. Dilution is necessary to overcome potential inhibitory substances or metabolites, including antibiotics, which may be present in the body fluid or tissue, and to facilitate quantitative estimation of the number of organisms present. In theory, greater isolation sensitivity may be obtained by centrifugation of urine and by performing serial dilutions

on an aliquot from the sediment. Tissues are preferably minced rather than ground for cultivation to circumvent potential growth inhibitors that are more likely to be released with grinding.

M. hominis, U. urealyticum, and M. genitalium are very different organisms with their own unique metabolic properties and cultivation requirements. They have different pH ranges for optimal growth, as well as different biochemical substrates from which they derive energy. U. urealyticum generates ATP by urea hydrolysis, M. hominis metabolizes arginine to ammonia, and M. genitalium metabolizes glucose. No single medium formulation will optimally support the growth of all three organisms. Mycoplasmal growth medium ordinarily contains animal serum, peptones, yeast extract, and metabolic substrates such as glucose, arginine, or urea. Shepard's 10 B broth and A8 agar have been successfully employed for several years for cultivation of both M. hominis and U. urealyticum (Fig. 7.20). SP-4 broth and agar will support the growth of M. hominis, U. urealyticum, and M. genitalium with appropriate pH and additives (Fig. 7.21). Antibiotics such as penicillin or nystatin are routinely incorporated into the media to inhibit bacterial and fungal contamination.

Very little information is available concerning the recovery of M. genitalium from clinical material. It is thought to grow best in an atmosphere containing 95% nitrogen and CO_2, but its extremely slow multiplication requires prolonged incubation over a period of weeks.

M. hominis and U. urealyticum are much easier to recover from clinical specimens. Their relatively rapid growth rates make identification of most positive cultures possible within two to five days. Broth cultures may be incubated at 37°C under atmospheric conditions and agar plates under 95% N_2 and 5% CO_2. Ureaplasmas, in particular, are susceptible to a rapid, steep death phase in culture, which is likely to result from a combination of urea depletion, ammonia production, and elevated pH due to urease activity. The presence of growth in 10 B medium is suggested by an alkaline shift due to the urease activity of ureaplasmas or arginine hydrolysis by M. hominis, causing the phenol red indicator to turn from yellow to pink (Fig. 7.20). The presence of growth in SP-4 broth is evident by a red to yellow (acidic) shift due to metabolism of glucose, or red to deeper red (alkaline) by arginine hydrolysis (Fig. 7.21). Broth

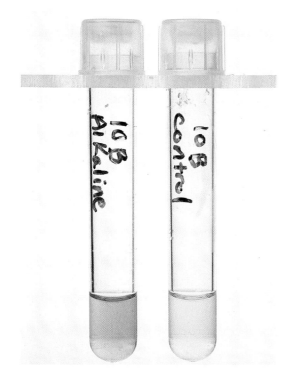

Fig. 7.20 Shepard's 10 B broth. This broth, containing phenol red pH indicator, is used to cultivate *M. hominis* and *U. urealyticum*. At a pH of 6.0 the broth is yellow. Growth of *U. urealyticum* or *M. hominis* with hydrolysis of urea or arginine, respectively, results in elevation of the pH and change in color from yellow to pink without significant increase in turbidity.

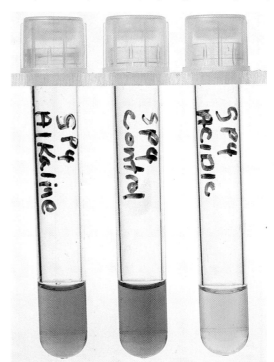

Fig. 7.21 SP-4 broth. This broth may be used for cultivation of *M. hominis*, *U. urealyticum*, or *M. genitalium*. It is normally prepared at a pH of 7.4 to 7.5. Growth of *M. hominis* with arginine hydrolysis elevates the pH, resulting in a color change from red to deep fuschia, while growth of a glucose-metabolizing mycoplasma such as *M. genitalium* results in a decrease in pH due to acidic end products and a change in color from red to yellow.

cultures showing color changes should be subcultured to agar. This combination of broth-to-agar inoculation technique has been shown to be the most sensitive for recovery of genital mycoplasmas.

SPECIES IDENTIFICATION

Colonies of U. *urealyticum* can be identified readily on A8 agar by urease production in the presence of CaCl$_2$ indicator. M. *hominis* colonies are urease-negative and have a typical "fried egg" appearance (Figs. 7.22 to 7.25). Unlike conventional bacteria, minute mycoplasmal colonies require a stereomicroscope to determine their presence and characterize their morphology.

In addition to M. *hominis*, other mycoplasmal species that may have similar growth requirements can also be present in clinical specimens and be morphologically indistinguishable. There are no biochemical tests that can readily distinguish between the large-colony mycoplasmal species, so serologic identification methods must be used. The tests are of two basic types. In the first group are procedures using living organisms, in which antiserum inhibits the growth or metabolic functions of the mycoplasma species or type against which it has been prepared. Examples include growth-inhibition, metabolism-inhibition (Fig. 7.26), and mycoplasmacidal methods.

The growth-inhibition method is specific but rather insensitive, making it useful for speciation of mycoplasmas but of limited, if any, value for antibody measurement. Metabolism-inhibition and mycoplasmacidal tests are sufficiently specific to use in organism identification and also are sensitive enough to be useful in antibody detection. The second broad group of serologic methods is that in which identification of organisms is accomplished by demonstrating reaction of specific antibody with whole fixed organisms or their antigens. The most widely used of these procedures is colony immunofluorescence.

A problem with any of these techniques is the existence of multiple serotypes of M. *hominis* and U. *urealyticum*. The many serotypes react specifically with antibody, requiring preparation of batteries of antisera if all strains are to be correctly identified.

SEROTYPING

There is some suggestion that certain serotypes of U. *urealyticum* are more likely to be associated with disease, but definitive evidence is lacking. Furthermore, the currently available methods of serotyping are not practical for routine use.

STAINS

Stains that bind to DNA can often aid in detection of mycoplasmas prior to culture results (see Fig. 7.15). Extranuclear fluorescence in fluid specimens treated with DNA fluorochrome stains such as Hoechst 33258 can be used to identify the presence of microorganisms. DNA fluorochrome will stain any pro-

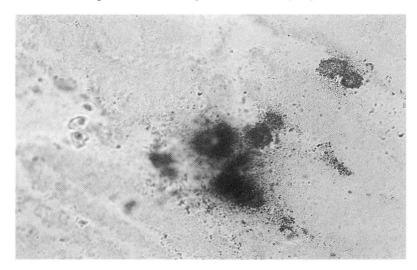

Fig. 7.22 Colonies of *U. urealyticum* growing on A8 agar. The granular brown appearance is due to urease activity in the presence of CaCl$_2$ indicator. The colonies are rather amorphous, as is often the case with ureaplasma colonies produced as a result of an initial isolation attempt from clinical material.

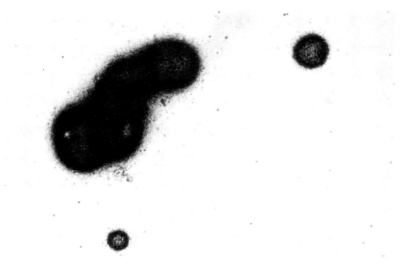

Fig. 7.23 Colonies of *U. urealyticum* growing on A8 agar after several passages on artificial media. Note the characteristics of these discrete colonies compared with those on the initial isolation plate shown in Figure 7.22.

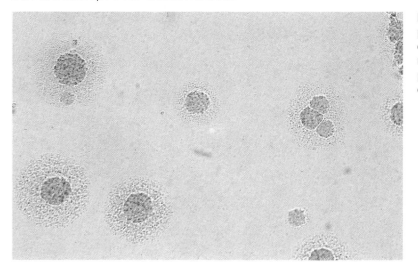

Fig. 7.24 Unstained colonies of *M. hominis* on A8 agar. Mycoplasmal colonies on agar typically exhibit a "fried egg" appearance due to growth in the agar in the center of the colony. Colonies measure 50 to 500 μm in diameter. Colonial morphology is dependent to a large extent on local growth conditions and media components.

karyotic DNA present. A Gram stain can be performed to exclude bacteria. Comparison of the specimen with a known positive control will help establish the presence of a mycoplasma, but confirmation with culture is essential for definitive diagnosis.

Mycoplasmas in exudates can be stained with Giemsa but most often such preparations are difficult to interpret due to cellular debris and artifacts. Colonies on agar can be more easily visualized by using the Dienes stain (see Fig. 7.25).

SEROLOGIC DIAGNOSIS

Patients with invasive M. *hominis* infections almost without exception seroconvert or have a significant rise in existing antibody. This response can be measured by the metabolism-inhibition assay (see Fig. 7.26), enzyme-linked immunosorbent assays, or other serologic procedures. Both acute and convalescent sera should be evaluated, results based on single specimens being difficult or impossible to interpret. Due to the ubiquity of most mycoplasmas in humans, it should be realized that detection of antibodies alone cannot be considered significant.

The assays mentioned are available for detection of antibodies to U. *urealyticum*. At present, however, determination of serologic responses is limited to research laboratories. Until more specific information is available concerning the value of antibody detection, serodiagnosis cannot be recommended for routine diagnostic purposes.

Treatment

Recognition that M. *hominis* and U. *urealyticum* are indeed causes of some genital and extragenital disease entities requires that some mention be made of what constitutes optimal chemotherapy. It is appropriate to perform diagnostic evaluations for mycoplasmas in patients who are suspected of having a condition for which mycoplasmas have been shown to be of etiologic significance (i.e., urethritis in men, PID in women, meningitis in newborns). A positive culture for either M. *hominis* or U. *urealyticum*, particularly in the absence of other microorganisms, is sufficient justification for treatment in most instances. Conditions such as PID in which cultures of the affected site may not be readily available, as well as the general lack of suitable mycoplasmal diagnostic facilities in many areas, make empiric treatment necessary in some instances. However, antibiotic resistance among clinical isolates of both M. *hominis* and U. *urealyticum* makes chemotherapy without validation by in vitro susceptibility testing risky. The most widely used technique to test the drug susceptibility of mycoplasmas and ureaplasmas is the microtiter broth-dilution method (Fig. 7.27).

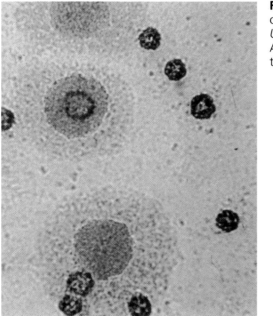

Fig. 7.25 Colonies of *M. hominis* and *U. urealyticum* on A8 agar stained by the Dienes method.

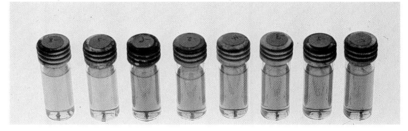

Fig. 7.26 Example of metabolism-inhibition test results. This test is essentially a growth-inhibition technique carried out in liquid medium. Organisms that multiply in liquid medium containing a specific substrate metabolize the substrate, and the products alter the pH of the medium as indicated by a change in color of an appropriate pH indicator. Specific antibody inhibits multiplication of the organisms and therefore indirectly prevents the color change from occurring. The test may be used for determining levels of specific antibody by using a constant number of organisms and multiple dilutions of serum. The titer of the serum is recorded as the highest dilution that prevents the change in color of the medium. In addition, the test can be used for classification and characterization of clinical isolates by using antisera with known titers.

Fig. 7.27 Example of microtiter broth-dilution antibiotic sensitivity test results. This test allows large numbers of isolates to be tested simultaneously against several antibiotics and provides reproducible results. The method depends on the inhibition of mycoplasmal growth by specific dilutions of antibiotic, growth and inhibition of growth being indicated by the presence and absence, respectively, of a color change in culture medium containing phenol red pH indicator.

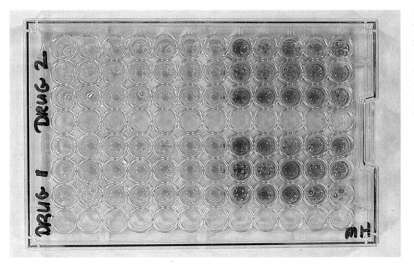

SUSCEPTIBILITIES OF *UREAPLASMA UREALYTICUM* AND *MYCOPLASMA HOMINIS* TO VARIOUS ANTIMICROBIALS

Fig. 7.28 Susceptibilities of *U. urealyticum* and *M. hominis* to various antimicrobials.

ANTIMICROBIAL	*U. UREALYTICUM* MIC*(μg/mL)	*M. HOMINIS* MIC*(μg/mL)
Doxycycline	0.05–1	0.1–0.4
Minocycline	0.03	0.4–0.8
Oxytetracycline	0.4–2	0.5–6.4
Tetracycline	0.05–8	0.2–6.8
Erythromycin	0.1–1.6	>1000
Clindamycin	1–50	0.2–1.6
Lincomycin	25–>500	0.2–1.6
Rosaramicin	0.008–4	<0.025–0.4
Spiramycin	32	2–16
Chloramphenicol	0.4–3.1	4–25
Gentamicin	3.1–12.5	1.6–12.5
Kanamycin	1.6–12.5	1.6–12.5
Streptomycin	0.4–3.1	4–32
Spectinomycin	16	<0.3–10
Nitrofurantoin	12.5–>1000	500
Polymixin	12.5–>1000	1000
Rifampicin	>1000	>100–7100
Vancomycin	500–>1000	500–>1000
Penicillin	>4000	>1000
Trimethoprim/ sulfamethoxazole	Inactive	Inactive

*MIC = minimal inhibitory concentration.

ORAL TREATMENT OPTIONS FOR MYCOPLASMAL AND UREAPLASMAL INFECTIONS

Fig. 7.29 Oral treatment options for mycoplasmal and ureaplasmal infections.

DRUG	ADULTS	CHILDREN
Tetracycline	250–500 mg QID	25–50 mg/kg/day, divided into 4 equal doses
Doxycycline	Loading dose of 200 mg; then 100 mg/day	Loading dose of 4 mg/kg, then 2 mg/kg/day
Clindamycin*	300–450 mg QID	8–16 mg/kg/day, divided into three to four equal doses
Erythromycin**	250–500 mg QID	30–50 mg/kg/day, divided into four equal doses

*Effective only for *M. hominis.*
**Effective only for *U. urealyticum.*

A summary of antimicrobial susceptibilities of U. urealyticum and M. hominis is given in Figure 7.28. M. hominis and U. urealyticum are resistant to sulfonamides, trimethoprim, and all antibiotics acting by inhibition of cell wall synthesis. Both organisms are often resistant to aminoglycosides and chloramphenicol as well. M. hominis is susceptible to clindamycin and resistant to erythromycin, while the reverse is true for ureaplasmas. This differential susceptibility is sometimes useful in separating mixed cultures in order to test additional drug susceptibilities of each mycoplasmal component. Tetracyclines are the drugs of choice for M. hominis and U. urealyticum infections if there are no contraindications. However, as many as 40% of clinical isolates of M. hominis may be tetracycline-resistant. Approximately 80 to 90% of ureaplasmal strains are sensitive to tetracycline, although the incidence of resistant strains may be increasing. If a mycoplasma is resistant to one drug in the tetracycline group, it is usually resistant to others as well. Erythromycin-resistant strains also occur, and there may be a correlation between tetracycline resistance and erythromycin resistance. Doxycycline is better absorbed than tetracycline and has a longer half-life. However, it is considerably more expensive and has not been shown to be clinically superior to other tetracyclines.

Tetracyclines given in standard doses usually penetrate the meninges and synovial fluid and achieve levels exceeding the minimal inhibitory concentration for susceptible mycoplasmal or ureaplasmal strains. Clindamycin provides alternative therapy for M. hominis infections not involving the central nervous system in which there is a contraindication to using tetracycline, or in case of tetracycline resistance. In treating conditions known to be sexually transmitted such as urethritis, the index case as well as all sexual contacts should receive antibiotics to prevent reinfection.

The infant with M. hominis meningitis presents a difficult therapeutic situation. Normally, tetracycline therapy is contraindicated in children less than 8 years of age, but no other currently available drug is approved for use or shown to be effective in this condition. There are precedents for using intravenous tetracycline or doxycycline to treat infants with mycoplasmal or ureaplasmal meningitis in which the organisms were eradicated.

Erythromycin is the drug of choice for ureaplasmal infections in neonates. Although erythromycin penetrates poorly into the central nervous system, U. urealyticum has been eradicated from CSF with erythromycin in one instance following treatment failure with doxycycline.

The development of resistance of many strains of U. urealyticum and M. hominis to the aforementioned "first-line" antibiotics has prompted investigation of many new antimicrobial compounds as they become available. Preliminary in vitro studies suggest that some of the newer quinolones may possibly be effective against some isolates, although none have been widely tested in vivo.

Guidelines for duration and routes of drug administration have not been systematically evaluated for either local urogenital or extragenital systemic mycoplasmal or ureaplasmal infections; these should be determined individually according to the type and location of infection, as well as the age and clinical condition of the patient. Figure 7.29 outlines various oral treatment options. In general, treatment for 10 to 14 days is recommended. For neonates with meningitis or other sys-temic infections, parenteral therapy using the same dosage guidelines is advisable, with follow-up cultures to ensure eradication of the organisms. Immunosuppressed persons with systemic mycoplasmal infections, including the joints and the urinary or respiratory tract, may harbor multiply resistant strains. Prolonged parenteral therapy, possibly requiring increased dosages, followed by weeks to months of oral therapy may be necessary. This may seem overly aggressive, but previously published cases and personal experience indicate that such infections can be extremely difficult to eradicate. Arthritis due to these organisms can eventually lead to progressive, irreversible joint damage if left alone or treated inadequately.

BIBLIOGRAPHY

Cassell GH, Clyde WA, Kenny GE, McCormack WM, Taylor-Robinson D: Ureaplasmas of humans: With emphasis upon maternal and neonatal infections. Pediatr Infect Dis 5:S221, 1986.

Cassell GH, Cole BC: Mycoplasmas as agents of human disease. N Engl J Med 304:80, 1981.

Cassell GH, Crouse DT, Waites KB, Rudd PT, Davis JK: Does Ureaplasma urealyticum cause respiratory disease in newborns? Pediatr Infect Dis 7:535, 1988.

Cassell GH, Waites KB, Crouse DT, Rudd PT, Canupp K, Stagno S, Cutter G: Association of Ureaplasma urealyticum infection of the lower respiratory tract with chronic lung disease and death in very low birth weight infants. Lancet 1:240, 1988.

Cassell GH, Davis JK, Waites KB, Rudd PT, Talkington D, Crouse D, Horowitz SA: Pathogenesis and significance of urogenital mycoplasmal infections, in Bondi A, Stieritz DD, Campos JM, Miller LA (eds): Urogenital Infections: New Developments in Laboratory Diagnosis and Treatment. Adv Exp Med Biol 224:93, 1987.

Mardh PA, Moller BR, McCormack WM: Mycoplasma hominis: A human pathogen. Sex Transm Dis 10:S225, 1983.

McCormack WM, Taylor-Robinson D: The genital mycoplasmas, in Holmes KK, Mardh PA, Sparling F, Wiesner PJ (eds): Sexually Transmitted Diseases. New York, McGraw-Hill Book Co., 1984, pp 408–419.

Senterfit LB: Antibiotic susceptibility testing of mycoplasmas, in Tully JG, Razin S (eds): Methods in Mycoplasmology. New York, Academic Press, 1983, vol 2, pp 397–401.

Shepard MC: Culture media for ureaplasmas, in Razin S, Tully JG (eds): Methods in Mycoplasmology. New York, Academic Press, 1983, vol 1, pp 137–146.

Taylor-Robinson D: Recovery of mycoplasmas from the genitourinary tract, in Tully JG, Razin S (eds): Methods in Mycoplasmology. New York, Academic Press, 1983, vol 2, pp 19–26.

Taylor-Robinson D: Serological identification of ureaplasmas from humans, in Tully JG, Razin S (eds): Methods in Mycoplasmology. New York, Academic Press, 1983, vol 2, pp 57–66.

Taylor-Robinson D, McCormack WM: The genital mycoplasmas. N Engl J Med 302:1003, 1063, 1980.

Tully JG, Taylor-Robinson D, Cole RM, et al: A newly discovered mycoplasma in the human urogenital tract. Lancet 1:1288, 1981.

Waites KB, Rudd PT, Crouse DT, Canupp KC, Nelson KG, Ramsey C, Cassell GH: Chronic Ureaplasma urealyticum and Mycoplasma hominis infections of central nervous system in preterm infants. Lancet 2:17, 1988.

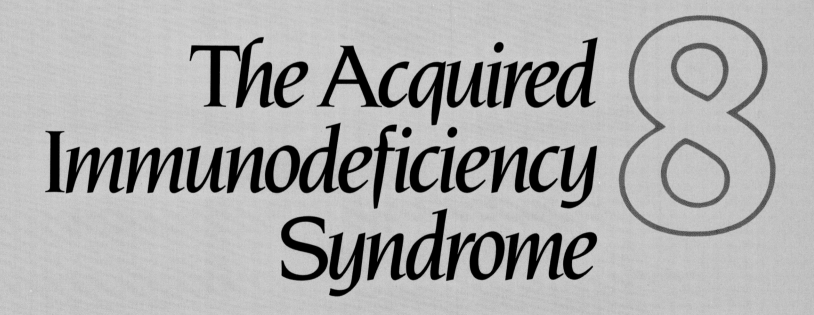

The Acquired Immunodeficiency Syndrome 8

P. E. KOZARSKY, H.M. BLUMBERG, M.H. DuPUIS

Introduction

The acquired immunodeficiency syndrome (AIDS) was first recognized in the spring of 1981 when the Centers for Disease Control (CDC) received multiple reports from New York and California of Pneumocystis carinii pneumonia and Kaposi's sarcoma occurring in previously healthy male homosexuals. Because these individuals were noted to have underlying immunosuppression with no apparent cause, the CDC formulated a case definition for AIDS: any disease that is moderately predictive of a defect in cell-mediated immunity occurring in a person with no documented cause for immune deficiency. The human immunodeficiency virus (HIV), a retrovirus, was identified as the etiologic agent for this disease, and the CDC surveillance definition was revised to include additional infections and malignancies in conjunction with a positive serologic test for HIV antibody. Further revision of the CDC definition to include numerous HIV-infected patients who have serious, disabling, or fatal conditions (e.g., encephalopathy or wasting syndrome) took place on September 1, 1987. For reporting purposes this revision adds to the surveillance definition most of those severe noninfectious, noncancerous HIV-associated conditions that are categorized in the CDC clinical classification

---

SUMMARY OF CDC CLASSIFICATION SYSTEM FOR HUMAN IMMUNODEFICIENCY VIRUS (HIV)

GROUP

I   Acute infection
Mononucleosis-like syndrome associated with seroconversion

II Asymptomatic infection*
Positive HIV antibody test

III Persistent generalized lymphadenopathy*
Palpable lymphadenopathy at two or more extrainguinal sites for >3 months duration in the absence of a concurrent illness or infection to explain findings

IV Other disease

SUBGROUP

A Constitutional disease[†]
For example, fever or diarrhea persisting > 1 month; or involuntary weight loss >10% of baseline; and absence of a concurrent illness to explain findings

B Neurologic disease[†]
Dementia, myelopathy, or peripheral neuropathy and an absence of a concurrent illness or condition

C Secondary infectious diseases

CATEGORY

C-1 Specified secondary infectious diseases listed in the CDC surveillance definition of AIDS[†]

C-2 Other specified secondary infectious diseases (oral hairy leukoplakia, multidermatomal herpes zoster, recurrent Salmonella bacteremia, nocardiosis, tuberculosis, and oral candidiasis)

D Secondary cancers[†]
Kaposi's sarcoma, non-Hodgkin's lymphoma, or primary lymphoma of the brain

E Other conditions
Clinical findings or diseases, not classifiable above, may be attributable to HIV infection and are indicative of a defect in cell-mediated immunity; symptoms attributable to either HIV infection or a coexisting disease not classified elsewhere; or clinical illnesses that may be complicated or altered by HIV infection. These include chronic lymphoid interstitial pneumonitis and constitutional symptoms, secondary infectious diseases, and neoplasms not listed above.

*Patients in Groups II and III may be subclassified on the basis of a laboratory evaluation.
[†]Includes those patients whose clinical presentation fulfills the definition of AIDS used by the CDC for national reporting.

Figure 8.1 Summary of CDC classification system for human immunodeficiency virus (HIV).

DISEASES INDICATIVE OF AIDS, IN CONJUNCTION WITH POSITIVE SEROLOGIC OR VIROLOGIC TEST FOR HIV

PROTOZOAN INFECTIONS

Pneumocystis carinii pneumonia (may be classified as a fungus)

Toxoplasma gondii encephalitis or disseminated infection

Chronic Cryptosporidium enteritis

Chronic Isospora enteritis

NONCONGENITAL VIRAL INFECTIONS

Chronic mucocutaneous herpes simplex

CMV infection of an organ other than liver or lymph node

Progressive multifocal leukoencephalopathy

BACTERIAL INFECTIONS

Disseminated Mycobacterium avium-intracellulare infection

Disseminated Mycobacterium tuberculosis infection

Salmonella (nontyphoid) septicemia, recurrent

FUNGAL INFECTIONS

Candidiasis—esophageal, pulmonary, or bronchial

Cryptococcal meningitis or disseminated infection

Disseminated histoplasmosis

Disseminated coccidioidomycosis

MALIGNANCIES

Kaposi's sarcoma

Primary brain lymphoma

Non-Hodgkin's lymphoma

OTHER

Chronic lymphoid interstitial pneumonitis in children (<13 years old)

HIV encephalopathy (AIDS or HIV dementia)

HIV wasting syndrome (emaciation or slim disease)

Figure 8.2 Diseases indicative of AIDS, in conjunction with positive serologic or virologic test for HIV.

for HIV infection (Fig. 8.1). Figure 8.2 lists a summary of diseases indicative of AIDS.

Known as human T-cell lymphotropic virus type III (HTLV-III), lymphadenopathy-associated virus (LAV), and AIDS-associated virus (ARV), HIV produces a spectrum of illness from asymptomatic or subclinical to the severe, fatal disease, AIDS. It is important to note that AIDS represents only the "tip of the iceberg" of HIV-related disease (Fig. 8.3) and should be used exclusively for cases that meet the CDC surveillance criteria.

Patients with manifestations of HIV-related disease who do not meet the CDC surveillance definition for AIDS are diagnosed with AIDS-related complex, or ARC (Fig. 8.4). This ARC subgroup encompasses patients with a wide range of clinical symptoms and manifestations, from mild to severe. Current estimates place the number of patients with ARC in the U.S. at several hundred thousand.

Finally, there is a third group of individuals infected with HIV who are asymptomatic, often without immunologic abnormalities. This last group is by far the largest, with current estimates ranging from 1 to 2 million persons.

The true risk of developing AIDS for HIV-infected individuals is unknown, but it is estimated that each year 7% of seropositive patients with ARC will progress to AIDS. The Public Health Service estimates that 30% of seropositive individuals will eventually develop AIDS over the next 5 to 10 years. The mean interval between infection with HIV and the onset of AIDS exceeds 7 years.

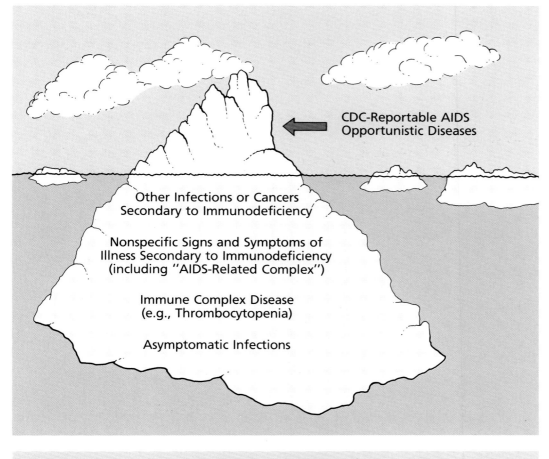

Figure 8.3 The clinical spectrum of HIV infection. AIDS represents only the "tip of the iceberg" of HIV-related disease.

Figure 8.4 AIDS-related complex: clinical manifestations and laboratory abnormalities.

AIDS-RELATED COMPLEX*

CLINICAL MANIFESTATIONS	LABORATORY ABNORMALITY
Lymphadenopathy in 2 or more noninguinal sites for >3 months	Helper T-cells <400/mm³
Fever >100°F for 3 months	T4 helper/T8 suppressor ratio <1.0
Weight loss >10%	Leukopenia
Persistent diarrhea	Thrombocytopenia
Fatigue	Anemia
Night sweats	Elevated serum globulins
Oral candidiasis	Anergy to skin tests
Oral hairy leukoplakia	Reduced blastogenesis
Herpes zoster	

*Most physicians make the diagnosis of ARC on the basis of clinical manifestations and a positive HIV serology.

Epidemiology

By May of 1988, over 60,000 cases of AIDS had been reported in the U.S., with more than half of them fatal. Cases have been reported from every state (Fig. 8.5), but the greatest number of reports have come from large metropolitan areas that have numerous homosexual men and intravenous drug abusers such as New York City, San Francisco, Los Angeles, Miami, and Houston. In addition, large numbers of cases have been reported from Washington, D.C., Newark, Chicago, Philadelphia, Atlanta, Dallas, and Boston.

The incidence of AIDS continues to increase, with the number of cases doubling approximately every 13 months (Fig. 8.6). By 1991, it is estimated that 270,000 individuals in the U.S. will have the disease or will have died from it (Fig. 8.7). Prior to the use of zidovudine (azidothymidine, or AZT), which may prolong survival in some patients, the median survival was one year. No patient with AIDS has had complete recovery of the immune system, although a small percentage of patients with

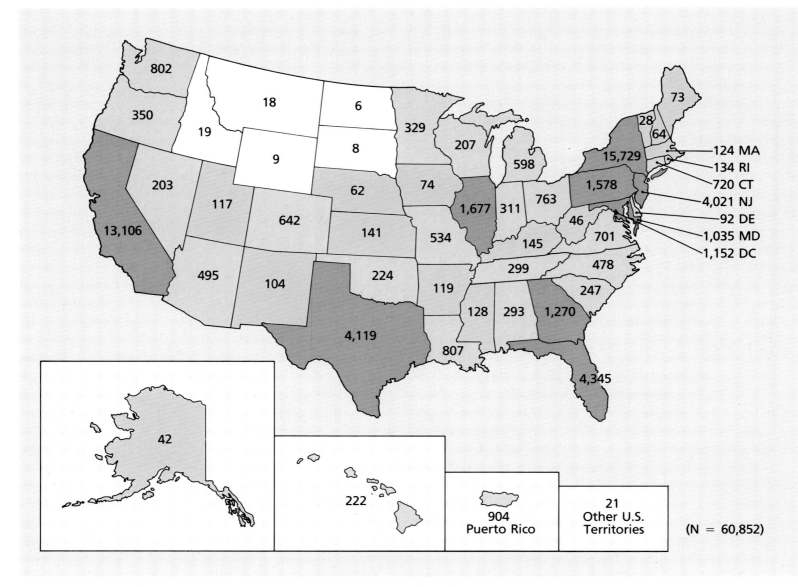

Figure 8.5 Cases of AIDS in the U.S. reported to the CDC by state through May 2, 1988.

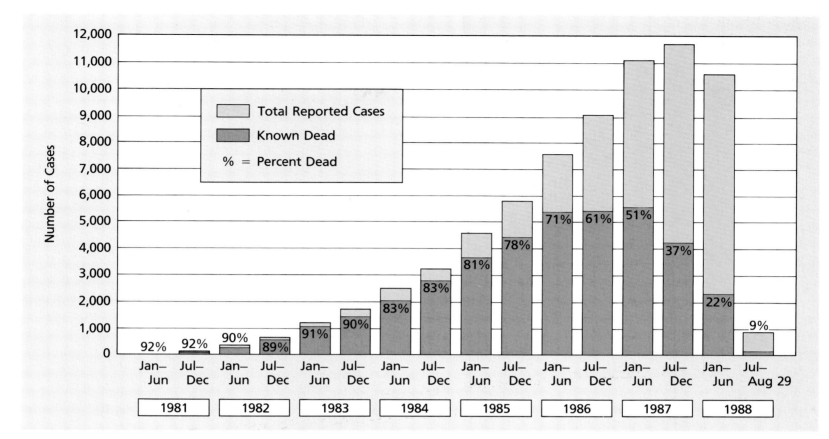

Figure 8.6 Reported cases of AIDS and case-fatality rates in the U.S. by half-year of diagnosis through August 29, 1988.

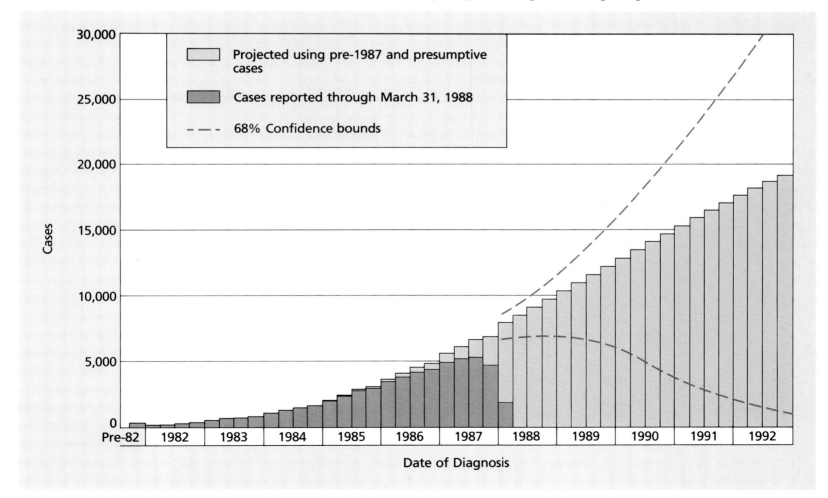

Figure 8.7 Incidence of AIDS in the United States, by quarter-year of diagnosis, projected from cases reported as of March 31, 1988 and diagnosed as of June 30, 1987.

Kaposi's sarcoma has survived up to 5 years. The major disease categories of presentation in adults with AIDS are listed in Figure 8.8.

The original CDC surveillance definition for AIDS in children was more stringent than that for adults due to the other commonly recognized causes of immunodeficiency in this group. Because of this, it is felt that the number of cases of pediatric AIDS has been grossly underestimated. Therefore, a new pediatric case definition and classification system has been formulated by the CDC, which may help to clarify HIV-related disease in this group of patients.

The demographic patterns for AIDS in the U.S. and Europe are generally quite similar. Nearly 90% of reported cases have occurred in individuals between the ages of 20 and 49, and approximately 90% of those affected have been males. In Africa and the Caribbean area, however, the picture is different. Central Africa and to a lesser degree adjacent countries in eastern and southern regions of Africa have been the most severerly affected areas. Millions of Africans are thought to be infected with HIV, and the seropositive rate is estimated to be as high as 10% of the population in some central African countries. Additional human retroviruses that cause AIDS have been identified, but at present they appear to account for only a small number of AIDS cases worldwide. In western Africa AIDS has been caused by a virus known as HIV-2. This virus is closely related to HIV-1 and has a similar mode of transmission. However, serologic tests for HIV-1 often fail to detect HIV-2. In western Africa HIV-2 is more prevalent than HIV-1 (Fig. 8.9). Unlike the demographic patterns in the U.S. and Europe, in both Africa and the Caribbean region the male-to-female ratio of reported cases of AIDS is nearly 1:1. In Africa, HIV infection is transmitted primarily through heterosexual rather than homosexual activity.

In addition, parenteral exposure by blood transfusions, the use of unsterilized needles (often in hospitals or medical clinics), and perinatal transfer from infected mothers to their newborns all play a significant role in transmission of the virus.

MODES OF TRANSMISSION

There is no evidence to suggest that HIV infection is spread by nonsexual close contact, by the airborne route, by water, or by food handlers. Although HIV can be isolated from many body fluids, transmission of the virus has been documented by only four routes: sexual contact (heterosexual or homosexual), exposure to body fluids (mainly blood) or blood-contaminated needles, receipt of infected blood or blood products, and perinatal infection. Since sexual contact has been responsible for transmission of 78% of all AIDS cases, widespread educational efforts are currently underway to promote "safer sex" among both the heterosexual and the homosexual populations. Other steps being taken in the U.S. to reduce the spread of the virus include screening blood for HIV-1 antibody and heat-treating plasma products to inactivate HIV.

As pregnancy may increase the risk of a seropositive mother developing ARC or AIDS, HIV antibody testing and counseling regarding the potential hazards of HIV infection to both the newborn and the mother should be offered to women at high risk. It is believed that 50 to 60% of pregnant HIV-positive women will transmit the virus to their offspring either in utero or at delivery.

The risk of acquiring HIV infection in health care workers is low. Indeed, the estimated risk of acquiring HIV through needlestick exposure is less than 1%, much less than that for acquiring hepatitis B where the risk of infection is 6 to 30%.

REPORTED CASES OF AIDS IN THE UNITED STATES BY DISEASE CATEGORY AND SEX FROM 1981 THROUGH AUGUST 29, 1988

Figure 8.8 Reported cases of AIDS in the U.S. by disease category and sex from 1981 through August 29, 1988.

DISEASE CATEGORY	MALES (%) (N = 65,656)	FEMALES (%) (N = 6,362)	TOTAL (%) (N = 72,018)
Kaposi's sarcoma only	10	1	9
Pneumocystis carinii pneumonia only	61	58	61
Other opportunistic diseases	29	41	30
Total	100	100	100

Despite thousands of needlesticks with needles from HIV-seropositive patients, seroconversion has been clearly documented in only a few health care workers who have been exposed either to a rather large innoculum of blood/body fluids or by direct exposure to blood.

HIV and other retroviruses are susceptible to common disinfectants such as alcohol, phenol, formalin, sodium hypochlorite (household bleach), and glutaraldehyde. Customary dishwashing and laundering procedures are felt to provide adequate decontamination of food service items and linens.

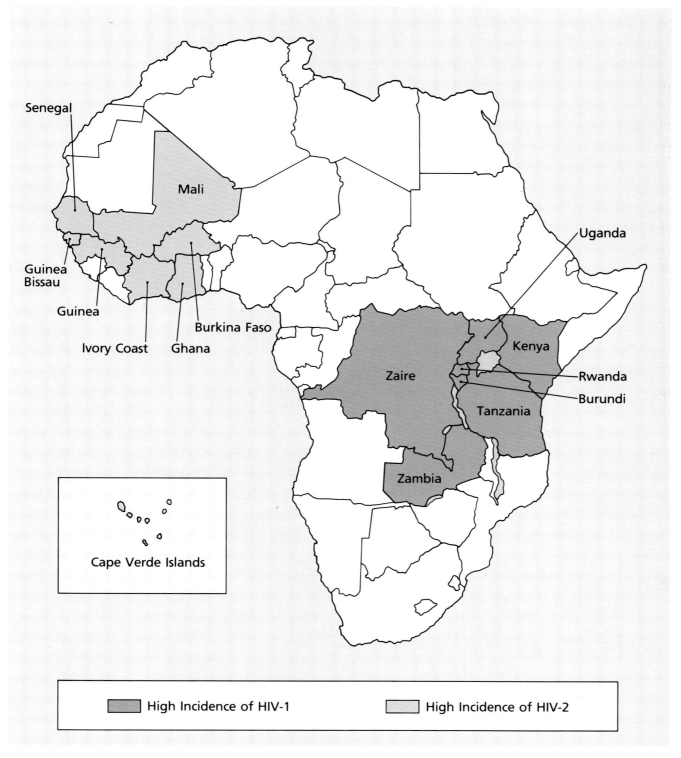

Figure 8.9 HIV infection in Africa. The highest incidences of HIV-1 and HIV-2 infection and AIDS have been reported from central Africa as shown within the outlined areas.

High Incidence of HIV-1   High Incidence of HIV-2

Serologic Testing

For clinical purposes, serologic testing is the primary mode of detecting HIV infection. Infection with HIV causes a serologic response consisting of the production of a number of antibodies to various components of HIV. The most commonly used diagnostic test is the enzyme-linked immunosorbent assay (ELISA), which generally becomes positive within 3 months after an individual is infected (Figs. 8.10 and 8.11). The sensitivity of the different ELISA test kits ranges from 93.4 to 99.6%, while the specificity range is estimated to be 99.2 to 99.8%. However, in a population with a low prevalence of infection, even a spec- ificity of 99.8% does not provide the desired predictive value for a positive test. For this reason the Western Blot test, which has a high specificity, is used as a confirmatory test (Fig. 8.12). Other methods of HIV detection include HIV culture and direct detection of HIV antigens. Current HIV culture techniques are cumbersome, time consuming, of low sensitivity, and generally only available at research facilities. HIV antigen tests show clinical promise; the p24 antigen test may become quite useful in diagnosing patients with acute HIV infection who are in a "window period" and have not yet developed antibodies to HIV.

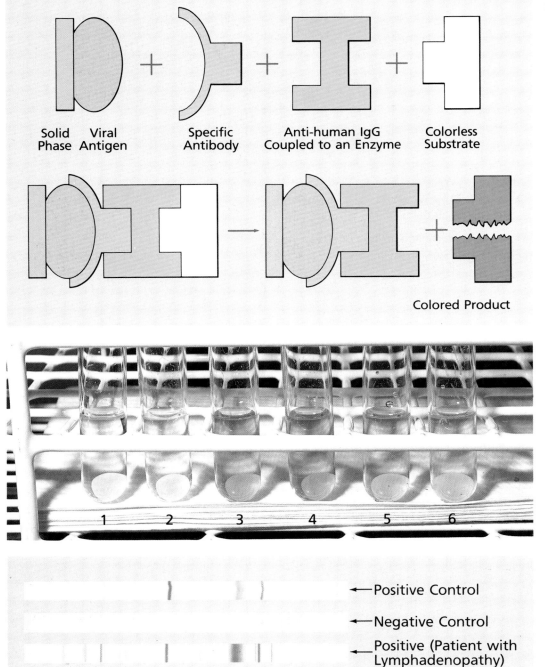

Figure 8.10 The enzyme-linked immunosorbent assay (ELISA), the antibody assay for HIV.

Solid Phase   Viral Antigen   Specific Antibody   Anti-human IgG Coupled to an Enzyme   Colorless Substrate

Colored Product

Figure 8.11 Color reaction produced by HIV ELISA test. Color reaction signifies presence of antibody to HIV. Tubes 1 and 2: Negative control and nonreactive HIV antibody test from a patient. Tube 3: Positive control. Tube 4: Strongly reactive test. Tubes 5 and 6: Weakly reactive tests. Tubes are placed in a spectrophotometer, and an optical density reading is obtained.

1   2   3   4   5   6

Figure 8.12 The Western Blot Confirmatory Test. The presence of the antibody to the core protein P24 and membrane glycoprotein (GP) 41 determines the positivity of the Western Blot.

←Positive Control

←Negative Control

←Positive (Patient with Lymphadenopathy)

←Weakly Positive

←Negative

←Reagent Blank

P24   GP-41/45

The Virus and Immunology

The human immunodeficiency virus is a retrovirus, the structure of which is shown in Figure 8.13. Other members of the retrovirus family are feline leukemia virus, Rous sarcoma virus of chickens, and visna virus of sheep. The hallmark of this virus class is the enzyme reverse transcriptase, which catalyzes the synthesis of DNA that corresponds to the viral RNA. This viral DNA copy is then integrated into the host's genome and can remain latent. When the T-cell is immunologically activated, viral DNA becomes transcribed into RNA and translated into proteins that form the new virions that bud from the cell (Fig. 8.14). The HIV

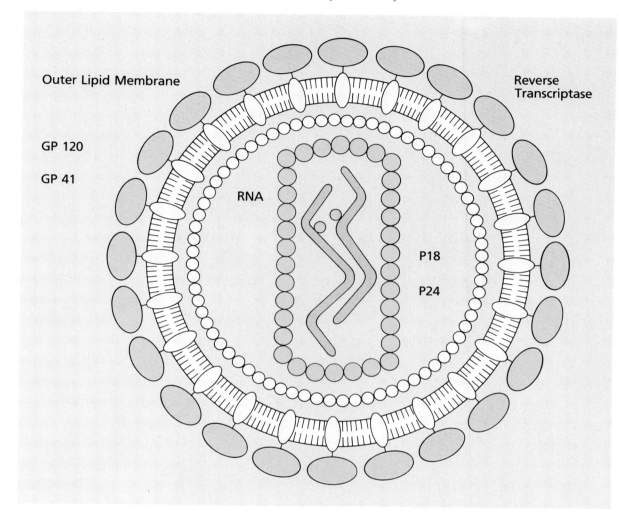

Outer Lipid Membrane

GP 120

GP 41

RNA

Reverse Transcriptase

P18

P24

Figure 8.13 The HIV virion. The retrovirus consists of an outer lipid membrane studded with glycoprotein molecules, each of which consists of two subunits, GP120 and GP41. The membrane lipids are derived from the host cells. The major viral core protein is P24, and P18 is another core protein. The RNA is in the core along with the enzyme reverse transcriptase.

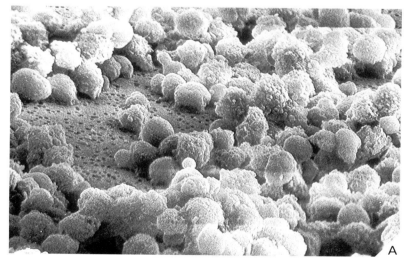

A

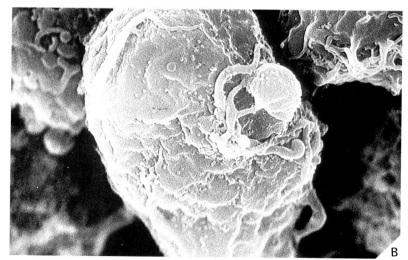

B

Figure 8.14 A Scanning electron micrograph (SEM) (low magnification) of a population of HIV-infected lymphocytes. B SEM of HIV-infected T4 lymphocyte showing virus budding from its plasma membrane.

genome is complex. The integrated form of the viral DNA is called the provirus (Fig. 8.15).

A major effect of HIV is on the T-cell branch of the immune system (Fig. 8.16). Two major subsets of T-cells based on cell surface markers are the T4 and T8 cells. HIV binds to cells with T4 (or CD4) cell receptors. The predominant cell infected is the T4 lymphocyte, but other cells including monocytes, macrophages, some B-cells, endothelial cells lining blood and lymph vessels, epithelial cells of skin and other tissues, and neural cells may bear the CD4 receptor marker and thus become infected by HIV.

T4 cells have the "inducer" function of aiding the maturation of other T-lymphocytes from their precursors. Their "helper" activity refers to the fact that they enable cytotoxic T-cells to destroy other cells bearing antigens, and they enable B-cells to mature and secrete antibody. T8 cells have "suppressor" or "cytotoxic" functions and dampen the immune response of B-cells and of other T-cells. The normal ratio of T4 to T8 cells is

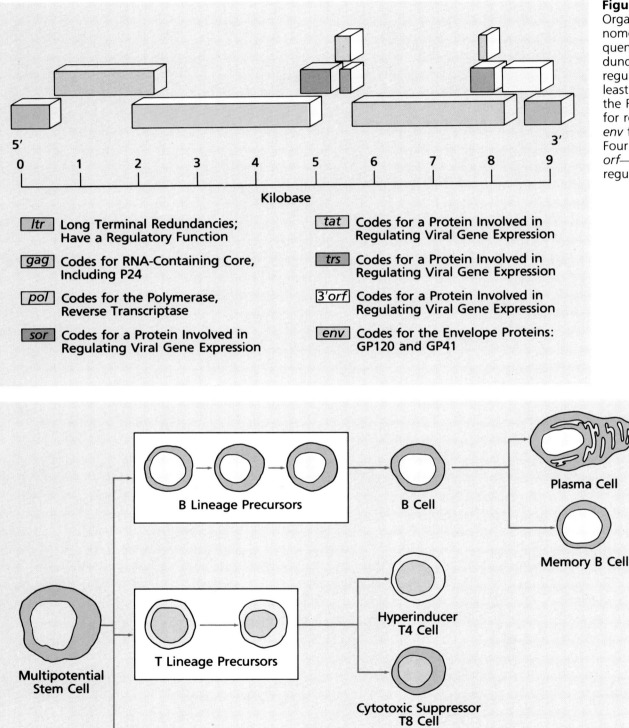

Figure 8.15 The HIV provirus. Organization of the HIV genome. At each end are DNA sequences called long terminal redundancies (ltr), which have a regulatory function. There are at least seven genes. *gag* codes for the RNA-containing core, *pol* for reverse transcriptase, and *env* for the envelope proteins. Four others—*tat, trs, sor,* and *3' orf*—encode small proteins that regulate gene expression.

Figure 8.16 The mononuclear cell lineage. Cellular participants in the immune defense diverge from common precursors—the multipotential stem cells found in the bone marrow.

ltr	Long Terminal Redundancies; Have a Regulatory Function
gag	Codes for RNA-Containing Core, Including P24
pol	Codes for the Polymerase, Reverse Transcriptase
sor	Codes for a Protein Involved in Regulating Viral Gene Expression
tat	Codes for a Protein Involved in Regulating Viral Gene Expression
trs	Codes for a Protein Involved in Regulating Viral Gene Expression
3'orf	Codes for a Protein Involved in Regulating Viral Gene Expression
env	Codes for the Envelope Proteins: GP120 and GP41

approximately 2:1. With HIV infection, this ratio gradually decreases, first from an increase in T8 cells, then from a decrease in T8 cells along with a profound decrease in T4 cells. This decrease in T4 cells is felt in large part to account for the development of the clinical manifestations in AIDS, although all wings of the immune system are eventually impaired (Fig. 8.17).

Clinical Manifestations

The clinical manifestations of AIDS vary and may point to a particular organ system or may be nonspecific (i.e., fever, weight loss, malaise, anorexia). Many patients will present with multiple problems at the same time, such as pneumonia and enteritis. Patients with acute HIV infection may be asymptomatic or may present with a viral-like syndrome, a mononucleosis syndrome, or aseptic meningitis. Patients with these presentations may be in the process of seroconverting and may initially be seronegative for HIV.

PULMONARY
The most common initial presentation of AIDS is pulmonary disease (Fig. 8.18). Over half of all patients with AIDS present

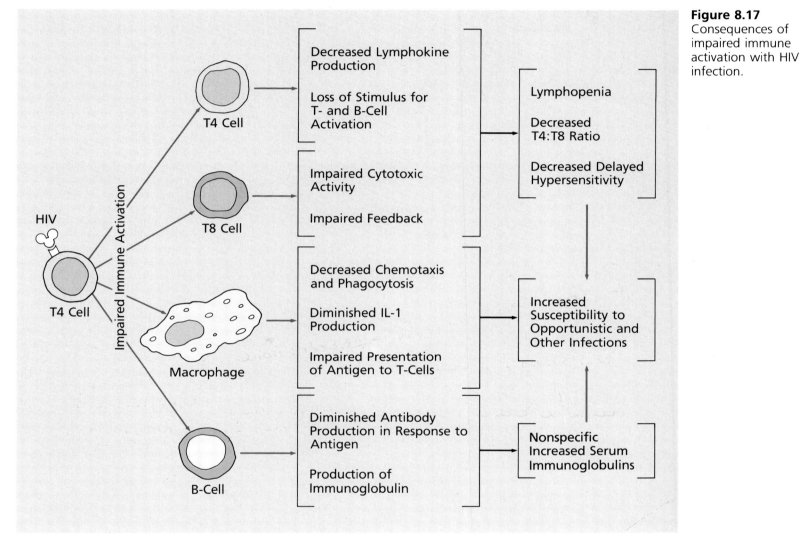

Figure 8.17 Consequences of impaired immune activation with HIV infection.

Figure 8.18 Causes of pulmonary disease in AIDS.

CAUSES OF PULMONARY DISEASE IN AIDS

Pneumocystis carinii	Kaposi's sarcoma
Mycobacterium tuberculosis	Streptococcus pneumoniae
Mycobacterium avium-intracellulare (and other atypical mycobacteria)	Hemophilus influenzae
	Lymphoma
Cytomegalovirus	Lymphoid interstitial pneumonitis (in children)
Cryptococcus neoformans	
Histoplasma capsulatum	

with pneumonia caused by *Pneumocystis carinii* (PCP). The signs and symptoms of PCP are listed in Figure 8.19. These symptoms may be short-lived or may develop over weeks to months. Examination may reveal rales or rhonchi but is often unremarkable. Chest x-ray usually shows bilateral interstitial infiltrates that may progress (Fig. 8.20); however, chest films can occasionally be normal, in which case an abnormal arterial blood gas, abnormal pulmonary function as measured by a decrease in the carbon monoxide diffusing capacity, or an abnormal gallium scan of the lungs may indicate infection (Fig. 8.21). In addition, PCP can appear as an alveolar infiltrate more characteristic of a bacterial pneumonia (Fig. 8.22). Figure 8.23 presents an algorithm on the evaluation of pulmonary problems in patients with AIDS.

The definitive diagnosis of PCP is made by bronchoscopy, although some have found the organism in induced, expectorated sputum. The organisms may be stained by Gomori methenamine-silver stain, by Giemsa stain, and by other stains from material obtained by bronchoalveolar lavage (BAL) in >90% of cases. Sometimes, however, a transbronchial biopsy

Figure 8.19   Signs and symptoms of *Pneumocystis carinii* pneumonia.

SIGNS AND SYMPTOMS OF *PNEUMOCYSTIS CARINII* PNEUMONIA

Shortness of breath	Night sweats
Dry cough	Weakness
Chest discomfort	Malaise
Fever	

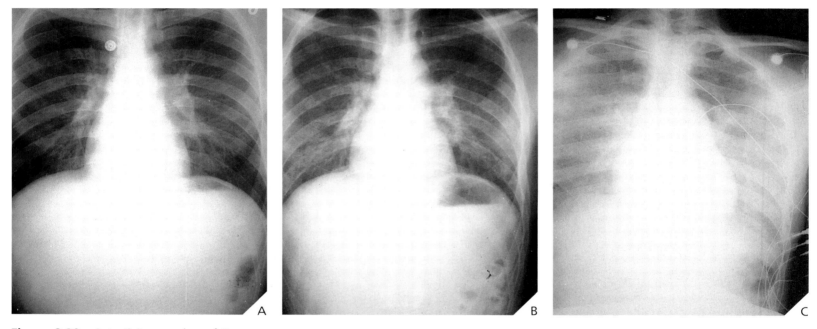

Figure 8.20   A to C Progression of *Pneumocystis carinii* pneumonia despite treatment in a patient with AIDS.

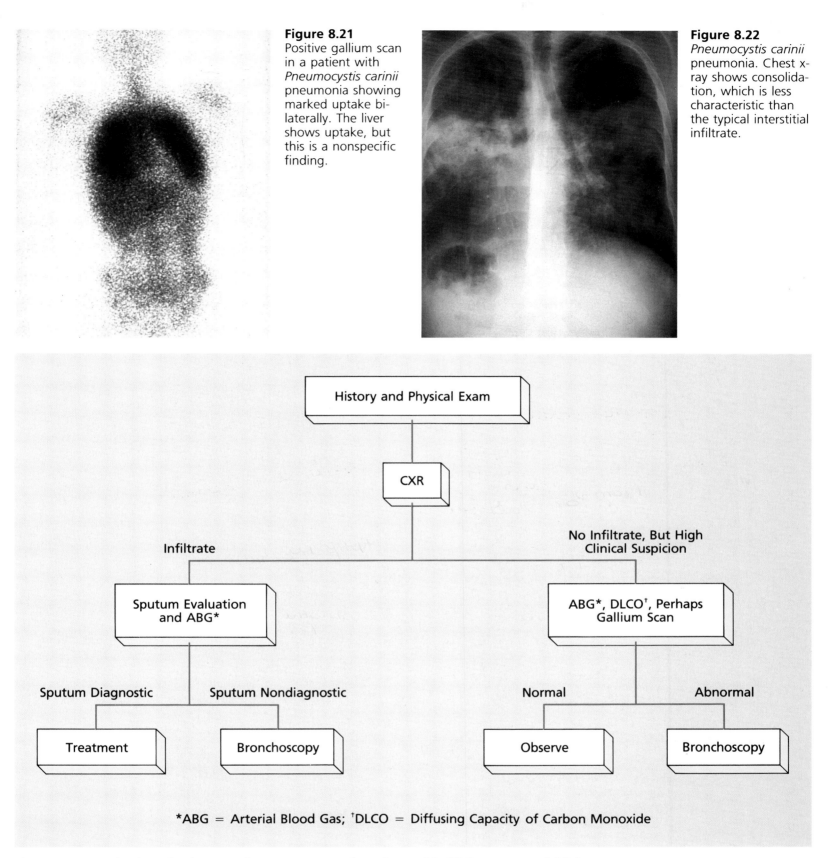

Figure 8.21
Positive gallium scan in a patient with *Pneumocystis carinii* pneumonia showing marked uptake bilaterally. The liver shows uptake, but this is a nonspecific finding.

Figure 8.22
Pneumocystis carinii pneumonia. Chest x-ray shows consolidation, which is less characteristic than the typical interstitial infiltrate.

History and Physical Exam

CXR

Infiltrate

No Infiltrate, But High Clinical Suspicion

Sputum Evaluation and ABG*

ABG*, DLCO†, Perhaps Gallium Scan

Sputum Diagnostic

Sputum Nondiagnostic

Normal

Abnormal

Treatment

Bronchoscopy

Observe

Bronchoscopy

*ABG = Arterial Blood Gas; †DLCO = Diffusing Capacity of Carbon Monoxide

Figure 8.23 Evaluation of pulmonary signs or symptoms in patients with AIDS or suspected AIDS.

is necessary. The photomicrographs in Figure 8.24 show the organism in lavage and biopsy material. The electron micrograph shows the organism in greater detail (Fig. 8.25). An autopsy specimen is shown in Figure 8.26.

Other "opportunistic" infections may also involve the lung. Patients with AIDS may develop pulmonary mycobacterial disease. This may be due to typical Mycobacterium tuberculosis or to an atypical organism such as Mycobacterium avium-intracellulare. The diagnosis may be made by sputum examination or by examination of BAL or biopsy specimens. Skin testing may not be helpful, since many patients with AIDS are anergic. Interestingly, individuals who are HIV-positive but do not have AIDS may develop M. tuberculosis infection months or longer before severe signs of immunodeficiency arise. In many U.S. cities the rate of M. tuberculosis infection is increasing, in large part due to reactivation of the disease in HIV-infected patients. The x-ray in Figure 8.27 shows left upper lobe tuberculosis in a patient

with ARC. Sputum examination revealed the characteristic "red snappers" (Fig. 8.28).

Patients with AIDS who have pulmonary involvement with M. avium-intracellulare may present with or without signs and symptoms of pulmonary disease. Many will have only malaise, fever, and weight loss, and the chest x-ray may be normal. The organism may be isolated from a BAL, or it may be isolated from a culture of sputum or lung tissue. The significance of these incidental findings is unknown. When examining any tissue specimens from patients with AIDS, it is important to do a Ziehl-Neilsen stain for acid-fast organisms, since typical granulomas are often not seen.

The lung may also be involved in disseminated cytomegalovirus (CMV) infection. Again, signs and symptoms of pulmonary involvement may be absent, or the patient may present with fever, shortness of breath, and/or cough (Figs. 8.29 and

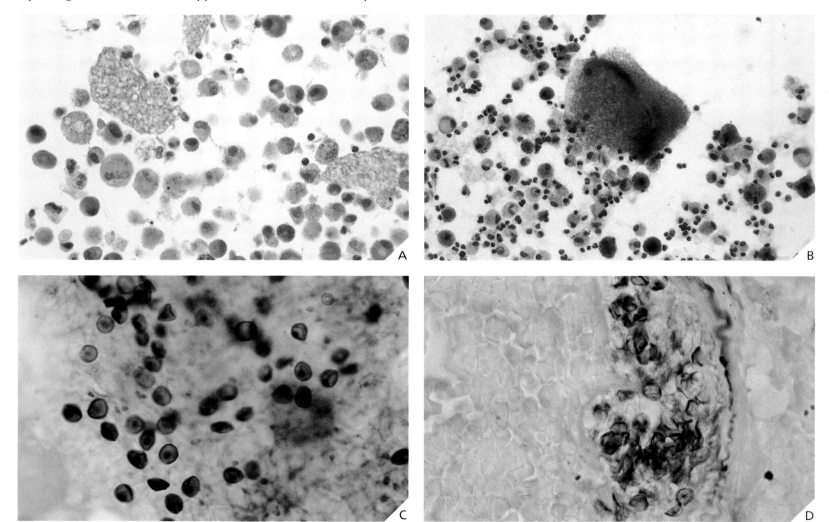

Figure 8.24 *Pneumocystis carinii* pneumonia (PCP) bronchoalveolar lavage, cytospin preps. **A** and **B** Appearance of PCP with routine histologic stains. **A** Mass of *Pneumocystis* organisms having a foamy, exudative appearance with hematoxylin and eosin (H&E) stain (×250). **B** Similar mass of organisms having a "dirty" green-brown appearance with Papanicolaou stain (×250). With both stains individual cysts are not readily discernible. Note adjacent large pigmented alveolar macrophages. **C** Morphology of individual

Pneumocystis carinii cysts with Gomori methanamine silver (GMS) stain, which stains cyst walls. The cysts are often round to ovoid, but helmet-, comma-, or sickle-shaped forms are also common. Note the characteristic central "dot" seen in many as well as occasional transverse grooves (×1000). **D** Transbronchial lung biopsy of PCP. The morphology of the cysts in tissue sections may appear somewhat more distorted than in smear preparations (GMS, ×1000).

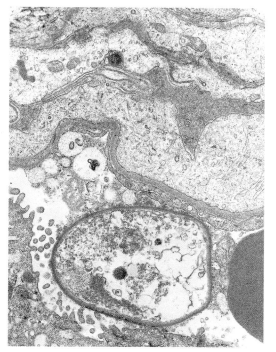

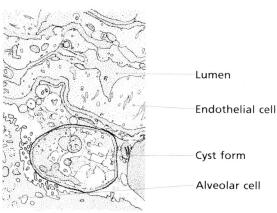

Lumen

Endothelial cell

Cyst form

Alveolar cell

Figure 8.25 An electron micrograph of the cyst form of *Pneumocystis carinii* in the lung.

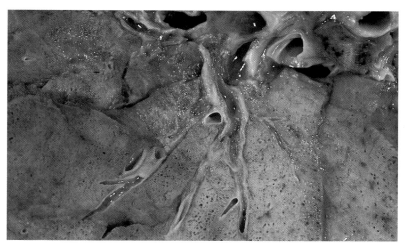

Figure 8.26 Autopsy lung tissue from an AIDS patient with diffuse *Pneumocystis* pneumonitis. Diffuse consolidation is present with patchy areas of induration and mucus plugging of bronchioles.

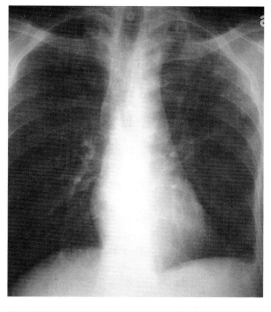

Figure 8.27 Left upper lobe infiltrate due to *Mycobacterium tuberculosis* in a patient with ARC. HIV-infected patients usually will not have cavitary tuberculosis and often have disseminated disease.

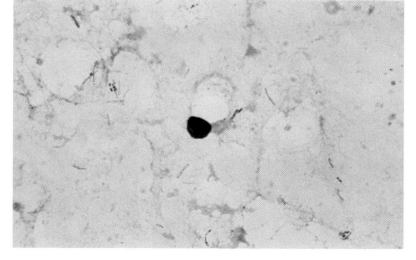

Figure 8.28 Sputum. Numerous acid-fast bacilli are present in the background, several of which demonstrate the typical beaded morphology (Kinyoun stain, × 1000).

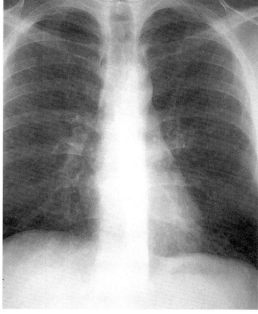

Figure 8.29 Chest x-ray in a patient with AIDS showing a fine interstitial pneumonitis. Biopsy revealed cytomegalovirus.

8.30). Many times when CMV is found in the lung, it can be isolated from other tissues, as well as from urine and semen. Results of serologic tests for CMV in AIDS often show an elevated IgG antibody titer to the virus, and classical titer changes of acute and convalescent sera may not be detected. Microscopic examination for evidence of intranuclear inclusions is a recommended method for diagnosis of significant infection.

Although neurologic disease caused by *Cryptococcus neoformans* is more common than other manifestations of the fungus, some patients with AIDS do present with pulmonary cryptococcosis (Fig. 8.31). Patients usually present with fever and pulmonary symptoms. The diagnosis depends on identification of the organism from fluid or tissue specimens. In addition, when cryptococcus is found in one organ system, it often can be found in others such as the lymph nodes or the meninges. Test results for serum cryptococcal antigen may be positive.

Disseminated histoplasmosis is a more recently recognized

opportunistic infection seen in patients with AIDS (Fig. 8.32). Other common pulmonary infections in these patients are bacterial pneumonias, in particular those due to *Streptococcus pneumoniae* and *Hemophilus influenzae*.

Although one usually associates Kaposi's sarcoma with cutaneous disease, the tumor may also be found in the lung. It may present as a pleural effusion or in an interstitial pattern on the chest x-ray similar to PCP (Fig. 8.33). Patients with pulmonary Kaposi's sarcoma usually experience a rapidly progressive deterioration. They need not have cutaneous disease to have lung involvement.

GASTROINTESTINAL

Gastrointestinal manifestations are also quite frequent. The most common complaint is diarrhea, but patients also have nausea, vomiting, bloating, and gastrointestinal bleeding. Perforation may even occur. The diagnosis of the offending path-

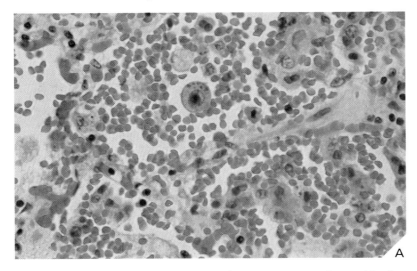

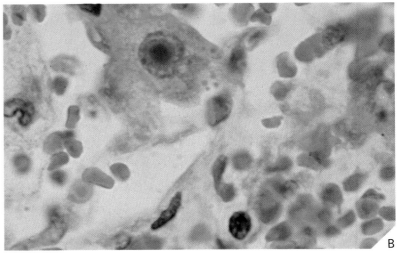

Figure 8.30 **A** Autopsy lung tissue from an AIDS patient with disseminated cytomegalovirus (CMV). The infected alveolar macrophage demonstrates overall cellular enlargement ("cytomegaly"), a large central, darkly staining intranuclear inclusion, a surrounding clear halo, and several smaller basophilic cytoplasmic inclusions

(H&E, ×400). **B** Higher magnification of another CMV-infected alveolar macrophage, again demonstrating the large intranuclear inclusion with several small, peripherally located cytoplasmic inclusions. Not all CMV-infected cells will demonstrate discernible cytoplasmic inclusions (H&E, ×1000).

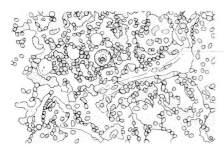

CMV-infected cell

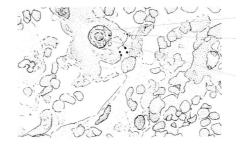

Clear halo

Cytoplasmic inclusions

Intranuclear inclusion

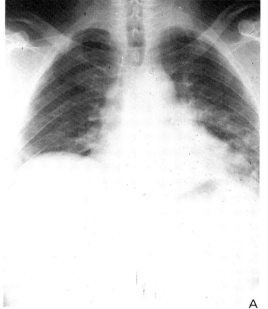

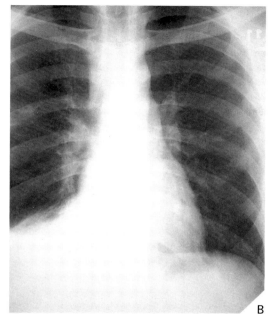

A

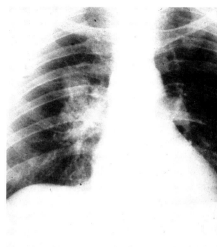

Figure 8.32 Chest x-ray showing pulmonary histoplasmosis. The diagnosis is made by bronchoscopy and biopsy.

B

Figure 8.31 **A** Chest x-ray showing a nodular pulmonary infiltrate due to *Cryptococcus neoformans.* **B** Chest x-ray showing a right pleural effusion, which on culture grew *Cryptococcus neoformans;* in addition, this patient had disseminated cryptococcal infection with positive blood cultures.

Figure 8.33 Chest x-ray showing Kaposi's sarcoma of the lung. The bilateral interstitial and nodular infiltrates were proven by transbronchial biopsy to be Kaposi's sarcoma. **A** PA view. **B** Lateral view.

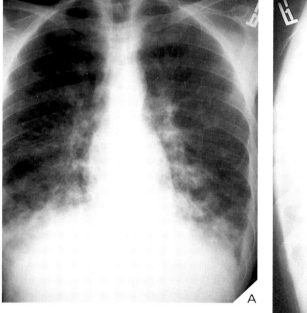

A

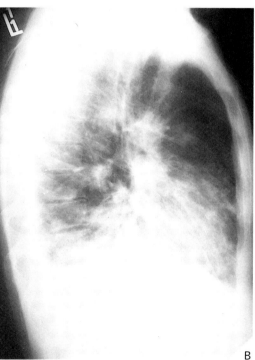

B

ogen requires a stepwise approach as outlined in Figure 8.34. Symptoms of proctitis, perirectal pain, and/or discharge in the homosexual male require careful evaluation of the anal area for the problems outlined in Figure 8.35. Rarer causes of proctitis include *Enterobius vermicularis* (pinworms), *Phthirus pubis* (crabs), *Sarcoptes scabei* (scabies), and trauma.

Diarrhea in the patient with AIDS causes significant morbidity and mortality. The differential diagnosis is long, but should be considered for each patient in an effort to find a treatable problem. The more common causes of intestinal disease and diarrhea are listed in Figure 8.36.

EVALUATION OF DIARRHEA IN PATIENTS WITH AIDS

INITIAL STUDIES

Microscopic evaluation of stool for white blood cells

Stool culture (for *Salmonella, Shigella,* and *Campylobacter*)

Modified acid-fast stain (for *Cryptosporidium*)

Microscopic evaluation of stool for ova and parasites x 3

Evaluation of stool for *Clostridium difficile* toxin (if patient has been taking antibiotics recently)

IF ABOVE STUDIES ARE NONDIAGNOSTIC, CONSIDER THE FOLLOWING

Sigmoidoscopy with biopsy

Upper endoscopy with duodenal drainage or small bowel biopsy

Viral and/or chlamydial cultures

Barium studies

Figure 8.34
Evaluation of diarrhea in patients with AIDS.

ETIOLOGIES OF PROCTITIS IN HOMOSEXUAL MEN

DISEASE	SIGNS AND SYMPTOMS	DIAGNOSIS
Herpes simplex	Atypical and ulcerative lesions, pain.	Tzanck prep (or Wright's stain) of base of lesion. Look for multinucleated giant cells. Viral culture.
Syphilis	Atypical and multiple chancres.	Rapid Plasma Reagin (RPR)/Venereal Disease Research Laboratory (VDRL) tests, darkfield microscopy.
Chlamydia trachomatis	Rectal discharge, fistula, pain.	*Chlamydia* cultures, rapid diagnostic tests.
Genital warts	Raised, fleshy lesions.	Clinical exam, biopsy.
Gonorrhea	Rectal discharge, pain.	Gram stain and culture.

Figure 8.35
Etiologies of proctitis in homosexual men

CAUSES OF GASTROINTESTINAL DISEASE AND DIARRHEA IN PATIENTS WITH AIDS

BACTERIAL	VIRAL	PARASITIC	NEOPLASTIC
Salmonella sp.	Cytomegalovirus	*Cryptosporidium muris*	Kaposi's sarcoma
Shigella sp.	Herpes simplex	*Entamoeba histolytica*	
Campylobacter sp.		*Giardia lamblia*	
Mycobacterium avium-intracellulare		*Isospora belli*	
Mycobacterium tuberculosis			
Clostridium difficile			

Figure 8.36
Causes of gastrointestinal disease and diarrhea in patients with AIDS

The usual enteric pathogens, *Salmonella*, *Shigella*, and *Campylobacter* spp., are found more frequently in patients with AIDS than in the normal population. Severe infection due to *Salmonella typhimurium* is common. These patients present with diarrhea and fever and usually have positive stool and blood cultures. Relapses, despite therapy, are common.

Cytomegalovirus (CMV) may involve any part of the gastrointestinal tract and cause disease ranging from diarrhea to bleeding and perforation. Barium studies are often abnormal (Fig. 8.37). Appearance at endoscopy is also variable, showing either normal mucosa or discrete lesions. Serologic evidence of prior CMV infection is almost universal in this population so that an elevated IgG antibody titer to CMV is not helpful. The diagnosis is made by biopsy. Patients with CMV colitis will often have evidence of CMV elsewhere, and culture of urine and buffy coat of blood may be positive. Photomicrographs in Figures 8.38 and 8.39 show CMV lesions in the esophagus and in the colon, respectively.

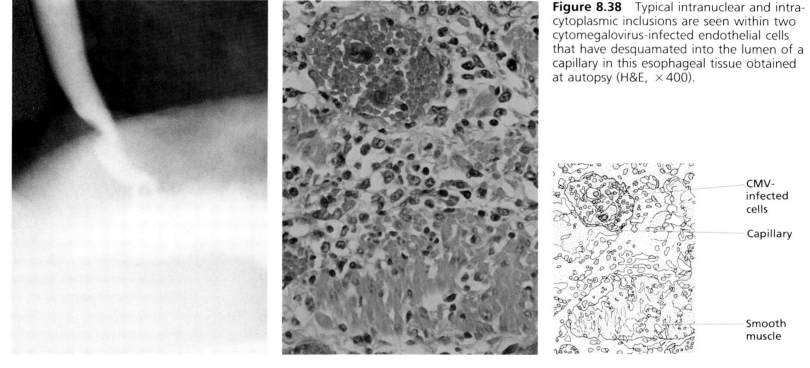

Figure 8.38 Typical intranuclear and intracytoplasmic inclusions are seen within two cytomegalovirus-infected endothelial cells that have desquamated into the lumen of a capillary in this esophageal tissue obtained at autopsy (H&E, ×400).

CMV-infected cells

Capillary

Smooth muscle

Figure 8.37 Upper gastrointestinal series showing a lower esophageal ulcer, which on biopsy revealed cytomegalovirus. This patient with AIDS had complained of severe dyspepsia.

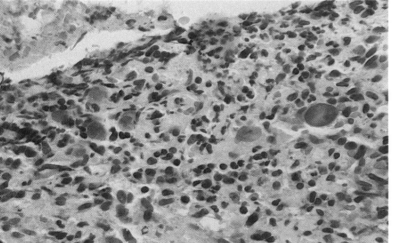

Figure 8.39 Numerous cytomegalovirus-infected cells are present within the lamina propria of this colon biopsy. Kaposi's sarcoma was also present in several other of the tissue fragments from this biopsy. The neoplasm, however, is not present in this photomicrograph (H&E, ×400).

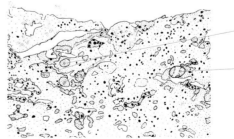

Cluster of CMV-infected cells

CMV-infected cell

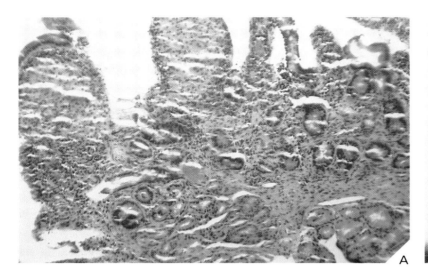

A

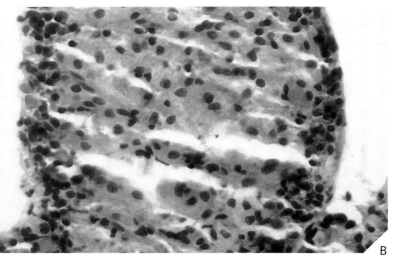

B

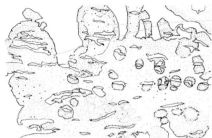

Markedly thickened intestinal villi

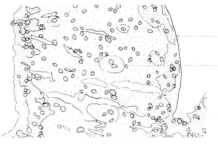

Surface epithelium

Numerous foamy histiocytes within lamina propria

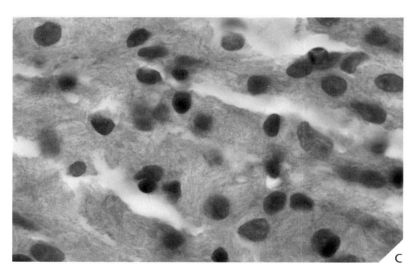

C

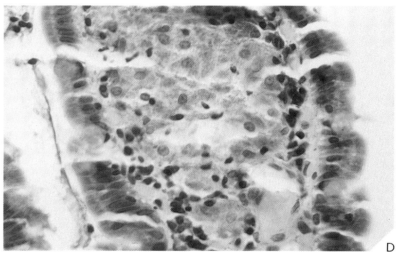

D

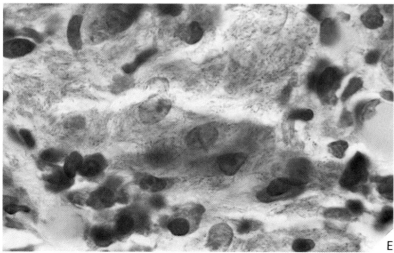

E

Figure 8.40 A Small bowel biopsy demonstrating several enlarged and thickened villi due to *Mycobacterium avium-intracellulare* infection (H&E, × 100). **B** Higher magnification of a thickened intestinal villus demonstrating prominent expansion of the lamina propria by numerous histiocytes having pale, eosinophilic cytoplasm (H&E, × 400). **C** High magnification of foamy histiocytes. This appearance is due to the presence of large numbers of intracytoplasmic mycobacteria. However, the appearance with routine H&E-stained sections is essentially identical to that seen in Whipple's disease, and an acid-fast stain is requisite to confirm the presence of mycobacteria (H&E, × 1000). **D** The cytoplasm of the histiocytes appears red due to the large numbers of intracytoplasmic mycobacteria with this acid-fast stain (Ziehl-Nelson stain, × 400). **E** Numerous acid-fast bacilli filling cytoplasm of histiocytes (Ziehl-Nielson stain, × 1000).

M. *avium-intracellulare* is another important cause of gastrointestinal symptomatology. Manifestations include abdominal pain, diarrhea, anemia, and weight loss. Diagnosis of intestinal M. *avium-intracellulare* can be made from stool smears or culture. Barium studies may show nonspecific mucosal abnormalities, and abdominal CAT scan may reveal associated enlarged retroperitoneal nodes. Diagnosis is best made by biopsy of the small or large bowel (Fig. 8.40). M. *avium-intracellulare* is also frequently found in liver biopsies, bone marrow biopsies, lymph node biopsies, and blood cultures.

The parasite *Cryptosporidium*, a coccidian protozoan, causes severe, watery, cholera-like diarrhea with cramps and sometimes nausea and vomiting. Long known to be a veterinary pathogen, it has more recently been found to cause a self-limited diarrhea in the normal host and an unremitting and untreatable diarrhea in patients with AIDS. Its life cycle is shown in Figure 8.41. In one study, cryptosporidia were found in 21% of patients with AIDS and diarrhea. Diagnosis can be made by looking for oocysts in the stool using a modified acid-fast stain

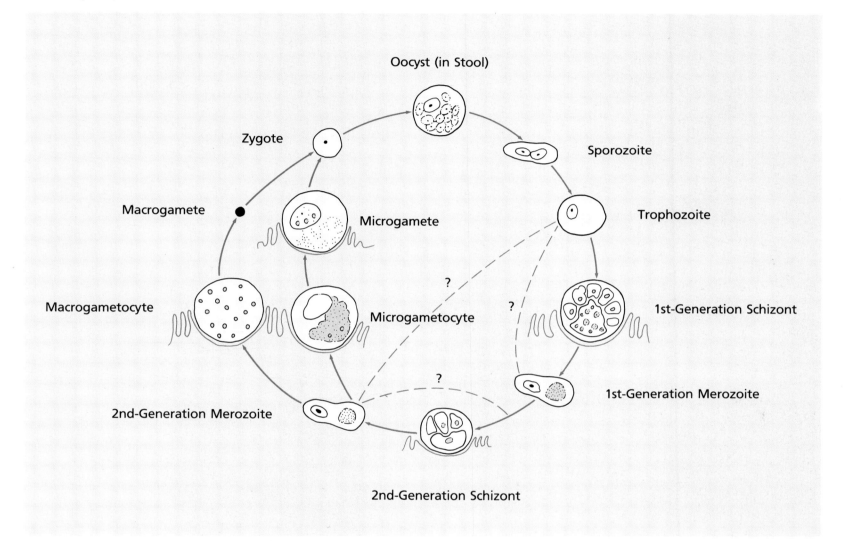

Figure 8.41 Life cycle of *Cryptosporidium*.

as shown in Figure 8.42. Diagnosis can also be made by biopsy, especially of the small bowel (Fig. 8.43). Cryptosporidia have also been reported to cause infection in the stomach, as well as in the biliary tree, presenting as acalculous cholecystitis.

Another coccidian protozoan, *Isospora belli*, has recently been reported to cause significant diarrhea in patients with AIDS, particularly in Haitians. Stool examination may reveal the oocysts (Fig. 8.44).

Two other important causes of diarrhea in patients with AIDS are *Entamoeba histolytica* and *Giardia lamblia*. Amebiasis is found commonly in the homosexual male population and may cause proctocolitis with diarrhea, tenesmus, cramps, abdominal pain, and rectal discharge. Multiple stool samples for ova and parasites should be collected and, if negative, biopsies should be done for diagnosis. Stool specimens showing both an amebic cyst and motile trophozoite are shown in Figure 8.45. Figure 8.46 demonstrates that what may appear to be ulcerative colitis on a barium enema may actually be amebic colitis.

G. lamblia is a common pathogen in patients with AIDS and causes problems ranging from asymptomatic infection to se-

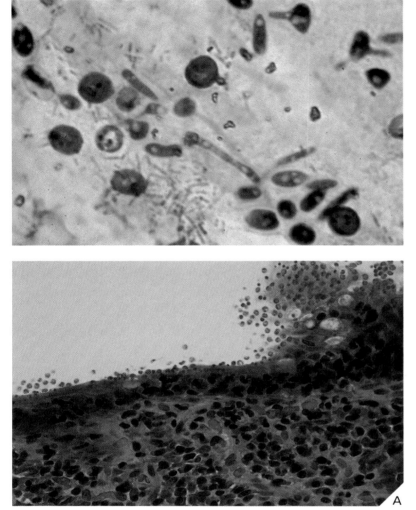

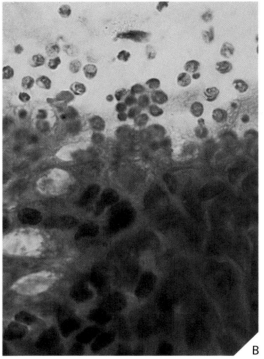

Figure 8.42 Although cryptosporidia can be identified in unstained and iodine-stained concentrated wet mounts, their detection is facilitated by staining smears with a modified acid-fast stain. Oocysts measuring 4 to 6 μm are acid-fast (red), while yeast (of similar size) and other fecal matter are not. Sporozoites can occasionally be seen in some oocysts. (Modified acid-fast stain, × 1000).

Figure 8.43 **A** Innumerable cryptosporidia seen infecting the mucosal brush border in this duodenal biopsy. The organisms appear as small, 4-to-6-mm, round basophilic bodies adherent to the mucosal surface on routine H&E-stained histologic sections (H&E, × 40). **B** Higher magnification demonstrates numerous cryptosporidia adherent to the brush border of duodenal mucosa. In histologic sections, the organisms are not acid-fast perhaps because the organisms seen infecting the brush border of small bowel mucosa represent a different stage in the life cycle of cryptosporidia than is passed in stool (H&E, × 400).

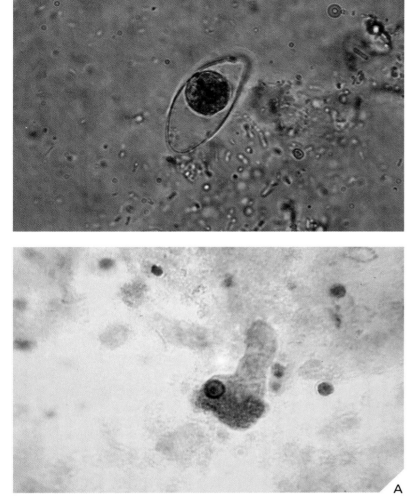

Figure 8.44 Iodine-stained wet mount of fecal concentrate demonstrating the coccidian protozoa *Isospora belli*. Seen in this photomicrograph is an immature oocyst (approximately 25 to 30 μm) with a single central granular zygote (×1000).

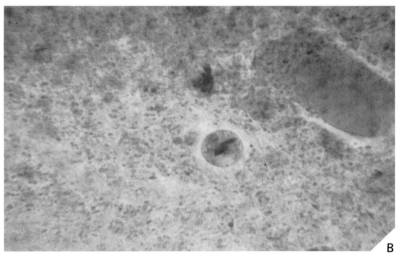

A   B

Figure 8.45 A *Entamoeba histolytica* trophozoite. Note the single nucleus with evenly distributed peripheral chromatin, a central karyosome, and granular cytoplasm with a suggestion of an ingested erythrocyte within the peripheral cytoplasm (Trichrome stain,

×1000). **B** *Entamoeba histolytica* cyst. Spherical cyst with only one visible nucleus (immature cyst) and several cytoplasmic chromatoidal bodies (iodine wet mount, ×400).

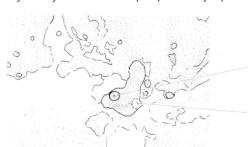

Nucleus with central karyosome

Possible ingested erythrocyte

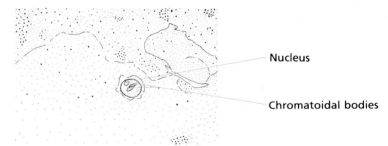

Nucleus

Chromatoidal bodies

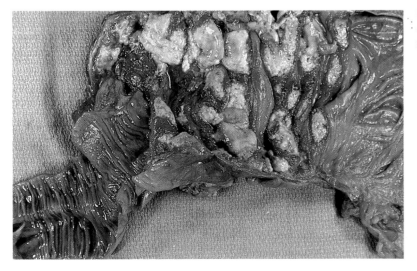

Figure 8.46 Markedly dilated segment of proximal large bowel demonstrating numerous ulcers (whitish-green mucosal defects) secondary to *Entamoeba histolytica* infection.

vere, watery diarrhea, abdominal cramps, bloating, nausea, and severe malabsorption. Stool examation may reveal trophozoites or cysts (Fig. 8.47); however, if the stool exam is negative, either the string test or upper endoscopy with duodenal drainage and biopsy may detect the parasites that live in the proximal small bowel (Fig. 8.48).

Candidiasis is the most common infection of the digestive tract in patients with AIDS. Oral candidiasis is frequently seen in patients with ARC and AIDS (Fig. 8.49). Patients with AIDS and esophageal candidiasis may present with dysphagia or odynophagia, which may prevent eating. The diagnosis may be suggested by a barium swallow as seen in Figure 8.50. Occasionally *Candida* will cause enteritis with ulceration of the bowel.

Herpes simplex is also a major cause of esophagitis in AIDS, and herpetic ulcerations may be found throughout the esophagus, causing severe pain.

A number of tumors of the gastrointestinal tract have been described in patients with AIDS. Kaposi's sarcoma is the most

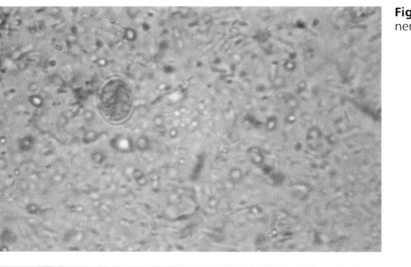

Figure 8.47 Cyst of *Giardia lamblia* showing ovoid shape, prominent cyst wall, granular cytoplasm, and at least two nuclei.

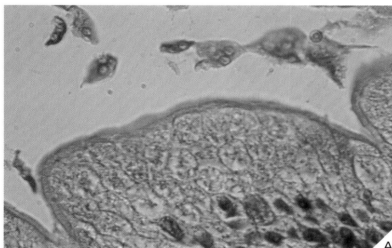

A

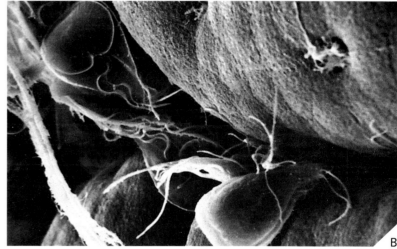

B

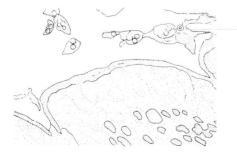

Giardia with "owl's eye" appearance of nuclei

Figure 8.48 **A** Duodenal biopsy demonstrating multiple *Giardia* organisms overlying the brush border of the surface mucosal epithelium. Note the classic "owl's eye" appearance of the two nuclei in several of the organisms (H&E, × 1000). **B** Scanning electron micrograph of *Giardia* trophozoites in a crevice of a human jejunal villus (× 1550).

common, with nearly one-half of patients with dermatologic Kaposi's sarcoma also having gastrointestinal lesions. These lesions are commonly seen in the oral cavity on the palate or gums (Fig. 8.61G). Lesions may also be seen throughout the stomach, small bowel, and large bowel, particularly in the ano-rectal area. The lesions are usually asymptomatic; however, they can bleed or cause obstruction or perforation. Biopsies are sometimes negative because the tumors are submucosal, and the biopsy may be too superficial to be diagnostic.

One of the most important features of gastrointestinal illness in AIDS, and certainly the most obvious, is cachexia. In one study, 96% of patients experienced weight loss, with a mean loss of 34 lbs. The term "slim disease" has been used to de-scribe African patients with AIDS who are chronically ill with watery diarrhea, vomiting, abdominal pain, and severe weight loss.

NEUROLOGIC

Neurologic problems are extremely common in AIDS (Fig. 8.51). Any patient with AIDS who presents with neurologic signs and/or symptoms should have an evaluation that includes a complete physical examination, as well as the examinations outlined in Figure 8.52.

The most common central nervous system (CNS) infection is cryptococcal meningitis. This may be seen in the face of disseminated disease or it may be an isolated problem. The pre-

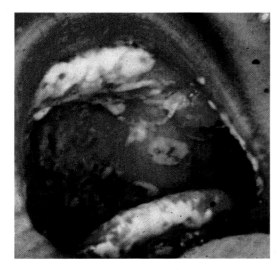

Figure 8.49 White plaques of oral candidiasis in a patient with AIDS.

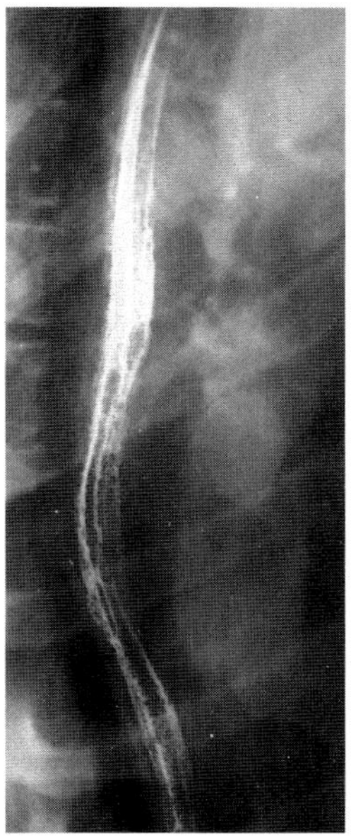

Figure 8.50 Barium swallow showing mucosal irregularities, plaque formation, and ulceration suggestive of esophageal candidiasis. Endoscopy with biopsy confirmed the diagnosis.

COMMON NEUROLOGIC PROBLEMS IN PATIENTS WITH AIDS

Figure 8.51 Common neurologic problems in patients with AIDS.

Cryptococcal meningitis

Toxoplasmosis

Primary CNS lymphoma

Progressive multifocal leukoencephalopathy

Neurosyphilis

Peripheral neuropathy or myelopathy

HIV infection of the CNS: Aseptic meningitis, "AIDS encephalopathy"

EVALUATION OF NEUROLOGIC PROBLEMS IN PATIENTS WITH AIDS

Figure 8.52 Evaluation of neurologic problems in patients with AIDS.

CAT scan with contrast (and/or MRI)

Lumbar puncture (if no mass effect on CAT scan) with CSF sent for:

  Gram stain

  Cell count

  Glucose

  Protein

  India ink stain

  Cryptococcal antigen

  Venereal Disease Research Laboratory (VDRL) Slide Test

  Cytology

  Culture—routine, acid-fast, and fungal (viral, if available)

sentation is usually subacute to chronic with variable symptoms including headache and fever without meningismus. Because cryptococcal meningitis involves the base of the brain, cranial nerves may be involved, and the patients may present with a nerve palsy. The diagnosis of cryptococcal meningitis is made by spinal fluid examination and/or culture (Fig. 8.53). The India ink smear may be positive; however, detection of cryptococcal antigen is the most sensitive diagnostic test. The organism may also invade the brain, as noted in an autopsy specimen in Figure 8.54.

The parasite *Toxoplasma gondii* causes problems ranging from a mononucleosis-like syndrome in the normal host to disseminated disease in the immunocompromised host. Patients with AIDS frequently present with CNS disease manifested by headache, by seizures, or by focal neurologic deficits. Computerized axial tomography (CAT scan) helps to make a presumptive diagnosis of toxoplasmosis (Fig. 8.55). If patients do not respond to the usual therapy for toxoplasmosis in several weeks or if they deteriorate despite treatment, a brain biopsy may be indicated (Fig. 8.56). Spinal fluid examination is nonspecific and

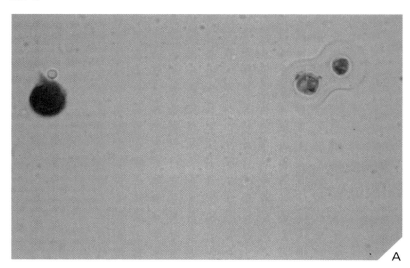

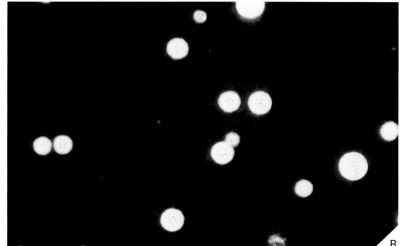

Figure 8.53 **A** Irregular violet-staining budding yeast with prominent clear-to-slightly opaque capsule typical of *Cryptococcus* present in a cerebrospinal fluid (CSF) cytology specimen. A darkly staining, poorly preserved small lymphocyte is also present (Cytospin prep, Wright's stain, ×1000). **B** India ink preparation of CSF speci-

men demonstrating numerous yeast, some of which are budding. These are seen as clear spaces against the dark background. This appearance is largely due to displacement of the ink by large amounts of capsular material and is characteristic of *Cryptococcus* (×400).

Budding yeast

Prominent capsule

Lymphocyte

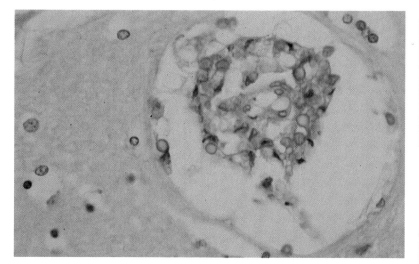

Figure 8.54 Cryptococcal organisms present within a perivascular space in autopsy brain tissue from a patient with AIDS. A mucicarmine stain was used, which stains the polysaccharide capsule of *Cryptococcus* red and is specific for encapsulated forms of *Cryptococcus*. Other yeast will not stain with mucicarmine (×400).

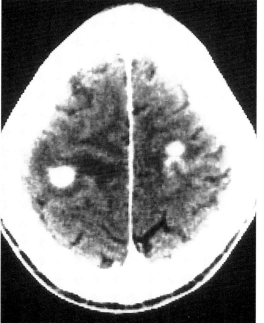

Figure 8.55 Computerized axial tomography scan with contrast of the brain in a patient with AIDS showing two enhancing lesions compatible with CNS toxoplasmosis.

may be normal. Serology is not helpful because the IgG is often elevated and indicates previous exposure, which is common in the general population. The IgM does not rise even in the face of acute infection in patients with AIDS.

Primary CNS lymphoma is one of the tumors found in these patients. Presentation, such as headache or focal neurologic deficits, is similar to that of any space-occupying lesion of the CNS. Figure 8.57 shows a CAT scan and magnetic resonance imaging (MRI) of large lesions, which on biopsy proved to be lymphoma.

Progressive multifocal leukoencephalopathy (PML) is a rare, progressive, demyelinating disease caused by a papovavirus that has been described in patients who have underlying diseases affecting humoral and cell-mediated immunity. More recently it has been seen in patients with AIDS. Signs and symptoms are diverse and reflect different areas of demyelination.

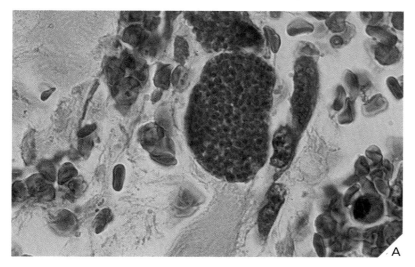

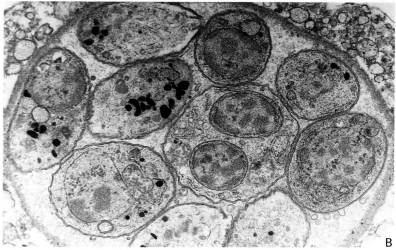

Figure 8.56 **A** Brain biopsy showing extracellular *Toxoplasma* cysts containing large numbers of trophozoites. Cysts can also be intracellular (H&E, × 1000). **B** Transmission electron photomicrograph of an intracellular *Toxoplasma* cyst containing portions of 10 intracystic organisms. The cyst wall appears slightly more dense peripherally and less dense, granular, and slightly irregular internally. The wall of the individual organism is composed of a double-layered pellicle. Nuclei can be seen within some of the organisms, as well as a variety of cytoplasmic organelles including dense bodies, endoplasmic reticulum, and finely granular material.

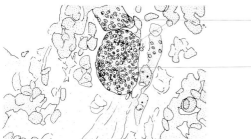

Cysts

Intracystic trophozoites

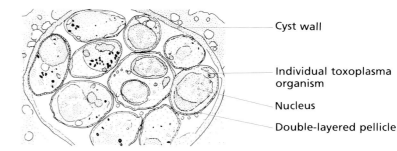

Cyst wall

Individual toxoplasma organism

Nucleus

Double-layered pellicle

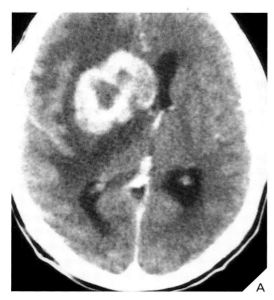

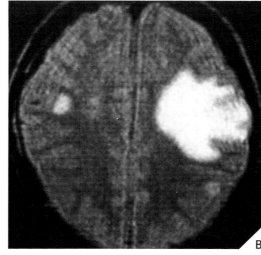

Figure 8.57 **A** Computerized axial tomography scan with contrast showing a large lesion impinging on the ventricle with shift of midline structures. Biopsy of this lesion revealed lymphoma. **B** Magnetic resonance imaging scan showing a large lesion in another patient, which on biopsy also showed lymphoma.

There may be paresis, behavioral changes, mental impairment and dementia, ataxia, and dysarthria. The electroencephalogram is diffusely slow. Spinal fluid findings are normal, but occasionally the CAT scan or MRI can be useful in making the diagnosis (Fig. 8.58).

Neurosyphilis (e.g., meningovascular) recently has been recognized as not uncommon in patients with HIV disease. In addition, other advanced manifestations of syphilis have been noted in patients with AIDS and ARC.

HIV itself may also cause significant neurologic disease. Patients may develop peripheral neuropathy, aseptic meningitis, or what is commonly termed "AIDS encephalopathy." Encephalopathy is one of the most common and puzzling changes that is noted in patients with AIDS and includes anything from inappropriate affect, progressive dementia, aphasia and paresis, to mutism. The head CAT scan may show atrophy and dilated ventricles, and brain biopsy, when performed, may show HIV (Fig. 8.59). The diagnosis is often made clinically, however.

DERMATOLOGIC

There are many kinds of cutaneous lesions seen in patients with AIDS, as noted in Figure 8.60. Kaposi's sarcoma is an asymptomatic purple papule or nodule. It is a malignancy of the endothelial cells of blood vessels and therefore may appear anywhere on the body or in various organ systems. Figures 8.61

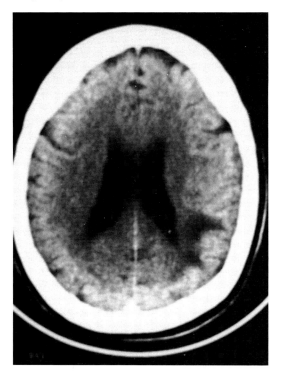

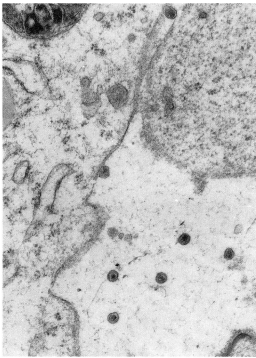

COMMON SKIN FINDINGS IN PATIENTS WITH AIDS

Kaposi's sarcoma

Chronic herpes simplex

Herpes zoster

Candida albicans

Seborrheic dermatitis

Hairy leukoplakia

Ichthyosis

Pityrosporum

Molluscum contagiosum

Scabies

Disseminated *Cryptococcus*

Folliculitis (including eosinophilic folliculitis)

Psoriasis

Figure 8.58 Computerized axial tomography scan showing markedly dilated ventricles. A brain biopsy revealed progressive multifocal leukoencephalopathy.

Figure 8.59 HIV virions in extracellular space of brain from case of AIDS encephalitis in 38-year-old homosexual man with acute onset dementia.

Figure 8.60 Common skin findings in patients with AIDS.

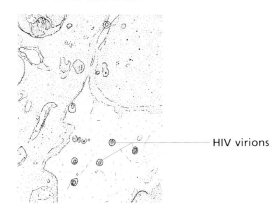

HIV virions

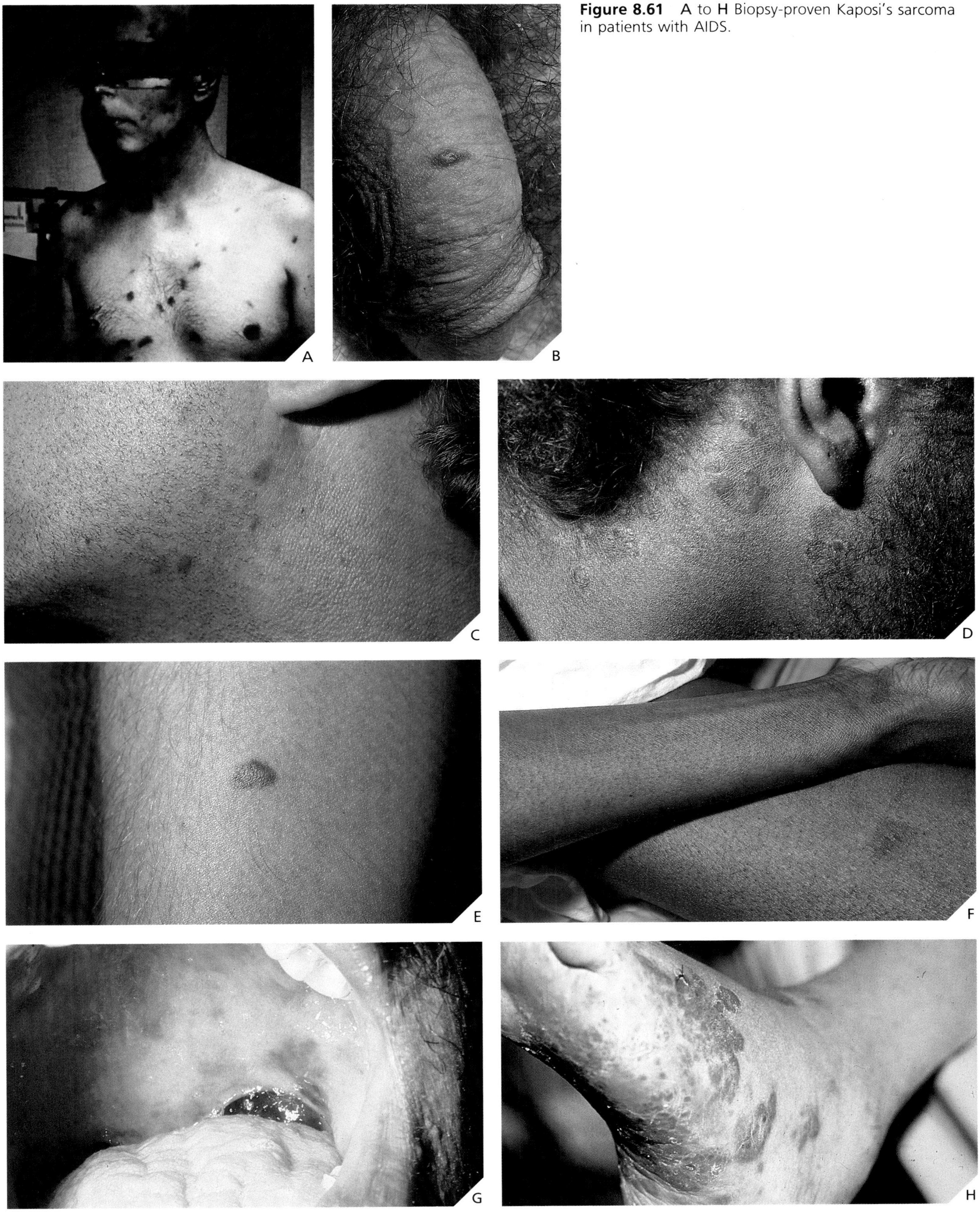

Figure 8.61 A to H Biopsy-proven Kaposi's sarcoma in patients with AIDS.

and 8.62 show several examples of skin lesions and their histology.

Oral candidiasis is extremely common in HIV-infected individuals (Fig. 8.49). The white plaques are usually asymptomatic, unless they involve the pharynx and cause odynophagia. Appearing similar to oral thrush is hairy leukoplakia of the mouth (Fig. 8.63). This, too, is asymptomatic but, unlike yeast, scraping does not remove these lesions.

Also very common in HIV-infected patients is seborrheic dermatitis (Fig. 8.64). Interestingly, the seborrhea tends to worsen during exacerbations of opportunistic infection.

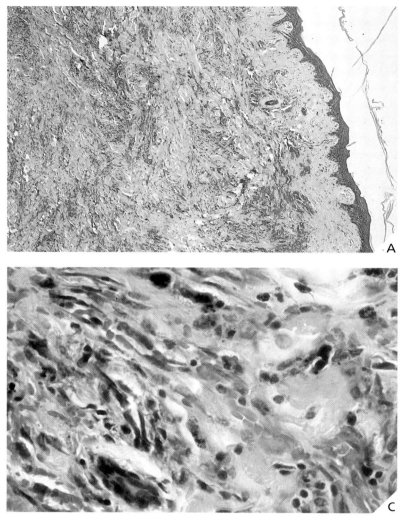

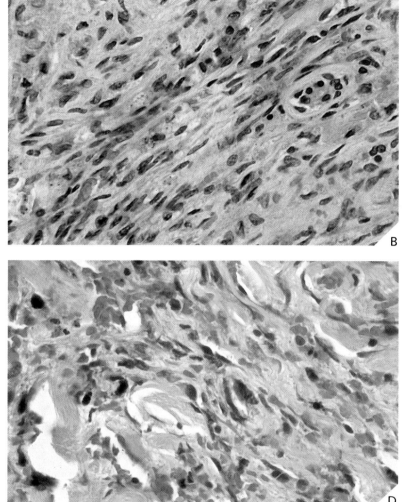

Figure 8.62 **A** Low-power photomicrograph of cutaneous Kaposi's sarcoma. The neoplasm is poorly circumscribed and diffusely involves the reticular dermis. Both the vascular and spindle cell features are readily apparent. Very early lesions often contain a chronic inflammatory infiltrate, demonstrate little cytologic atypia, and strongly resemble benign reactive granulation tissue, making the diagnosis exceedingly difficult if not impossible at that stage (H&E, ×40). **B** Kaposi's sarcoma. The spindle cell neoplastic component predominates in this photomicrograph. Occasional extravasated erythrocytes are present (H&E, ×400). **C** and **D** Kaposi's sarcoma. Neoplastic vessels, multiple abnormal slit-like vascular spaces, marked cytologic atypia, extravasated erythrocytes, and a small amount of brownish granular hemosiderin pigment can be seen. These features are characteristic of this sarcoma of endothelial cell origin (H&E, ×400).

Figure 8.63 Fine, reticulate, white plaques characteristic of oral hairy leukoplakia in a patient with AIDS.

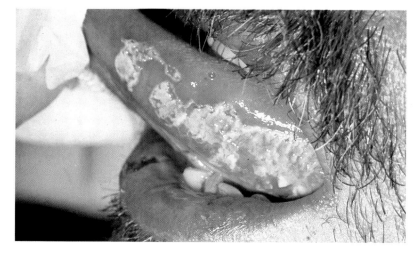

Herpesvirus infections (including herpes simplex, herpes zoster, Epstein-Barr virus, and cytomegalovirus) are severe problems in those with impaired cellular immunity. Mucocutaneous herpes simplex can be chronic and appears around the mouth, nose, and anus (Fig. 8.65). The lesions are often extremely painful and may be ulcerative rather than vesicular.

The diagnosis of herpes infection is made by viral culture, by Tzanck smear (or Wright's stain) of the base of the lesions, or by biopsy (Fig. 8.66).

Herpes zoster is seen commonly in HIV-infected patients. This infection is usually seen in the months preceding the diagnosis of AIDS. Typical lesions cause irritation and pain in a

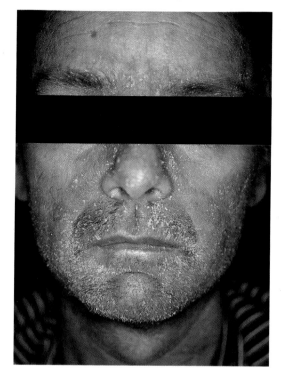

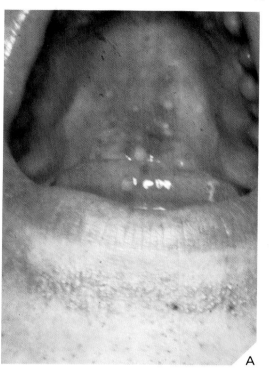

A

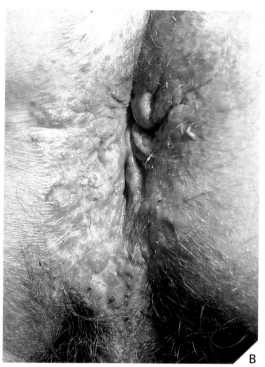

B

Figure 8.64 Typical seborrheic dermatitis found in nasolabial folds, in facial creases, and between eyebrows.

Figure 8.65 **A** Vesicles of herpes simplex on the palate in a patient with AIDS. **B** Peri- anal vesicular and ulcerative lesions of herpes simplex.

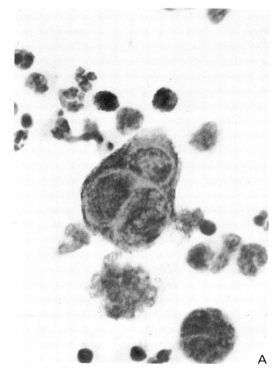

A

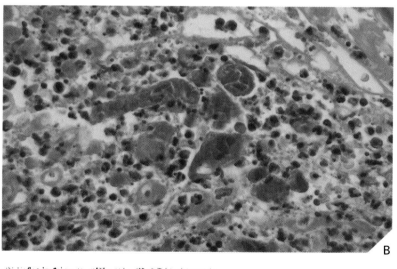

B

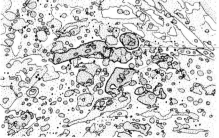

Herpes-infected multinucleated giant cells

Figure 8.66 **A** Tzank smear (made from the base of an early vesicular herpetic lesion) demonstrating a huge multinucleated giant cell with ground glass Cowdry type A intranuclear inclusions characteristic of herpetic infection (Giemsa stain, ×400). **B** Skin biopsy from an early herpetic lesion demonstrating prominent acantholysis, ballooning degeneration of epidermal cells, neutrophils (some of which are fragmented and karyorrhectic), and scattered multinucleated giant cells with eosinophilic glassy viral inclusions typical of herpes infection (H&E, ×400).

dermatomal distribution (Fig. 8.67). Figures 8.68–8.70 show other common dermatologic problems in patients with AIDS.

OPHTHALMIC

There are many ocular manifestations of AIDS (Fig. 8.71). Early HIV infection may be detected by the appearance of cotton wool spots in the retinas of high-risk patients (Fig. 8.72). It is unknown why these occur, and they may come and go. The most ominous ophthalmic finding in AIDS is necrotizing retinitis due to cytomegalovirus (Fig. 8.73). Patients may complain of blurred vision or "floaters." Unfortunately, despite treatment, blindness may occur. *T. gondii* chorioretinal lesions may reactivate in patients with AIDS (Fig. 8.74).

Reiter's syndrome has been described in patients with AIDS who present with conjunctivitis in addition to arthritis and urethritis (Fig. 8.75).

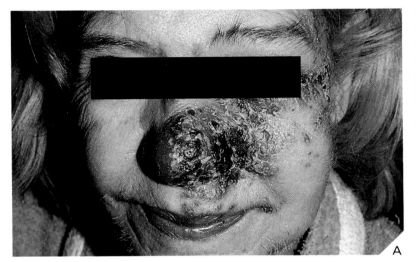

A

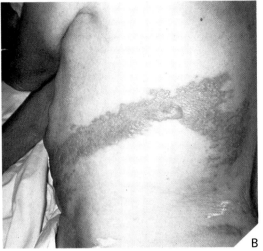

B

Figure 8.67 A Herpes zoster involving cranial nerve V. B Herpes zoster involving a thoracic dermatome in a patient with AIDS.

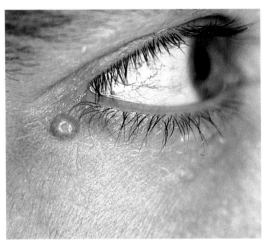

Figure 8.68 Molluscum contagiosum in a patient with AIDS.

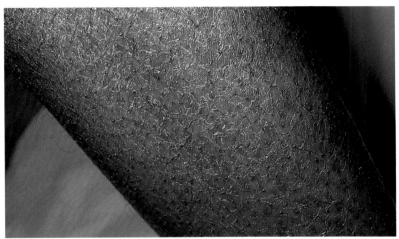

Figure 8.69 Icthyosis in a patient with AIDS.

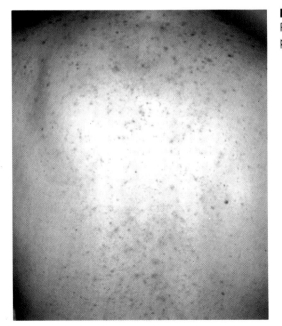

Figure 8.70 Pityrosporum in a patient with AIDS.

OCULAR FINDINGS IN PATIENTS WITH AIDS

COMMON	LESS COMMON
Cotton wool spots	Conjunctivitis (Reiter's syndrome)
Cytomegalovirus retinitis	Histoplasmosis
Toxoplasma chorioretinitis	Cryptococcosis
	Candidiasis
	Pneumocystis
	Mycobacterium avium-intracellulare

Figure 8.71 Ocular findings in patients with AIDS.

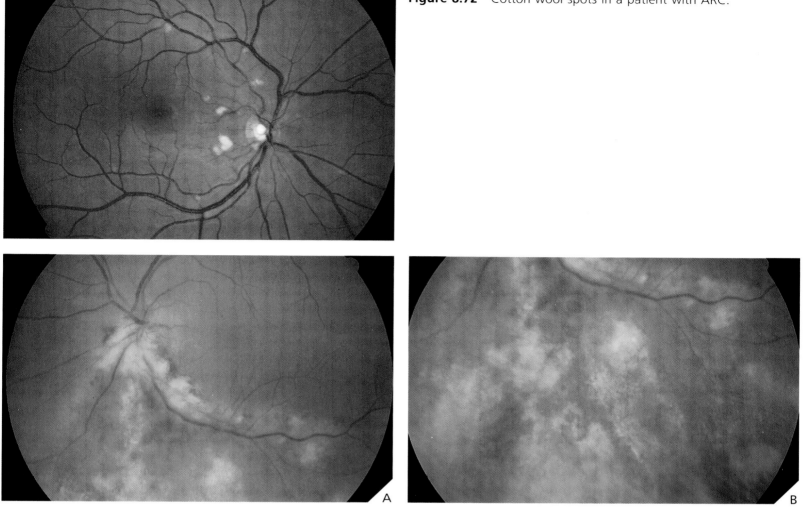

Figure 8.72 Cotton wool spots in a patient with ARC.

Figure 8.73 A and B Cytomegalovirus retinitis. Note typical retinal swelling, hemorrhage, and necrosis.

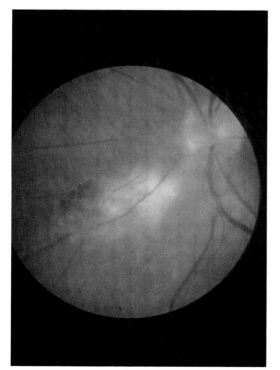

Figure 8.74 Reactivation of ocular *Toxoplasma* chorioretinitis in an area of previous scarring.

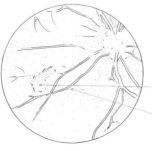

Old pigmentation

Fresh infiltrate

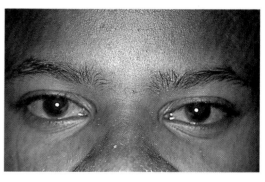

Figure 8.75 Conjunctivitis of Reiter's syndrome. The patient complained of tearing, itching, and redness of the eyes. In addition, he had arthritis and urethritis.

HEMATOLOGIC/ONCOLOGIC

There are many lymphohematologic disorders in patients with AIDS. Patients who are HIV antibody-positive may present with lymphadenopathy. If it does not resolve or if the patient has other signs or symptoms, a biopsy should be done. In some cases the node will show hyperplasia, and with progression of immunosuppression the node architecture may change (Fig. 8.76).

More serious pathology may also be detected in enlarged peripheral nodes as well as visceral ones. The abdominal CAT scan (Fig. 8.77) was performed on an HIV-positive patient with a persistent fever. Because other investigated sites revealed no pathology, the patient required a laparotomy for diagnosis. The enlarged retroperitoneal nodes revealed both Hodgkin's and non-Hodgkin's lymphomas (Fig. 8.78). Figure 8.79 lists some of the more common tumors seen in patients with AIDS.

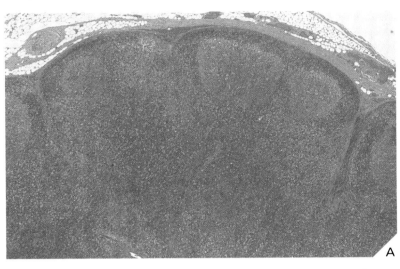

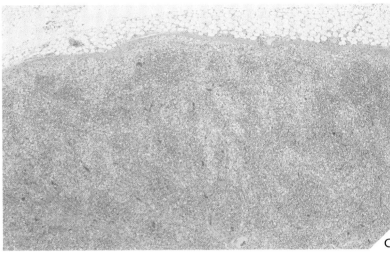

Figure 8.76 **A** Low-power photomicrograph demonstrating prominent follicular hyperplasia with multiple large and somewhat irregular follicles that are occasionally confluent. Focal effacement of the mantle zone of small lymphocytes surrounding the germinal centers can be seen. Additionally, there is paracortical hyperplasia and irregular sheets of pale histiocytic or epithelioid cells (H&E, ×40). **B** Prominent effacement of the normal lymph node architecture. There are scattered "burnt out" germinal centers and vascularity is prominent (H&E, ×40). **C** Severe lymph node effacement. The node has a "pale" quality due to the complete loss of follicles and marked lymphoid depletion (H&E, ×40).

Figure 8.77 Abdominal CAT scan showing retroperitoneal lymphadenopathy in a patient wtih AIDS.

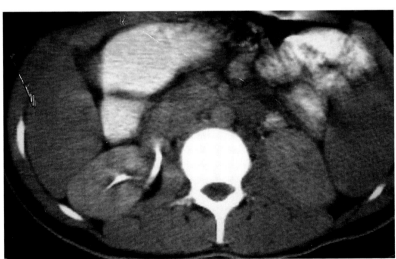

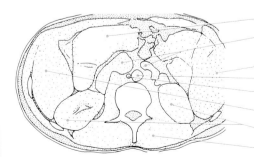

- Stomach
- Mass of enlarged lymph nodes
- Spleen
- Aorta
- Inferior vena cava
- Liver
- Kidneys
- Psoas muscle

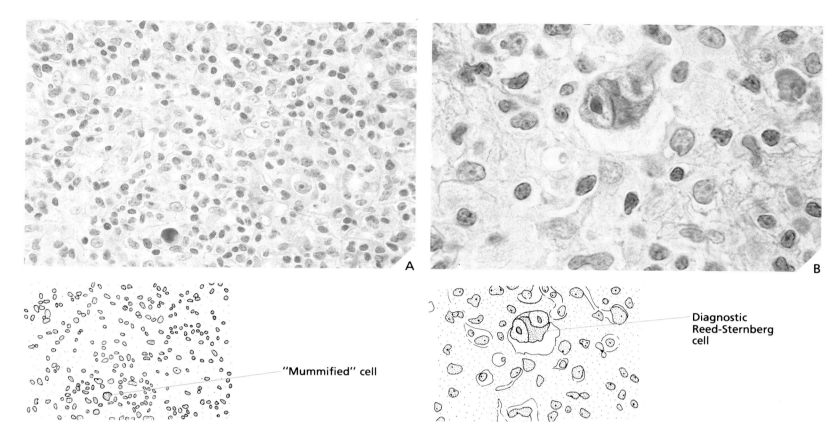

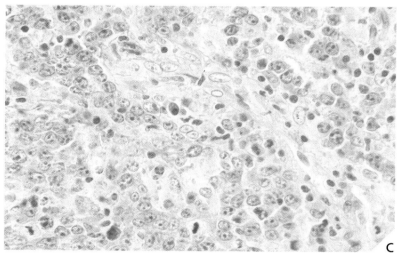

Figure 8.78 **A** Hodgkin's lymphoma, mixed cellularity type, retroperitoneal lymph nodes. Note effacement of the normal nodal architecture (absence of typical germinal centers and other normal landmarks), numerous larger histiocytic cells, scattered large atypical mononuclear cells with prominent nucleoli, few lymphocytes, and plasma cells and a large cell with a darkly staining pyknotic nucleus and eosinophilic cytoplasm—the so-called "mummified cell" of Hodgkin's lymphoma (H&E, ×250). **B** Hodgkin's lymphoma, mixed cellularity type. Note the Reed-Sternberg cell (binucleated cell with large eosinophilic nucleoli) requisite for a diagnosis of Hodgkin's disease (H&E, ×1000). **C** Malignant non-Hodgkin's lymphoma, diffuse, large cell type (histiocytic lymphoma, Rappaport classification), retroperitoneal lymph node. Same patient as in **A** and **B** found to have both Hodgkin's and non-Hodgkin's lymphomas in separate retroperitoneal lymph nodes at laparotomy. Lymph node is effaced by large neoplastic lymphoid cells, some with prominent nucleoli (H&E, ×400).

Figure 8.79 Tumors in patients with AIDS.

TUMORS IN PATIENTS WITH AIDS

Kaposi's sarcoma

Small bowel lymphoma

Non-Hodgkin's lymphomas (small noncleaved lymphoma—either Burkitt or non-Burkitt type— and immunoblastic sarcoma)

Squamous cell carcinoma of the tongue

Squamous cell carcinoma of the rectum

Cloacogenic carcinoma of the rectum

Hodgkin's lymphoma

Enlarged lymph nodes may also contain opportunistic pathogens. Both the chest x-ray and the chest CAT scan seen in Figure 8.80 show mediastinal adenopathy, and biopsy in both cases revealed M. *avium-intracellulare* (Fig. 8.81). Evaluation of yet another high-risk patient with fever and lymphadenopathy revealed disseminated histoplasmosis. Figure 8.82 shows the organism in culture, as well as the node histology.

A bone marrow examination with aspirate, biopsy, and culture is a valuable diagnostic tool and often shows significant pathology in patients with AIDS. At times the marrow will show only nonspecific dysplasia (Fig. 8.83). The peripheral smear may reveal thrombocytopenia indicative of the idiopathic thrombocytopenic purpura-like syndrome seen in these patients. Interestingly, in infections such as disseminated histoplasmosis, the blood smear may reveal organisms packed inside leukocytes (Fig. 8.84). Patients with AIDS may also develop anemia secondary to malnutrition, bleeding, drug toxicity, or invasion of the bone marrow by lymphoma or by opportunistic infection.

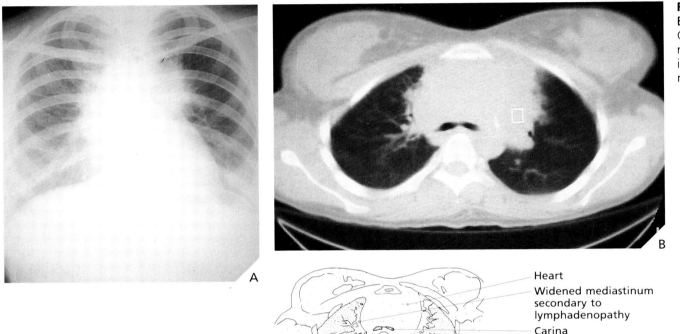

Figure 8.80 A and B Chest x-ray and CAT scan showing mediastinal widening due to lymphadenopathy.

Heart
Widened mediastinum secondary to lymphadenopathy
Carina
Lungs

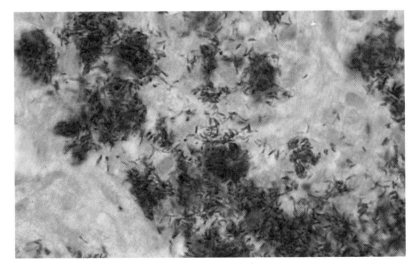

Figure 8.81 Large numbers of acid-fast bacilli are present predominantly within an intracellular location in histiocytes in this lymph node section. Although the pattern of large numbers of acid-fast bacilli completely filling and obscuring the cytoplasm is typical of *Mycobacterium avium-intracellulare*, it is not possible to speciate mycobacteria on a morphologic basis, and culture with identification is necessary (Ziehl-Nielson stain, × 1000).

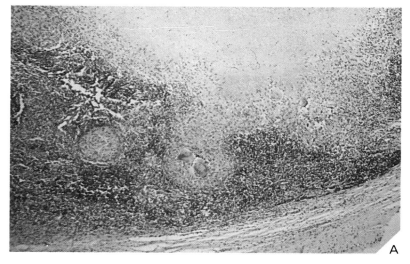

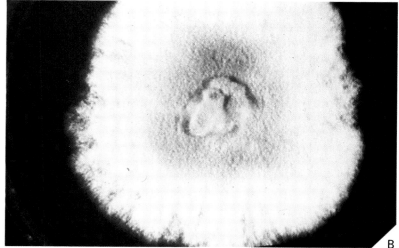

Figure 8.82 **A** Lymph node demonstrating caseating granulomatous inflammation in an AIDS patient with disseminated histoplasmosis. Histoplasma organisms were identified in tissue sections with fungal stains as well as in cultures from lymph node tissue (H&E,

× 100). **B** Colony of *Histoplasma capsulatum* on Sabouraud's agar cultured from the lymph node of the above patient (**A**). Note the white, fluffy, cottony aerial mycelium. With aging, the colony may turn gray-brown as seen centrally in this colony.

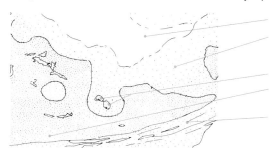

Caseous necrosis
"Wall" of granuloma composed of epithelioid histiocytes
Multinucleated giant cells
Unremarkable lymphoid tissue
Lymph node capsule

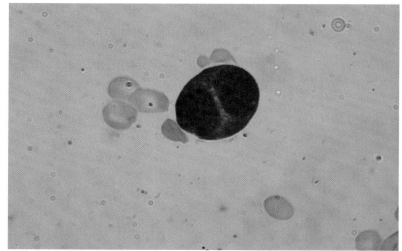

Figure 8.84
Numerous intracellular histoplasma organisms can be seen within the hematopoietic cells in the center of the photomicrograph. The yeast, which measure 2 to 5 μm, are usually seen intracellularly within macrophages, giant cells, or neutrophils. However, they can also be found extracellularly (Wright's stain, × 1000).

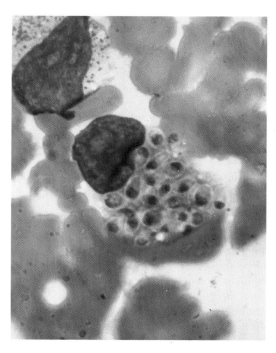

Figure 8.83 Myelodysplasia present in the bone marrow from a patient with AIDS. In this photomicrograph a dysplastic erythroid form demonstrating binucleation is seen. Scattered dysplastic myeloid forms were also seen elsewhere in the marrow aspirate smears (Wright's stain, × 1000).

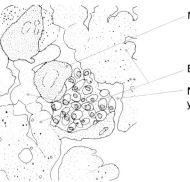

Nucleus

Erythrocytes

Numerous intracytoplasmic yeast

Figures 8.85 and 8.86 show bone marrow invaded by *Histoplasma capsulatum* and *Cryptococcus neoformans*, respectively.

MISCELLANEOUS CLINICAL PRESENTATIONS

As has become obvious, HIV can cause a myriad of clinical diseases. In addition to those listed above, there can be renal, endocrine, and cardiac manifestations of HIV infection.

Renal

A variety of renal lesions in patients with HIV infection has been described, consisting of both glomerular and tubular changes. AIDS-associated nephropathy, consisting of nephrotic range proteinuria and focal and segmental glomerulosclerosis, has been one of the most common renal syndromes. This entity usually results in end stage renal disease. Other HIV-related renal abnormalities include other glomerular morphologic changes as well as nonspecific lesions such as acute tubular necrosis, nephrocalcinosis, and interstitial nephritis.

Endocrine

Adrenal insufficiency has been described in a number of AIDS patients. The most frequent etiology has been CMV infection of the adrenal gland, but other microorganisms including M.

tuberculosis and *Histoplasma capsulatum* may produce a similar state.

Cardiac

The clinical spectrum of cardiac disorders in HIV-related disease includes HIV-induced viral myocarditis, congestive cardiomyopathy (presumed to be of viral origin), nonbacterial thrombotic endocarditis, and incidental Kaposi's sarcoma of the myocardium. In addition, potentially treatable conditions include tuberculosis and fungal (e.g., cryptococcal) pericarditis.

Treatment

Treatment of AIDS may be directed toward the virus itself or toward its complications (Fig. 8.87). Because of the underlying immune deficiency induced by HIV, relapses or new infections often occur and, once established, the acquired immunodeficient state is generally progressive and leads to death. The hope is that this progression can be controlled and even reversed by antiviral agents that prevent replication of the virus and its cytopathogenicity of the immune system.

Stages in the life cycle of HIV that may be targets for therapeutic intervention are listed in Figure 8.88. The first drug

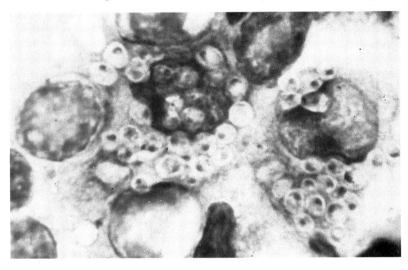

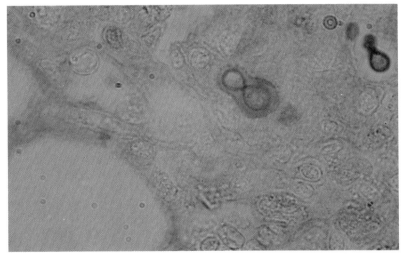

Figure 8.85 *Histoplasma capsulatum* present within the cytoplasm of several macrophages in this marrow aspirate smear (Wright's stain, × 1000).

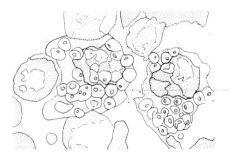

Intracellular *Histoplasma capsulatum*

Figure 8.86 *Cryptococcus neoformans* in bone marrow biopsy. Two yeast are seen demonstrating narrow based budding. In this Alcian blue/PAS-stained section, the cell wall stains faintly pink with PAS, typical of fungi. The Alcian blue component stains the polysaccharide capsule light blue and can be used as an equally effective alternative to the mucicarmine stain to demonstrate the capsule of *Cryptococcus neoformans* (Alcian blue/PAS, × 1000).

COMMON OPPORTUNISTIC INFECTIONS IN PATIENTS WITH AIDS: CLINICAL SYNDROME AND AVAILABLE THERAPY

ORGANISM	SYNDROME	TREATMENT
Protozoa		
Pneumocystis carinii (may be classified as a fungus)	Pneumonia	Trimethoprim-sulfamethoxazole (TMP-SMZ) (IV) or pentamidine isethionate (IV or IM) or trimethoprim (PO) and dapsone (PO)
Toxoplasma gondii	Encephalitis, brain abscess	Sulfadiazine and pyrimethamine and folinic acid (PO) or clindamycin and pyrimethamine
Cryptosporidium muris	Gastroenteritis	None
Isospora belli	Gastroenteritis	TMP-SMZ (PO)
Fungi		
Candida albicans	Oropharyngitis	Nystatin suspension (PO) or clotrimazole troches
	Esophagitis	Ketoconazole (PO) or low-dose amphotericin B (IV) (if no response to ketoconazole)
Cryptococcus neoformans	Meningitis, pneumonia, fungemia	Amphotericin B (IV)
Viruses		
Cytomegalovirus	Chorioretinitis, pneumonia, hepatitis, colitis, adrenalitis, disseminated infection	DHPG (gancyclovir (3-[1,3-dihydroxy-2-propoxymethyl] guanine)) (IV)
Herpes simplex	Mucocutaneous lesions, especially perianal (in homosexual men)	Acyclovir (PO or IV)
Varicella zoster	Primary varicella infection, local or disseminated herpes zoster	Acyclovir (PO or IV)
Mycobacteria		
M. avium-intracellulare	Gastroenteritis, disseminated infection (blood, liver, spleen, marrow, lung)	None of proven benefit
M. tuberculosis	Pneumonia, dissemination, FUO	Isoniazid (INH), rifampin with or without ethambutol

Figure 8.87 Common opportunistic infections in patients with AIDS: clinical syndrome and available therapy.

STAGES IN THE REPLICATIVE CYCLE OF A PATHOGENIC HUMAN RETROVIRUS THAT MAY BE TARGETS FOR THERAPEUTIC INTERVENTION

Figure 8.88 Stages in the replicative cycle of a pathogenic human retrovirus that may be targets for therapeutic intervention.

STAGE	POTENTIAL INTERVENTION
Binding to target cell	Antibodies to the virus or cell receptor
Early entry into target cell	Drugs that block fusion or interfere with retroviral uncoating
Transcription of RNA to DNA by reverse transcriptase	Reverse transcriptase inhibitors
Degradation of viral RNA in an RNA–DNA hybrid	Inhibitors of RNase H activity
Integration of DNA into host genome	Drugs that inhibit *pol* gene-mediated "integrase" function
Expression of viral genes	"Anti-sense" constructs; inhibitors of the *tat*-III protein or *art*/*trs* protein
Viral component production and assembly	Myristylation, glycosylation, and protease inhibitors or modifiers
Budding of virus	Interferons

specifically approved for use in the treatment of certain patients with AIDS and ARC is zidovudine (Retrovir) (formally known as azidothymidine, or AZT).

Zidovudine is a thymidine analog and, when incorporated into DNA, prevents viral DNA chain synthesis (Figs. 8.89 and 8.90). Severe toxicity may appear in the form of leukopenia and anemia. Further studies are ongoing to determine the usefulness of zidovudine, as well as other newer agents, in an attempt to halt the action of HIV in patients with AIDS and ARC.

In summary, AIDS is a fatal syndrome that occurs nearly worldwide and affects thousands of individuals. Because of profound immunodeficiency, patients characteristically develop numerous infections and malignancies. It is important to be familiar with the presentation of these illnesses in an effort to treat reversible problems. The hope is that better means of prevention and treatment will soon be available.

Picture credits for this chapter are as follows: Figs. 8.1, 8.3, 8.5 to 8.8, 8.10, 8.12, 8.15, and 8.41 adapted from and Figs. 8.14A and B, 8.42, 8.49, 8.56B, 8.61A, 8.61H, and 8.66A from the collection of the Centers for Disease Control in Atlanta, Georgia (Fig. 8.15 adapted from Gallo RC: The AIDS virus. Sci Am, January 1987, pp 48 and 54) (Fig. 8.42 courtesy of Pearl Ma, MD, Director of Microbiology, St. Vincent's Hospital, New York, New York [Taken from Ma P: Kinyoun acid-fast stain under oil immersion lens. Oocysts (acid-fast) stain red; yeast cells stain green— direct fecal smear. J Infect Dis 1983; 147:824–828]); Fig. 8.2 adapted from Centers for Disease Control: Revision of CDC surveillance case definition for acquired immunodeficiency syndrome. MMWR 36:suppl. no. 1S,1987; Fig. 8.4 adapted from Shulman JA, Blumberg HM, Kozarsky PE, Leaderman AL, Pinner R: Acquired immunodeficiency syndrome: An update for the clinician. Emory Univ J Med 1987;1:157–190; Fig.

8.16 adapted from Laurence J: The immune system in AIDS. Sci Am, December 1985, p 88; Fig. 8.17 adapted from Selwyn PA: AIDS: What is now known. Hosp Pract 1986;21:76; Figs. 8.25 and 8.59 courtesy of Suzanne S. Mirra, MD, Department of Pathology, Veterans Administration Medical Center, Atlanta, Georgia; Fig. 8.32 courtesy of Thomas F. Sellers, MD, Department of Medicine, Emory University School of Medicine; Figs. 8.47 and 8.48B courtesy of Lambert HP, Farrar WE: Infectious Diseases Illustrated. New York, Gower Medical Publishing, 1982; Figs. 8.53A and B, 8.54, 8.78A to C, 8.82A, and 8.85 courtesy of Lynn Hendrix, MD, Department of Pathology, Crawford Long Hospital of Emory University; Figs. 8.57B and 8.58 courtesy of Patricia Davis, MD, Department of Radiology, Emory University Hospital, Atlanta, Georgia; Fig. 8.61B courtesy of Marilynne McKay, MD; Figs. 8.61C to 8.61G, 8.65B, 8.68, 8.69, and 8.75 courtesy of Adele Moreland, MD; Fig. 8.63 courtesy of Carlos del Rio, MD, Department of Medicine (Infectious Diseases), Emory University School of Medicine; Figs. 8.64, 8.68, and 8.75 courtesy of Heidi Watts, PA-C, Atlanta, Georgia; Fig. 8.72 and 8.73A and B courtesy of Alan Kozarsky, MD; Fig. 8.74 courtesy of Spalton DJ, Hitchings RA, Hunter PA: Atlas of Clinical Ophthalmology. New York, Gower Medical Publishing, 1984; Fig. 8.76A to C courtesy of Thomas Spira, MD, Division of Host Factors, Centers for Disease Control, Atlanta, Georgia (Taken from Brynes RK, Chan WC, Spira TJ, et al: Value of lymph node biopsy in unexplained lymphadenopathy in homosexual men. JAMA 1983;250:1313–1317 ©1983 AMA); Fig. 8.84 courtesy of Carmelo Licitra, MD, Department of Medicine (Infectious Diseases), Emory University School of Medicine; Figs. 8.88 to 8.90 adapted from Mitsuya H, Broder S: Strategies for antiviral therapy in AIDS. Nature 1987;325:773–776 ©Macmillan Magazines Ltd.).

Acknowledgment for Editorial Assistance: Ms. Judy V. Wyndham, Department of Medicine, Crawford Long Hospital.

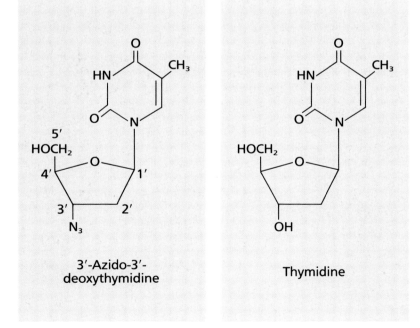

Figure 8.89 Structures of 3'-azido-3'-deoxythymidine and thymidine.

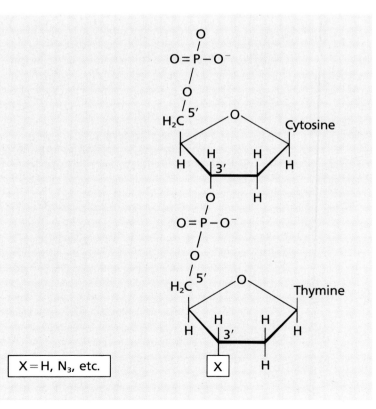

Figure 8.90 Possible mechanism of activity against HIV of 2', 3'-dideoxynucleosides as triphosphate products. When the 3'-carbon of the deoxyribose is modified by certain substitutions (shown by X) that replace the normal 3'-OH, it is not possible to form 5' → 3' phosphodiester linkages that are necessary for DNA elongation in the replication of the virus from an RNA form to a DNA form.

BIBLIOGRAPHY

Amman AJ: The acquired immunodeficiency syndrome in infants and children. Ann Intern Med 253:363, 1985.

Barnes DM: Grim projections for the AIDS epidemic. Science 232:1589, 1986.

Broaddus C, Duke M, Stulbarg MS, et al: Bronchoalveolar lavage and transbronchial biopsy for the diagnosis of pulmonary infection in the acquired immunodeficiency syndrome. Ann Intern Med 102:747, 1985.

Brynes RK, Chan WC, Spira TJ, Ewing EP Jr, Chandler FW: Value of lymph node biopsy in unexplained lymphadenopathy in homosexual men. JAMA 250:1313, 1983.

Castro KG, Hardy AM, Curran JW: The acquired immunodeficiency syndrome: epidemiology and risk factors for transmission. Med Clin N Am 70:635, 1986.

Centers for Disease Control: Pneumocystis pneumonia—Los Angeles. MMWR 30:250, 1981.

Centers for Disease Control: Kaposi's sarcoma and pneumocystis pneumonia among homosexual men—New York City and California. MMWR 30:305, 1981.

Centers for Disease Control: Update on acquired immunodeficiency syndrome (AIDS)—United States. MMWR 31:507, 1982.

Centers for Disease Control: Cryptosporidiosis: Assessment of chemotherapy of males with AIDS. MMWR 31:589, 1982.

Centers for Disease Control: Revision of the case definition of acquired immunodeficiency syndrome for national reporting—United States. MMWR 34:373, 1985.

Centers for Disease Control: Classification system for human T-lymphotropic virus type III/lymphadenopathy associated virus infection. MMWR 35:334, 1986.

Centers for Disease Control: AIDS weekly surveillance report. Atlanta: United States AIDS program. April 27, 1987.

Centers for Disease Control: Classification system for human immunodeficiency virus (HIV) infection in children under 13 years of age. MMWR 36:225, 1987.

Centers for Disease Control: Human immunodeficiency virus infections in the United States. MMWR 36:801, 1987.

Centers for Disease Control: Revision of the CDC surveillance case definition for acquired immunodeficiency syndrome. MMWR 36:suppl. no. 1S, 1987.

Centers for Disease Control: Update serologic testing for antibody to human immunodeficiency virus. MMWR 36:833, 1988.

Clavel F, Mansinko K, Chamaret S, et al: Immunodeficiency virus type 2 infection associated with AIDS in west Africa NEJM 316:1180, 1987.

Cohen IS, Anderson DW, Virmani R, et al: Cardiomyopathy, in association with the acquired immunodeficiency syndrome. NEJM 315:628, 1986.

Conant M, Hardy D, Sernatinger J, et al: Condoms prevent transmission of AIDS-associated retrovirus. JAMA 255:1706, 1986.

Conte JE Jr: Infection with human immunodeficiency virus in the hospital. Ann Intern Med 105:730, 1986.

Dworkin B, Wormser GP, Rosenthal WS, et al: Gastrointestinal manifestations of the acquired immunodeficiency syndrome: a review of 12 cases. Am J Gastroenterol 80:774, 1985.

Gallo RC: The first human retrovirus. Sci Am, December 1986, pp 88–98.

Gallo RC: The AIDS virus. Sci Am, January 1987, pp 47–56.

Ghatak NR, Zimmerman HM: Fine structure of toxoplasma in the human brain. Arch Pathol 95:276, 1973.

Glaser JB, Morton-Kute L, Berger SR, et al: Recurrent Salmonella typhimurium bacteremia associated with the acquired immunodeficiency syndrome. Ann Intern Med 102:189, 1985.

Goldschmidt RH, Mills J: Cardiomyopathy and AIDS, letter. NEJM 316:1158, 1987.

Hawkins A, Gold JW, Whimbley E, et al: Mycobacterium avium complex infection in patients with acquired immunodeficiency syndrome. Ann Intern Med 105:184, 1986.

Kovacs JA, Kovacs AA, Polis M, et al: Cryptococcosis in the acquired immunodeficiency syndrome. Ann Intern Med 103:533, 1985.

Konaman EW, Allen SD, Dowell VR Jr, Sommers HM: Color Atlas and Textbook of Diagnostic Microbiology. 2 ed. Philadelphia, J.B. Lippincott, 1983.

Krigel RL, Friedman-Kien AE: Kaposi's sarcoma in AIDS, in DeVita VT Jr, Hellman S, Rosenberg SA (eds): AIDS: Etiology, Diagnosis, Treatment, and Prevention. Philadelphia, J.B. Lippincott, 1985, pp 161–184.

Laurence J: The immune system in AIDS. Sci Am, December 1985, pp 84–93.

Lennette, EH (ed): Manual of Clinical Microbiology. 4 ed. Washington, D.C., American Society of Microbiology, 1985.

Lever WF, Schaumburg-Lever G: Histopathology of the Skin. 6 ed. Philadelphia, J.B. Lippincott, 1983.

Levy RM, Bredesen DE, Rosenblum ML: Neurological manifestations of the acquired immunodeficiency syndrome (AIDS): Experience at UCSF and review of the literature. J Neurology 62:475, 1985.

Martin LS, McDougal JS, Loskoski SL: Disinfection and inactivation of the HTLV-III/LAV. J Infect Dis 152:400, 1985.

McCray E: The cooperative needlestick surveillance group: Occupational risk of the acquired immunodeficiency syndrome among health care workers. NEJM 314:1127, 1986.

Mitsuya H, Broder S: Strategies for antiviral therapy in AIDS. Nature 325:773, 1987.

Murray JF, Felton CP, Garay SM, et al: Pulmonary complications of the acquired immunodeficiency syndrome. Report of the National Heart, Lung, and Blood Institute Workshop. NEJM 310:1682, 1984.

Myerowitz, RL: The Pathology of Opportunistic Infections with Pathogenetic, Diagnostic, and Clinical Correlations. New York, Raven Press, 1983.

Needlestick transmission of HTLV-III from a patient infected in Africa, editorial. Lancet 2:1376, 1984.

Okeenhendler E, Harzic M, LeRoux JM, et al: HIV infection with seroconversion after a superficial needlestick injury to the finger. NEJM 315:582, 1986.

Peterman TA, Drotman DP, Curran JW: Epidemiology of the acquired immunodeficiency syndrome (AIDS). Epidemiol Rev 7:1, 1985.

Peterman TA, Stenburner RL, Allen JR: Risk of HTLV-III/LAV transmission of families of persons with transfusion associated AIDS, abstract. Interscience Conference on Antimicrobial Agents and Chemotherapy. New Orleans, American Society for Microbiology, 1986.

Polsky B, Gold JW, Whimbley E, et al: Bacterial pneumonia in patients with the acquired immunodeficiency syndrome. Ann Intern Med 104:38, 1986.

Quinn TC, Corey L, Chaffee RG, Schoffler MD, Brancato FP, Holmes KK: The etiology of anorectal infections in homosexual men. Am J Med 71:395, 1981.

Quinn TC, Mann JM, Curran JW, Piot P: AIDS in Africa: An epidemiologic paradigm. Science 234:955, 1986.

Rao TKS, Friedman EA, Nicastri, AD: The types of renal disease in the acquired immunodeficiency syndrome. NEJM 316:1062, 1987.

Redfield RR, Wright DC, Tramont EC: The Walter Reed staging classification for HTLV-III/LAV infection. NEJM 314:131, 1986.

Safai B, Kozimer B: Malignant neoplasms in AIDS, in DeVita VT Jr, Hellman S, Rosenberg SA (eds): AIDS: Etiology, Diagnosis, Treatment, and Prevention. Philadelphia, J.B. Lippincott, 1985, pp 213–222.

Selwyn PA: AIDS: What is now known. I. Hosp. Prac 21:76, 1986.

Selwyn PA: AIDS: What is now known. II. Epidemiology. Hosp. Prac 21:127, 1986.

Selwyn PA: AIDS: What is now known. III. Clinical Aspects. Hosp Prac 21:119, 1986.

Shulman JA, Blumberg HM, Kozarsky PE, et al: Acquired immunodeficiency syndrome (AIDS): Update for the clinician. Emory Univ J Med 1:157, 1987.

Soave R, Danner RL, Honig CL, et al: Cryptosporidiosis in homosexual men. Ann Intern Med 100:504, 1984.

Spivak JL, Bender BS, Quinn TC: Hematologic abnormalities in the acquired immune deficiency syndrome. Am J Med 77:224, 1984.

Steckelberg JM, Cockerhill FR III: Serologic testing for human immunodeficiency virus antibodies. Mayo Clin Proc 63:373, 1988.

Stricot RL, Morse DL: HTLV-III/LAV seroconversion following a deep intramuscular needle injury. NEJM 314:1115, 1986.

Volberding P: The clinical spectrum of the acquired immunodeficiency syndrome: Implications for comprehensive patient care. Ann Intern Med 103:729, 1985.

Edman JC, Kovacs JA, Masur H, et al: Ribosomal RNA sequence shows Pneumocystis carinii to be a member of the fungi. Nature 334:519–522, 1988.

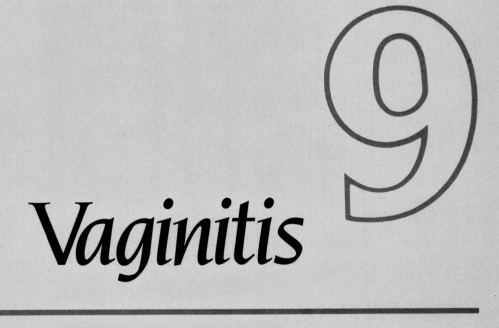

Vaginitis

G.P. SCHMID, R.J. ARKO

Introduction

Complaints referable to the vagina—vaginal discharge, odor, pruritis, and irritation—are extremely common. In 1976, a vaginal discharge was among the 25 most common reasons for consulting a physician in private practice in the United States, accounting for an estimated 4,377,000 office visits. Three infectious diseases of the adult vagina are recognized (although diseases affecting the cervix may also lead a woman to seek treatment for a vaginal discharge): bacterial vaginosis, trichomoniasis (caused by *Trichomonas vaginalis*), and candidiasis (usually caused by *Candida* spp.). Of the three, bacterial vaginosis is the most common, although its pathogenesis is the least understood and it is the only entity not caused by a single organism.

Normal Flora

The vagina is a dynamic ecosystem that is sterile at birth and becomes colonized within a few days with a predominantly gram-positive flora consisting of anaerobic bacteria, staphylococci, streptococci, and diphtheroids. The vaginal pH in premenarchal females is near neutral (pH, 7.0) until puberty. At that time, under the influence of estrogen, the vaginal epithelium increases to about 25 cells thick, glycogen levels in the epithelium and vagina increase, the predominant flora changes to lactobacilli, and the vaginal pH decreases to less than 4.5. This low pH is maintained until menopause, when the vaginal epithelium thins, a mixed flora of anaerobic bacteria, staphy-lococci, streptococci, and diphtheroids becomes reestablished, and the vaginal pH rises above 6.0 (Fig. 9.1).

An early hypothesis by Döderlein maintained that the predominant lactic acid-producing lactobacilli in the vagina serve a protective function against pathogenic bacteria and that an abnormal vaginal discharge results from a partial replacement of the normal flora by less acidophilic microorganisms. Consistent with this hypothesis, in vitro inhibitory effects of lactobacilli on other microorganisms have been shown. Similarly, the glycogen that appears in the vagina at puberty is an ideal substrate for the growth of lactobacilli, which, by converting glycogen to lactic acid, lower the vaginal pH to a level inhospitable to many other species of bacteria.

Lactobacilli vary greatly in size but generally are large, straight or curved rods (Fig. 9.2). They are gram-positive, but cells from older cultures may stain gram-negative or gram-variable. Lactobacilli are facultative or strictly anaerobic and usually are nonmotile. Although they have complex nutritional requirements, they produce lactic acid as their primary end product of carbohydrate metabolism.

BACTERIAL VAGINOSIS
Introduction

For many years, *nonspecific vaginitis* was loosely used to refer to vaginal discharges not caused by *T. vaginalis* or *Candida* spp. In 1955, Gardner and Dukes clinically defined this condition and entitled it "*Haemophilus vaginalis* vaginitis," believing the organ-

BACTERIA IN VAGINAL FLORA OF HEALTHY MENSTRUATING WOMEN, IN ORDER OF USUAL PREVALENCE	
AEROBIC/FACULTATIVE	ANAEROBIC
Lactobacilli	Lactobacilli
Diphtheroids	Peptococci
Gardnerella vaginalis	Peptostreptococci
Streptococci	*Bacteroides*
Staphylococci	*Eubacterium*

Figure 9.1 Bacteria in vaginal flora of healthy menstruating women, in order of usual prevalence.

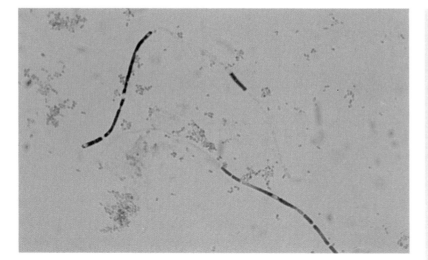

Figure 9.2 Large *L. acidophilus* cells showing gram-negative staining observed with older cultures. Small coccobacilli are *G. vaginalis* cells.

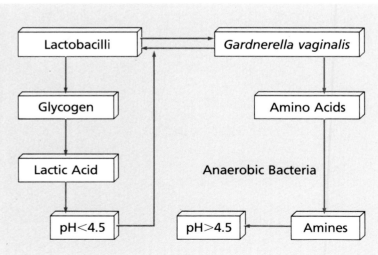

Figure 9.3 Hypothesized pathogenesis of bacterial vaginosis.

ism they described was causative. Today, H. *vaginalis* vaginitis is referred to as *bacterial vaginosis* (or, in Britain, as *anaerobic vaginosis*), reflecting both the lack of inflammation in the condition (hence, "-osis") and the recognition that H. *vaginalis* (subsequently, *Corynebacterium vaginale* and now named *Gardnerella vaginalis*, in honor of Gardner) is not the sole etiologic agent. Instead, bacterial vaginosis is thought to be a result of a complex interaction of multiple species of bacteria.

Gardner and Dukes believed the disease was caused by G. *vaginalis* because they identified the organism in women with bacterial vaginosis but not in women without the disease. In retrospect, they seem to have been unable to recover G. *vaginalis* from the latter group because the medium they used was insensitive and because women with bacterial vaginosis have far greater numbers of G. *vaginalis* organisms than do women without the condition. If current, sensitive media are used, as many as 50% of asymptomatic women are found to be colonized with G. *vaginalis*.

The involvement of bacterial species other than G. *vaginalis* in bacterial vaginosis was recognized by Pheifer et al. in 1978. They recognized that anaerobic bacteria—principally *Bacteroides* spp., *Peptococcus* spp., and *Peptostreptococcus* spp.—occur in increased numbers in the vaginal secretions of women with bacterial vaginosis and that metronidazole, which has high activity against anaerobic bacteria, provides effective therapy. Subsequently, *Mobiluncus* spp. have been found to be highly associated with bacterial vaginosis, as has *Mycoplasma hominis*.

The precise roles, if any, that these varying bacteria play in the etiology and pathogenesis of bacterial vaginosis are unclear. A hypothesized scheme of the pathogenesis of the disease, with resultant production of clinical symptoms, involves multiple microorganisms (Fig. 9.3). Under the influence of estrogen, the vaginal epithelial cells produce glycogen, which forms a substrate for the production of lactic acid by the predominant lactobacilli. The lactic acid produces a low pH, which is conducive to the growth of lactobacilli but not to many other bacterial species. If, for as yet unclear reasons, this symbiotic relationship is broken in one or more places, an overgrowth of bacteria associated with bacterial vaginosis (in particular, G. *vaginalis* and anaerobic species) occurs. G. *vaginalis* metabolically produces amino acids, which acts as a substrate for the production of volatile amines (e.g., putrescine) by anaerobic bacteria; these amines are responsible for the unpleasant odor associated with the disease. The amines, in turn, raise the vaginal pH, favoring the continued growth of G. *vaginalis* over lactobacilli.

Epidemiology

Bacterial vaginosis is the most common of the vaginitides, yet its epidemiology is not well understood. Although the disease is associated with sexual activity, being rare in women who are not sexually experienced, it is not considered an STD, and treatment of sexual partners is not routinely recommended. Although the use of an intrauterine device and a history of trichomoniasis have been associated with bacterial vaginosis, the majority of affected women have no identified risk factors. Without therapy, cases may be self-limited, intermittently recurrent, or chronic.

Clinical Manifestations

In 1983, an International Working Group on Bacterial Vaginosis formulated clinical criteria for the diagnosis of bacterial vaginosis (Fig. 9.4); using these criteria, as many as one-half of women in selected populations have the disease. Many cases are so mild that they are not recognized by patients, being found only on routine exams. Some of these women are only apparently asymptomatic, however, and following treatment will notice the disappearance of a previously inapparent vaginal discharge or odor.

Women with bacterial vaginosis may complain of a vaginal discharge or abnormal vaginal odor. The discharge, which typically is gray and smooth, clings to the vaginal walls (Fig. 9.5). The vaginal mucosa and vulva appear normal; this lack of inflammation has led to the use of the term *vaginosis* instead of *vaginitis*. The majority of women with bacterial vaginosis note a foul odor in the genital area, which initially may be noticed or intensified immediately following intercourse, when alkalinization of the vaginal secretions by semen occurs, leading to volatilization of polyamines.

Examination of a woman with a complaint of a vaginal discharge or odor should include an evaluation for the clinical criteria of bacterial vaginosis (see Fig. 9.4). The odor of the vaginal secretions should be tested by smelling the withdrawn

---

CLINICAL DIAGNOSTIC CRITERIA FOR BACTERIAL VAGINOSIS

Three of the following four criteria:

Thin, homogeneous discharge

pH > 4.5

Amine (fishlike) odor of vaginal secretions

Clue cells

Figure 9.4 Clinical diagnostic criteria for bacterial vaginosis.

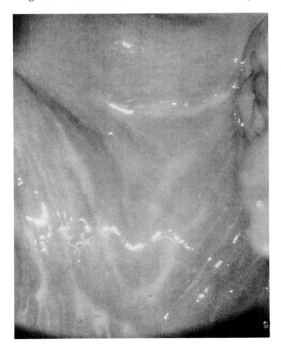

Figure 9.5 Vaginal discharge typical of bacterial vaginosis. Discharge is homogeneous and clings to vaginal wall, which is not inflamed.

speculum (the "whiff test"); normal vaginal secretions do not have an unpleasant odor. If this test is negative, a more sensitive procedure for detecting the amines is performed by adding a few drops of 10% potassium hydroxide (KOH) to a few drops of vaginal secretions and immediately smelling ("whiffing") the mixture for the transient, "dead fish" odor that is characteristic of bacterial vaginosis. The pH of vaginal secretions should be determined by using a strip of narrow-range pH paper (about pH 4.0 to 5.5), which may be applied to the withdrawn speculum or directly inserted into the vagina with a forceps. Last, a wet mount of vaginal secretions should be done to look for clue cells, epithelial cells covered with G. vaginalis that Gardner and Dukes called "clues" to the diagnosis of bacterial vaginosis. A Gram stain of vaginal secretions also can be done if it is to be used as a diagnostic test.

When examining a woman for bacterial vaginosis, potential diagnostic pitfalls must be avoided. The clinical or laboratory assessment may be affected by examination during menses, examination within two to three days of menses or sexual intercourse, recent douching, or the use of intravaginal products or systemic antimicrobials. Menses, semen, or douching may affect the pH, and a weakly positive whiff test may be produced by menstrual blood or semen. The pH paper should not sample water used to moisten the speculum, nor should cervical secretions, which are relatively alkaline, be sampled. Trichomoniasis, which also may have an elevated pH and a positive whiff test because of an accompanying overgrowth of anaerobes, must be excluded. Lastly, bacteria other than G. vaginalis, notably lactobacilli or Mobiluncus spp., can cling to epithelial cells so that the morphology of organisms on clue cells must be considered; if necessary, smears from women with possible clue cells should be Gram stained to distinguish gram-negative G. vaginalis from gram-positive Lactobacillus spp.

G. vaginalis, an opportunistic microorganism, infrequently is isolated from blood, from joint, amniotic, or spinal fluids, from semen, and from a variety of infected wounds of both men and women. Mobiluncus spp., an anaerobic curved rod often seen in association with G. vaginalis, also have been recovered from a number of extragenital sites.

Laboratory Tests

Although G. vaginalis can be isolated from the vagina of about 50% of all women, it is present in higher numbers ($>10^6$/mL) in vaginal secretions of bacterial vaginosis patients than in vaginal secretions from asymptomatic women (10^1/mL). Similarly, the change in flora in women with bacterial vaginosis (Fig. 9.6) can be appreciated by comparing it with the normal flora (see Fig. 9.1).

G. vaginalis shares many cultural and morphologic similarities with Haemophilus and Corynebacterium spp.; however, based on DNA homology studies, Gardnerella clearly is a separate genus. Although it is a fastidious, facultative bacterium, it can be grown in an atmosphere of 5 to 10% CO_2 (candle jar) or in an anaerobic chamber (Fig. 9.7). G. vaginalis organisms are gram-negative or gram-variable, pleomorphic coccobacilli or bacilli that average 0.4 by 1.5 μm in size (Fig. 9.8). In vaginal smears, they often are attached to epithelial cells (Fig. 9.9).

The primary isolation of G. vaginalis from specimens having mixed flora is best performed by using an enriched human or rabbit blood medium containing the selective antibiotics colistin and nalidixic acid (Fig. 9.10). The diffuse hemolysis that

---

BACTERIA IN VAGINAL FLORA OF WOMEN WITH BACTERIAL VAGINOSIS, IN ORDER OF USUAL PREVALENCE

AEROBIC/FACULTATIVE	ANAEROBIC
Gardnerella vaginalis	Bacteroides spp.
Lactobacillus spp.	Mobiluncus spp.
Diphtheroids	Gram-positive cocci (Peptococcus and Peptostreptococcus spp.

Figure 9.6 Bacteria in vaginal flora of women with bacterial vaginosis, in order of usual prevalence.

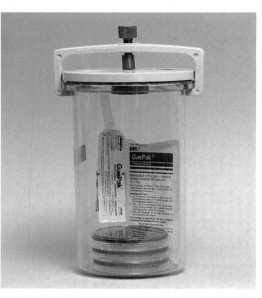

Figure 9.7 Anaerobic chamber (Gas Pac, BBL) utilizing disposable hydrogen and carbon dioxide generator envelopes and palladium catalyst.

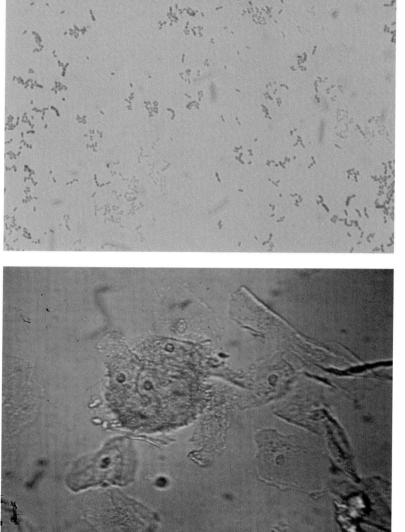

Figure 9.8 Gram stain of *G. vaginalis* from three-day culture showing gram-negative coccobacilli.

Figure 9.9 Clue cell—a vaginal epithelial cell with attached microorganisms. Clue cells are stippled (with attached bacteria), and to be called a clue cell should have a stippled border.

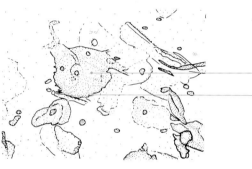

Clue cell

Stippled border

RECOMMENDED MEDIA FOR GROWTH AND IDENTIFICATION OF *GARDNERELLA VAGINALIS*

Primary isolation medium. Columbia CNA agar with colistin and nalidixic acid supplemented with 1% proteosepeptone #3 and 5% whole human, rabbit, or sheep blood.

Growth medium. Heart infusion agar supplemented with 5% defibrinated rabbit blood.

Growth medium. Chocolate agar II.

Starch hydrolysis medium. GC base agar supplemented with 1% IsoVitaleX and 0.1% cornstarch. This medium may develop peroxides that can be removed by treatment with catalase to improve sensitivity.

Starch hydrolysis medium. Purple agar base (Difco) plus 1% cornstarch.

Figure 9.10 Recommended media for growth and identification of *G. vaginalis.*

develops within one to three days around small, circular, grayish, colonies is diagnostically helpful (Fig. 9.11). Enhancement of the hemolytic zone around G. *vaginalis* colonies can be obtained by using a bilayer blood medium or by stabbing full-thickness blood plates with an inoculation loop in several areas (Figs. 9.12 and 9.13). Some *Gardnerella* strains produce wider hemolytic zones when incubated anaerobically.

G. *vaginalis* is biochemically active (Fig. 9.14). Routine laboratory identification, however, is usually determined by the appearance of typical colonies on human or rabbit blood agar, Gram stain characteristics, negative oxidase and catalase reactions, the presence or absence of hemolysis on varying types of blood agar, and hydrolysis of starch and/or hippurate (Fig. 9.15). Because G. *vaginalis* does not produce catalase, it may not grow sufficiently on some protein-enriched media where peroxides develop. Treatment of the surface of these media with sterile bovine liver catalase (5,000 U/mL) before inoculation can provide significant improvement in growth (Fig. 9.16). The hydrolysis of starch can be determined by inoculation onto a translucent starch medium.

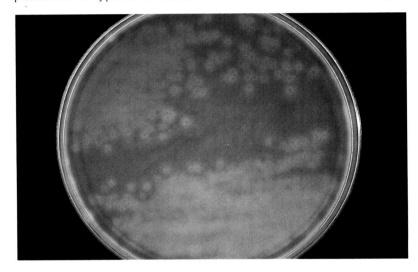

Figure 9.11 Human blood bilayer plate showing hemolysis surrounding G. *vaginalis* colonies incubated in 5% CO_2 for three days.

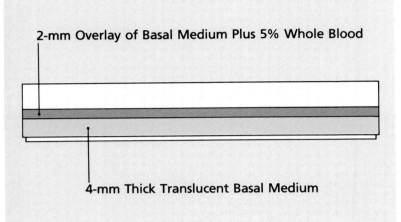

Figure 9.12 Human blood bilayer plate. A primary layer of basal medium is poured to an approximate thickness of 4 mm and allowed to solidify. A second layer of medium containing 5% red blood cells is poured to form a thin (2-mm) surface.

Figure 9.13 Full-thickness rabbit blood medium (heart infusion agar, BBL) with three-day culture of G. *vaginalis*. Note hemolysis around colonies and clearing around three stab inoculation areas.

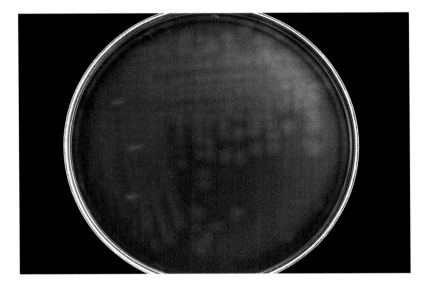

If specimens cannot be immediately inoculated onto culture plates, they should be placed in 0.5 mL of an enriched broth (e.g., trypticase-soy or Columbia) and either plated within a few hours or frozen at a temperature lower than $-50°C$. Pure cultures of G. vaginalis can be stored by freezing cells ($>10^8CFU/$ mL) in defibrinated rabbit blood at less than $-50°C$.

Mobiluncus ("motile hooks") spp. are a recently "rediscovered" group of anaerobic bacteria. These curved rods frequently are observed in vaginal smears from women with bacterial vagi-

nosis; like G. vaginalis, they can be found in vaginal smears from some asymptomatic women. Because culture techniques for Mobiluncus spp. are laborious and may be less sensitive than presumptive identification by vaginal smears or other means, such as DNA probes, the prevalence of Mobiluncus in vaginal secretions is difficult to determine. Consequently, the presence of Mobiluncus in the vagina is often based on microscopic results showing organisms with characteristic morphology.

BIOCHEMICAL TESTS USED IN THE IDENTIFICATION OF *GARDNERELLA VAGINALIS*

Figure 9.14 Biochemical tests used in the identification of G. vaginalis.

POSITIVE TESTS (>85% OF *GARDNERELLA VAGINALIS* STRAINS)

Beta-hemolysis of human and rabbit blood

Acid phosphatase

Beta-glucosidase

Hippurate hydrolysis

Starch hydrolysis

Inhibition of growth by metronidazole, 50 μg

Carbohydrate fermentations

NEGATIVE TESTS

Nonhemolytic on sheep or horse blood

Catalase

Oxidase

Indole

Urease

Nitrate reduction

Mannitol fermentation

MINIMAL TESTING FOR ROUTINE LABORATORY IDENTIFICATION OF *GARDNERELLA VAGINALIS*

Growth on human or rabbit blood agar with diffuse beta-hemolysis around small (1-to-3-mm), grayish colonies. No hemolysis on sheep or horse blood agar.

Gram stain shows small, pleomorphic rods, which are either gram-negative or gram-variable.

Negative oxidase and catalase reactions.

No discoloration of media on chocolate agar.

Hydrolysis of starch and/or hippurate.

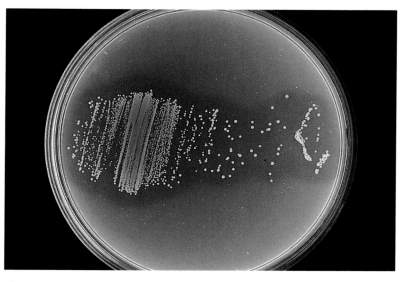

Figure 9.15 Minimal testing for routine laboratory identification of G. vaginalis.

Figure 9.16 G. vaginalis colonies growing on GC base medium supplemented with IsoVitaleX (BBL) and 0.1% cornstarch. Central areas of plate have been treated with bovine catalase to inhibit peroxides and improve growth, allowing starch hydrolysis around colonies to be observed.

Two species— M. *curtissi* (short form) and M. *mulieris* (long form) —have been distinguished based on size and subtle biologic differences (Figs. 9.17 to 9.19). Both species are motile by means of flagella originating from the concave aspect of the cell, and both have a laminated cell wall consistent with a gram-positive structure, even though they usually stain as gram-negative rods. When stained with methylene blue, terminal cytoplasmic inclusions can be observed in cells grown on a GC base medium (Fig. 9.20).

For primary isolation, freshly obtained specimens should be inoculated onto an enriched medium such as Columbia agar with 5% rabbit blood, supplemented with colistin and nalidixic acid to inhibit other bacteria. If clinical material must be transported for processing, an anaerobic, 35°C environment should be maintained. Culture plates should be incubated anaerobically for at least five days.

Mobiluncus colonies are small and gray. On chocolate agar, both *Mobiluncus* spp. appear as flattened colonies that do not discolor the media (Fig. 9.21). Oxidase and catalase tests are negative. Starch hydrolysis can be demonstrated by the growth of *Mobiluncus* on translucent GC Base agar supplemented with IsoVitaleX and 0.1% cornstarch, as for *Gardnerella*. Colonies of M. *mulieris* are differentiated from those of M. *curtissi* by growth, morphologic, and biochemical differences (see Fig. 9.19). On rabbit blood medium, M. *mulieris* produces a spotty hemolysis when incubated anaerobically for five days or longer, while M. *curtissi* produces very little or no hemolysis (Figs. 9.22 and 9.23). Storage of *Mobiluncus* cultures is similar to that used for *Gardnerella* cultures.

Because culture techniques for many organisms participating in the pathogenesis of bacterial vaginosis are difficult, and because simply isolating a specific organism from vaginal secretions of a woman with suspected bacterial vaginosis does not confirm the clinical diagnosis, Gram stain diagnosis is quite useful when used in conjunction with clinical criteria. Gram stains from women without bacterial vaginosis show a pre-

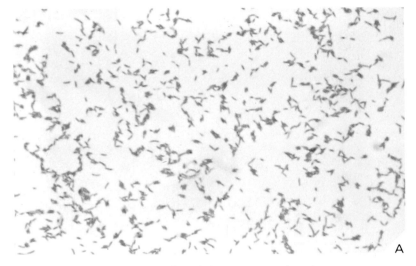
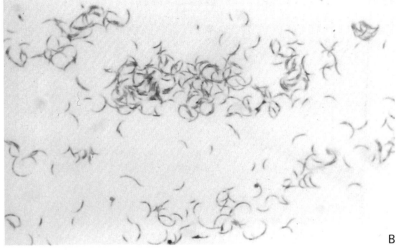

Figure 9.17 Gram stain of *Mobiluncus* spp., showing gram-negative staining of short and long forms. A M. *curtissi*. B M. *mulieris*.

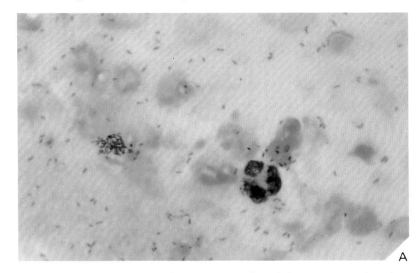
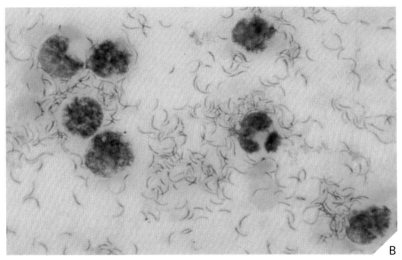

Figure 9.18 Methylene blue staining of *Mobiluncus* spp., showing their size in relation to that of white blood cells. A M. *curtissi*. B M. *mulieris*.

MOBILUNCUS: DISTINGUISHING FEATURES OF TWO SPECIES

Figure 9.19
Mobiluncus: Distinguishing features of two species.

	M. CURTISSI	M. MULIERIS
SIZE	Short (1-to-2-mm), curved rods	Long (2-to-4-mm), curved rods
GRAM STAIN	Variable	Negative
HEMOLYSIS OF RABBIT BLOOD	− (or weak)	+ (moderate beta)
LYSIS BY 3% KOH (STRING TEST)	−	+
BETA-GALACTOSIDASE	+ *	−
HIPPURATE HYDROLYSIS	+ *	−

*Positive in >85% of isolates.

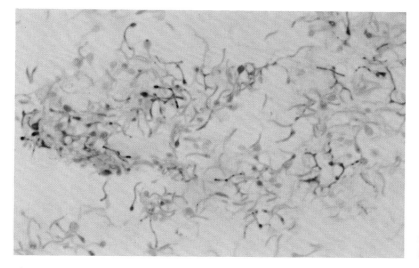

Figure 9.20 Methylene blue staining of *M. mulieris* grown for three days on a GC base medium supplemented with IsoVitaleX (BBL). Some cells show terminal enlargements or inclusions.

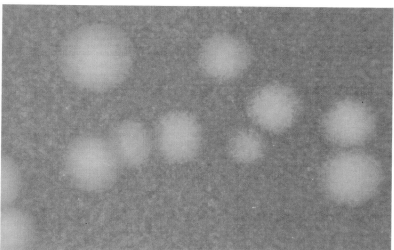

Figure 9.21 *Mobiluncus* sp. growing on chocolate agar medium (colonies, ×10).

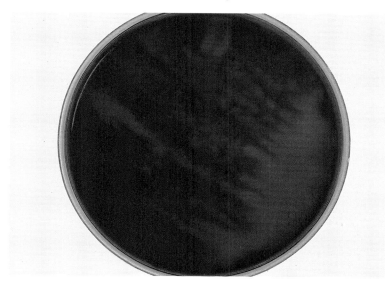

Figure 9.22 "Moth-eaten" hemolysis around colonies of *M. mulieris* growing on rabbit blood medium.

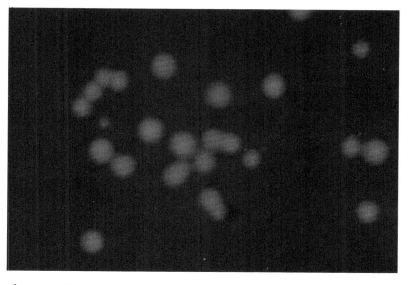

Figure 9.23 *M. curtissi* growing on rabbit blood agar (colonies, ×10).

dominance of lactobacilli and few other bacteria (Fig. 9.24A). Gram stains of vaginal secretions from affected women, however, show the replacement of lactobacilli by large numbers of small, gram-negative coccobacilli (consistent with G. *vaginalis*) and an increase in other flora (consistent with anaerobic species) (Fig. 9.24B). About half of the cases will have gram-negative or gram-variable, thin, curved rods consistent with *Mobiluncus* spp. (Fig. 9.25).

Laboratory diagnosis by gas–liquid chromatographic (GLC) identification of fatty acids is useful as a research tool. Normal vaginal secretions show only a lactate peak, consistent with the conversion of glycogen to lactic acid by lactobacilli. Secretions from patients with bacterial vaginosis, however, contain decreased levels of lactate but large amounts of acetate, butyrate, and succinate as a result of metabolism by bacteria that have largely replaced the lactobacilli (Fig. 9.26). A ratio of the succinate-to-lactate peaks of more than 0.4 is highly predictive of the disease (Fig. 9.27).

Treatment

Oral metronidazole is the drug most commonly used to treat bacterial vaginosis (Fig. 9.28). Varying doses are effective, with shorter courses having the advantage of ease of administration and lower total dose. The use of metronidazole is not recommended in pregnancy because of persistent fears of teratogenicity; during pregnancy, ampicillin or amoxicillin are most commonly used. Intravaginally administered metronidazole and clindamycin preparations are promising.

TRICHOMONIASIS
Introduction

T. *vaginalis* is a protozoan that infects specifically the genital tract. Although two other species of trichomonads colonize man (T. *tenax* in the mouth and *Pentatrichomonas hominis* in the large intestine), these organisms do not occur in the vagina. T. *va-*

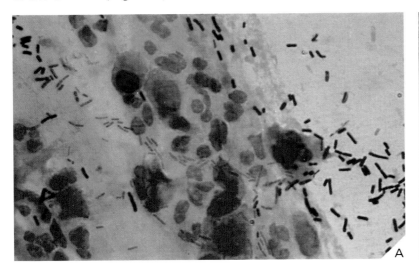

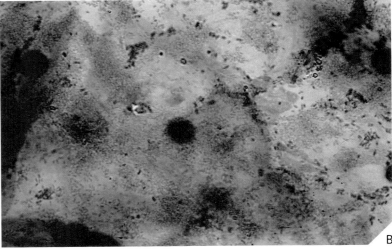

Figure 9.24 Gram stain of vaginal secretions. **A** From woman without bacterial vaginosis. **B** From woman with bacterial vaginosis.

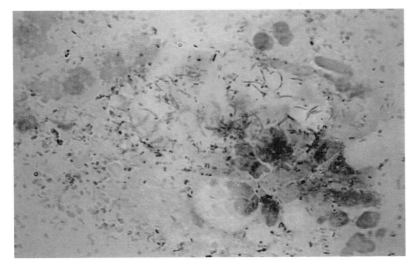

Figure 9.25 Gram stain of vaginal secretions from woman with bacterial vaginosis, showing presence of rods consistent with *M. mulieris*.

FATTY ACIDS PRODUCED BY COMMON VAGINAL BACTERIA

FATTY ACID	BACTERIA
Lactate	*Lactobacillus* spp.
Succinate	*Bacteroides* spp.
Acetate	*Gardnerella vaginalis*
	Peptococcus spp.
Butyrate	*Peptococcus* spp.

Figure 9.26 Fatty acids produced by common vaginal bacteria.

ginalis is ovoid, and approximately 10 to 20 μm wide (about the size of a white blood cell) (Fig. 9.29). The organism has four free, anterior flagella and a fifth flagellum embedded in an undulating membrane that extends around the anterior two-thirds of the cell. The flagella move the protozoan with a jerky movement.

Epidemiology

Women are the main carriers of disease. About one-third of men who are sexual partners of women with T. *vaginalis* are colonized in the urethra, but men, unlike women, rapidly clear the organism. One study found that 70% of men who had sex with an infected woman two days previously were infected, with this percentage dropping to 47% by 14 days or longer. Thus, transmission of disease depends upon relatively frequent in-tercourse of men with different partners, and/or occasional long-term infections in some men.

Clinical Manifestations

As many as one-half of women infected with T. *vaginalis* are asymptomatic. This number depends upon how women are selected for study, how closely the women are questioned for symptoms, and the sensitivity of diagnostic techniques. In symptomatic women, a vaginal discharge is the most common complaint. The discharge may be of any color, but appears purulent. As in bacterial vaginosis, some women notice a disagreeable odor, indicating the shared feature of these two diseases of overgrowth of anaerobic microorganisms with resultant amine production.

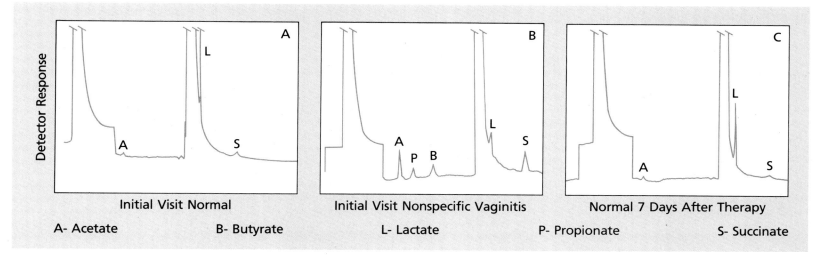

Figure 9.27 Gas–liquid chromatograph of vaginal secretions from a normal patient (**A**) and a patient with bacterial vaginosis before therapy (**B**) and after therapy (**C**).

EFFICACY OF ANTIMICROBIALS IN TREATING BACTERIAL VAGINOSIS

ANTIMICROBIAL	EFFICACY
Metronidazole, 500 mg, orally, twice a day for 7 days	95 to 100%
Metronidazole, 2 g, orally, once	85 to 90%
Metronidazole, 2 g, orally, once on Days 1 and 3	90 to 95%
Ampicillin, 500 mg, orally, 4 times a day for 7 days	48 to 100%

Figure 9.28 Efficacy of antimicrobials in treating bacterial vaginosis.

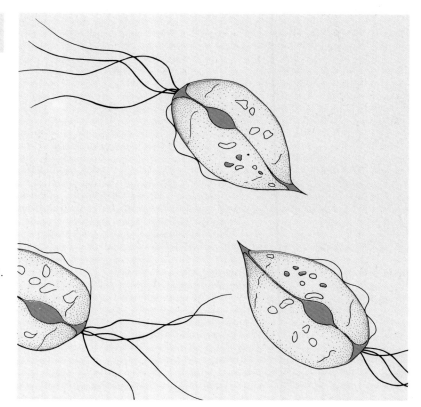

Figure 9.29 T. *vaginalis*.

On examination, the discharge may be profuse and visible externally. Frothiness of the discharge, along with a disagreeable odor, may be noticed. The vaginal mucosa is often erythematous, reflecting the inflammatory nature of the disease process (Fig. 9.30). In a small number of cases, the cervix is inflamed and has punctate hemorrhages (Fig. 9.31). Rarely, T. vaginalis has been found in the upper genital tract, but the significance of this occurrence is unknown.

Most men infected with T. vaginalis are asymptomatic. About 5 to 10% of men with nongonococcal urethritis are infected with T. vaginalis. The organism has been recovered from semen in association with an inflammatory semen analysis, but whether it is a cause of prostatitis is debatable.

Laboratory Tests

A variety of diagnostic techniques for T. vaginalis are available but none detect all infected women. The most commonly used and easiest technique is that of a wet mount of vaginal secretions. An aliquot of vaginal secretions, usually obtained with a swab, is mixed with a small amount of saline and examined with light- or phase-contrast microscopy under low power. Trichomonads are about the size of white blood cells and move with a jerky motion. Organisms tentatively identified under low power are examined under high power to confirm their motility and to visualize flagella (Fig. 9.32). The sensitivity of the wet mount varies with the concentration of trichomonads in the discharge, the dilution of secretions examined, the experience of the examiner, and the standard to which the wet mount is compared. The sensitivity may be as low as 50%, but most authorities consider it to be about 65 to 80%.

Culture is the most sensitive means of diagnosis; a variety of culture media are available. Although T. vaginalis can be cultured using solid media, all clinically useful media are liquid. Of media available in the United States, Diamond's medium (see Appendix 3) or a variant of it appears to be the best. An aliquot of vaginal secretions is placed into tubes and incubated at 33 to 37° C. A drop of fluid from the bottom of the tube, where the concentration of trichomonads is greatest, is examined by wet mount daily for seven days or until positive. If examination cannot be performed daily, examination at three to four days and again at seven days will detect almost all positive specimens.

Recently, fluorescein-labeled monoclonal antibodies have been used to detect trichomonads on vaginal smears (Fig. 9.33). The sensitivity of this procedure exceeds that of the wet mount but appears to be less than that of sensitive culture media. Compared with wet mount, this procedure requires more time and is more expensive, and thus may be most useful in situations where microscopy and/or culture is not available.

The Papanicolaou stain of exfoliated cervical cells may identify trichomonads (Fig. 9.34). Cytologic criteria for the diagnosis of trichomoniasis vary, however, from simply visualizing an inflammatory reaction thought to be typical of trichomoniasis to the necessity of visualizing flagella arising from a cell; the latter criteria are clearly more specific.

No widely accepted technique of differentiating strains of T. vaginalis exists. Reaction patterns based on panels of monoclonal antibodies and differences between in vitro hemolytic activity appear to offer the most promise in differentiating strains when necessary.

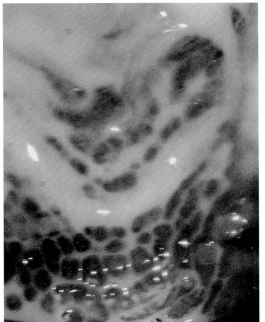

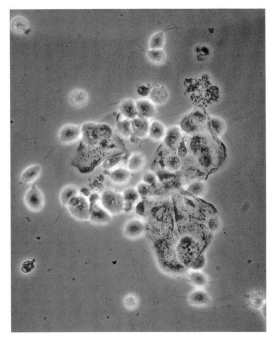

Figure 9.31 "Strawberry cervix," seen in about 10% of patients with trichomoniasis. Note frothiness of discharge.

Figure 9.30 Vaginal erythema and discharge from a patient with trichomoniasis. Note frothiness of discharge.

Figure 9.32 Trichomonads visualized by phase contrast microscopy (× 400).

Treatment

Metronidazole is the only antimicrobial widely recommended to treat trichomoniasis. Two regimens commonly are used. A single oral dose of 2 g, which is more than 90% effective, frequently is used because it is given as a single dose. Alternatively, 250 mg administered orally three times a day for seven days is slightly more effective. With both regimens, sexual partners are simultaneously treated.

Metronidazole-resistant strains of T. *vaginalis* have been reported from at least 26 states; the origin of their resistance is unclear. In resistant cases, high doses of oral or intravenous metronidazole have been required for cure.

CANDIDIASIS
Introduction

Vaginal disease caused by yeasts is common, with most women having at least one symptomatic, vaginal yeast infection during their lifetime. C. *albicans* causes 90% of vaginal infections (with other *Candida* spp. and *Torulopsis glabrata* causing most of the remainder); hence, vaginal yeast infections are often referred to as *candidiasis*. Recovery of the organism from, or identification

in, vaginal secretions is not sufficient to diagnose disease, however, because colonization of the vagina without symptoms occurs in approximately 10 to 15% of women.

Epidemiology

Although men can be colonized with *Candida* spp., and many male sexual partners of women with candidiasis are transiently colonized, candidiasis is not recognized as an STD. Instead, symptoms occur in women previously colonized with C. *albicans*. Although the reasons why symptomatic yeast infections occur are not completely understood, pregnancy, diabetes, use of birth control pills, steroid use, and systemic antimicrobial therapy (which eliminates competing vaginal flora) are recognized predisposing factors to symptomatic infection.

Clinical Manifestations

Candidiasis is a vulvovaginitis whose predominant symptom is pruritus. Typically, the onset is acute and occurs premenstrually. When seen by the clinician, the vulva and vagina may be erythematous and excoriated. Pruritus may occur without a discharge, and the opposite may occur (Fig. 9.35). The discharge,

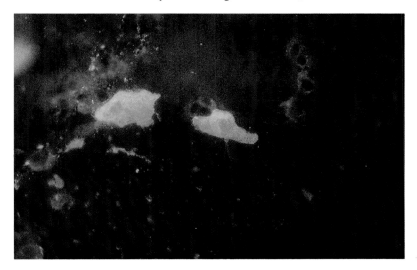

Figure 9.33 Trichomonad stained with fluorescein-labeled antibody (×1,000).

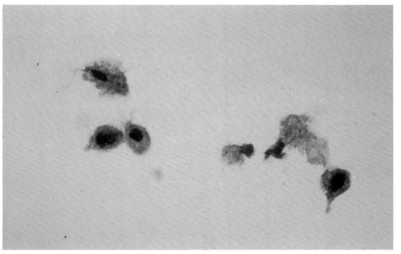

Figure 9.34 Trichomonads identified by Papanicolaou stain on exfoliated cervical cells.

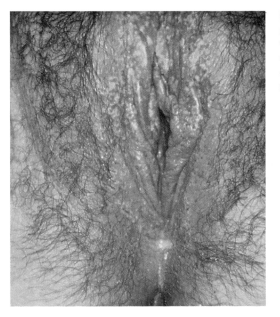

Figure 9.35 Mild discharge and inflammation of the vulva, commonly occurring in vulvovaginal candidiasis.

if present, usually is white, thick, and curdy (Fig. 9.36). Many women from whom *Candida* spp. are isolated may not complain of a discharge, and are thus asymptomatic. Nevertheless, women infected with *Candida* spp. are more likely to have a discharge the clinician considers abnormal (and thus have signs of disease) than women not colonized, indicating that the disease is inapparent to some women. There is no offensive odor to the vaginal secretions.

In men, *Candida* spp. may cause balanitis (inflammation of the glans penis) and balanoposthitis (inflammation of the glans penis and prepuce) (Fig. 9.37). *Candida* organisms have been recovered from semen and from the urethras of some men with nonspecific urethritis, but the significance of these findings is unclear.

Laboratory Tests

C. albicans occurs in both yeast and mycelial forms. Yeasts are oval cells about 4 to 8 μm in diameter (Fig. 9.38). In vaginal specimens, yeasts multiply asexually by forming buds (blastoconidia). If the buds keep forming and elongating, and do not detach from one another, they resemble hyphae and are called *pseudohyphae*. The constrictions between buds in the pseudohyphae differentiate them from true hyphae. Hyphae, which form a mycelium when they are abundant and inter-

twined, are rarely seen in vaginal secretions because they are formed only under poor growth conditions, while the vagina, rich in glycogen and oxygen, provides suitable growth conditions for *Candida* spp.

The diagnosis of candidiasis is most often made by wet-mount microscopy of vaginal secretions; this can be done when the vaginal secretions are examined for clue cells and trichomonads. Estimates of the sensitivity of the wet mount range from 40 to 85%, varying, as with trichomoniasis, with patient selection, observer experience, and sensitivity of the culture media to which the wet-mount results are compared. Symptoms appear to be directly correlated to the quantity of yeasts present, so that if symptomatic women are studied, the wet mount will appear highly sensitive.

The wet-mount specimen is examined for yeasts or pseudohyphae under low-power ($\times 100$) magnification; subsequent examination at high-power ($\times 400$) will detail the organism. Debris from epithelial cells or mucus may be mistaken for or may obscure yeasts, but this potential problem can be eliminated by adding a few drops of 10 to 15% KOH to the wet-mount specimen. The addition of KOH has been shown to improve both sensitivity and specificity.

Gram stain of vaginal secretions is as sensitive as wet mount in detecting infection. *Candida* spp. stain intensely gram-positive (see Fig. 9.38). *Candida* spp. may be seen on Papanicolaou-

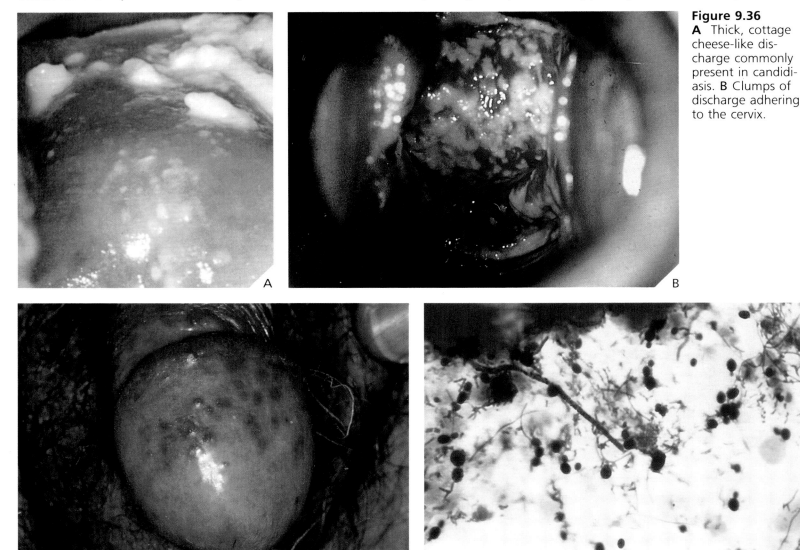

Figure 9.36
A Thick, cottage cheese-like discharge commonly present in candidiasis. **B** Clumps of discharge adhering to the cervix.

Figure 9.37 Balanitis of the penis, showing scattered inflamed areas.

Figure 9.38 Gram stain of vaginal secretions of woman with candidiasis. There are many gram-positive yeasts, occasionally with buds. Across the center of the slide is a long pseudohypha ($\times 1000$).

stained samples of exfoliated cervical cells. This method is not sensitive, however, detecting only about 50% of cases of symptomatic women.

Culture is the most sensitive diagnostic test. *Candida* spp. grow on many media, including blood agar, but special media for fungi are optimal. For greatest yield, at least two media, one with and one without antimicrobials inhibitory for competing microorganisms, should be used. Sabouraud's dextrose, the most widely used medium, supports the growth of all clinically important yeasts. *Candida* spp. grow at 25° C or 37° C—and in the yeast form at both temperatures—so using two temperatures offers no diagnostic advantage. Although *Candida* spp. grow most rapidly at 37° C, more rapidly growing bacteria may obscure fungal colonies at that temperature so that many authorities prefer 30° C. Pinpoint colonies may be visible at 24 hours but are more apparent at 48 to 72 hours. Nickerson's agar and its analogues may simplify identification of *Candida* spp. because the colonies are selectively dark, but identification in this manner is not totally reliable.

Treatment

Topical therapy for three to seven days with antifungal creams (e.g., clotrimazole, miconazole) is highly effective. In recurrent cases, risk factors should be considered, but a thorough search for subclinical diabetes mellitus is not warranted. Therapy for recurrent or intractable cases, which must be documented by laboratory tests, can be difficult. Although the gastrointestinal tract often is colonized and it has been hypothesized that such colonization acts as the source of recurrent vaginal disease, little evidence supports this position; thus, routine use of oral, nonabsorbable antifungal agents is unnecessary. Oral ketoconazole, 200 mg twice a day for five days, is useful for some recurrent or chronic cases. In some instances, intermittent premenstrual therapy has been successful.

Picture credits for this chapter are as follows: Fig. 9.5 courtesy of Dr. John Hawkinson, in Woodruff JD, Parmley TH: Atlas of Gynecologic Pathology. New York, Gower Medical Publishing, 1988; Fig. 9.27 courtesy of Spiegel CA, Amsel R, Eschenbach D, Schoenknecht F, Holmes KK: Anaerobic bacteria in nonspecific vaginitis. N Engl J Med 1980;303:601–607; Figs. 9.36B, 9.37, and 9.35 courtesy of Bingham JS: Pocket Picture Guide Series. Sexually Transmitted Diseases. London, Gower Medical Publishing Ltd., 1984.

BIBLIOGRAPHY

Amsel R, Totten PA, Spiegel CA, Chen KCS, Eschenbach D, Holmes KK: Nonspecific vaginitis: Diagnostic criteria and microbial and epidemiologic associations. Am J Med 74:14, 1983.

Bump RC, Zuspan FP, Buesching III WJ, Ayers LW, Stephens TJ: The prevalence, six month persistence, and predictive values of laboratory indicators of bacterial vaginosis (nonspecific vaginitis) in asymptomatic women. Am J Obstet Gynecol 150:917, 1984.

Chaltopadhyay B: The role of *Gardnerella vaginalis* in "non-specific" vaginitis. J Infect Dis 9:113, 1984.

Chen KCS, Amsel R, Eschenbach DA, Holmes KK: Biochemical diagnosis of vaginitis: determination of diamines in vaginal fluid. J Infect Dis 145:337, 1982.

Eschenbach DA, Hillier S, Critchlow C, Stevens C, DeRouen T, Holmes KK: Diagnosis and clinical manifestations of bacterial vaginosis. Am J Obstet Gynecol 158:819, 1988.

Gardner HL, Dukes CD: *Hemophilus vaginalis* vaginitis. Ann NY Acad Sci 83:280, 1959.

Gluperzynski Y, Labbe M, Crokaert F, Pepersack F, Van Der Auwera P, Yourassowsky E. Isolation of *Mobiluncus* in four cases of extragenital infection in adult women. Eur J Clin Microbiol 3:433, 1984.

Gravett MG, Nelson HP, DeRouen T, Critchlow C, Eschenbach DA, Holmes KK: Independent associations of bacterial vaginosis and *Chlamydia trachomatis* infection with adverse pregnancy outcome. JAMA 256:1899, 1986.

Greenwood JR: Current taxonomic status of *Gardnerella vaginalis*. Scand J Infect Dis Suppl 40:11, 1983.

Krieger JN, Tam MR, Stevens CE, et al.: Diagnosis of trichomoniasis: Comparison of conventional wet-mount examination with cytologic studies, cultures, and monoclonal antibody staining of direct specimens. JAMA 259:1223, 1988.

Lebherz TB, Ford LC: *Candida albicans* vaginitis: The problem is diagnosis, the enigma is treatment. Chemotherapy 28 (S 1):73, 1982.

Lossick JG: The diagnosis of vaginal trichomoniasis. JAMA 259:1230, 1988.

Mårdh P-A, Taylor-Robinson D (eds.): Bacterial Vaginosis. Stockholm, Sweden, Almqvist and Wiksell International, 1984.

Norrod PE, Morse SA: Presence of hydrogen peroxide in media used for cultivation of *Neisseria gonorrhoeae*. J Clin Microbiol 15:103, 1982.

O'Connor MI, Sobel JD: Epidemiology of recurrent vulvovaginal candidiasis: Identification and strain differentiation of *Candida albicans*. J Infect Dis 154:358, 1986.

Pheifer TA, Forsyth PS, Durfee MA, Pollock HM, Holmes KK: Nonspecific vaginitis: Role of *Haemophilus vaginalis* and treatment with metronidazole. N Engl J Med 298:1429, 1978.

Roberts MC, Hillier SL, Schoenknecht FD, Holmes KK: Comparison of Gram stain, DNA probe, and culture for the identification of species of *Mobiluncus* in female genital specimens. J Infect Dis 152:74, 1985.

Sobel JD: Vulvovaginal candidiasis—what we do and do not know. Ann Intern Med 101:390, 1984.

Spiegel CA, Amsel R, Eschenbach D, Schoenknecht F, Holmes KK: Anaerobic bacteria in nonspecific vaginitis. N Engl J Med 303; 601, 1980.

Spiegel CA, Amsel R, Holmes KK: Diagnosis of bacterial vaginosis by direct Gram stain of vaginal fluid. J Clin Microbiol 18:170, 1983.

Spiegel CA, Eschenbach DA, Amsel R, Holmes KK: Curved anaerobic bacteria in bacterial (nonspecific) vaginosis and their response to antimicrobial therapy. J Infect Dis 148:817, 1983.

Spiegel CA, Roberts M: *Mobiluncus* gen. nov., *Mobiluncus curtissi* subsp. *curtissi* sp. nov., *Mobiluncus curtissi* subsp. *holmesii* subsp. nov., and *Mobiluncus mulieris* sp. nov., curved rods from the human vagina. Int J Sys Bacteriol 34:177, 1984.

Thomason JL, Schreckenberger PC, Spellacy WN, Riff LJ, LeBeau LJ: Clinical and microbiological characterization of patients with nonspecific vaginosis associated with motile, curved anaerobic rods. J Infect Dis 149:801, 1984.

Totten PA, Amsel R, Hale J, Piot P, Holmes KK: Selective differential human blood bilayer media for isolation of *Gardnerella vaginalis*. J Clin Microbiol 15:141, 1982.

Venkataramani TK, Rathbun HK: *Corynebacterium vaginale* (*Hemophilus vaginalis*) bacteremia: Clinical study of 29 cases. Johns Hopkins Med J 139:93, 1976.

Weston TET, Nicol CS: Natural history of trichomonal infection in males. Brit J Vener Dis 39:251, 1963.

Wilson A, Ackers JP: Urine culture for the detection of *Trichomonas vaginalis* in men. Brit J Vener Dis 56:46, 1980.

Genital Human Papillomavirus Infections

10

A.A. MORELAND, K. STONE, B. MAJMUDAR

Introduction

Infection of the human genital tract with the human papillomavirus (HPV) is one of the most common sexually transmitted viral diseases. Genital warts (venereal warts, condylomata acuminata, fig warts) have long been recognized, but until recently were considered trivial; sexual transmission has even been questioned. Current understanding of this infection requires recognition that condylomata acuminata are only the most obvious manifestation of HPV infections of the anogenital region. A large body of evidence now supports the concept that subclinical HPV infections are much more common than was previously recognized. Additionally, current diagnosis and management of HPV infections must address the fact that some HPV types are frequently associated with squamous atypia and less frequently with invasive carcinoma of the anogenital tract.

The HPV is a 55-nm DNA virus that belongs to the papovavirus family (Fig. 10.1). It infects the skin and mucous membranes and replicates in the nuclei of infected epithelial cells. Production of the capsid antigens and virion assembly that are necessary for infectivity occur almost exclusively within the nuclei of the superficial layer of cells. The many clinically distinct variants correlate to a certain degree with the different HPV types identified by differences in DNA sequences. At least 12 of the more than 46 types of HPV have been described in lesions of the genital tract (Fig. 10.2). The HPV is very difficult to propagate and is not transmissible to other species. Inoculation experiments at the turn of the century and electron-microscopic evidence from 30 years ago offered the first direct and reproducible evidence of the viral etiology of condylomata. Recently, antigen detection using immunoperoxidase staining and molecular hybridization techniques has been used to confirm the presence of virus in tissues.

Epidemiology

Although cases of genital warts are not routinely reported, several limited surveys suggest that prevalence has increased in recent years (Fig. 10.3). A trend in increasing incidence has also been noted in a population-based study. New visits to private physicians' offices (Fig. 10.4) and many public STD clinics for genital warts outnumber those for genital herpes. Risk factors for genital warts or subclinical HPV infection have not been well studied, but probably differ from those for gonorrhea.

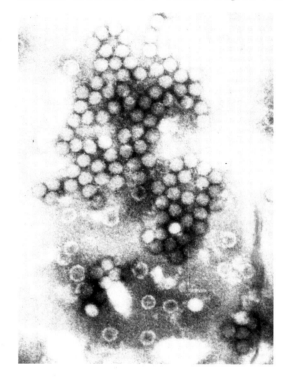

Figure 10.1
Electron micrograph of HPV (negative stain, phosphotungstic acid). The HPV has an icosahedral capsid 55 nm in diameter.

MOST FREQUENT CLINICAL MANIFESTATIONS OF COMMON HPV TYPES

HPV TYPE	GENITAL LESIONS
6,11	Anogenital condylomata
16,18,31,42	Bowenoid papulosis, vulvar intraepithelial neoplasia, Bowen's disease
6,11,16,18,31, 33,35	Cervical intraepithelial neoplasia, dysplasias of genital mucosa
16,18,31,33,35	Invasive cancer

Figure 10.2   HPV types frequently associated with genital lesions.

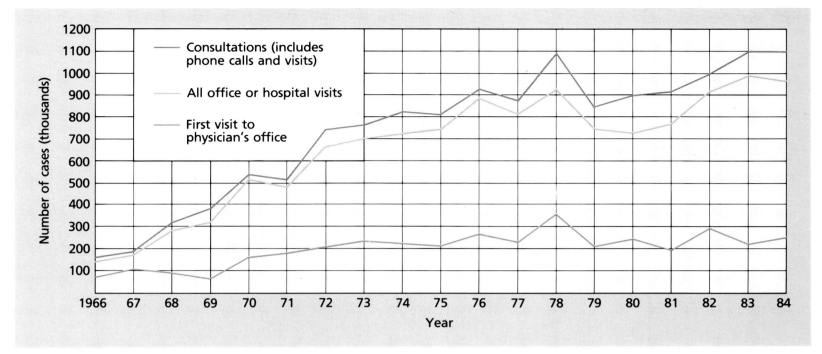

Figure 10.3 Visits to private physicians for genital warts. Genital warts are being diagnosed with increasing frequency in the United States. Total consultations (including telephone calls) increased seven-fold between 1966 and 1984. First visits—a more likely indicator of new cases—increased three-fold.

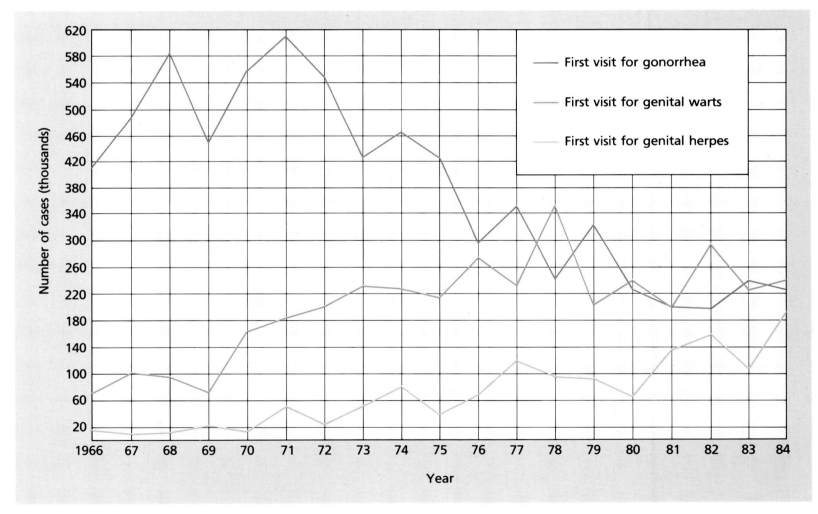

Figure 10.4 Comparison of visits to private physicians for warts, herpes, and gonorrhea. In recent years, new visits to private physicians for genital warts outnumber those for genital herpes or gonorrhea. However, new visits to many public STD clinics for gonorrhea greatly outnumber those for genital warts.

Genital warts are most commonly seen in persons aged 20 to 24 and appear to be more common in whites than blacks. Use of oral contraceptives and cigarette smoking may also be associated risk factors.

Cervical HPV infection is almost always asymptomatic and is much more common than clinically apparent genital warts. Many women with genital warts have coexistent cervical infection. In the U.S. and Canada, 0.5 to 3% of routine screening Papanicolaou smears show evidence of HPV infection, and prevalence generally decreases with age. However, prevalence is much higher in the few STD clinic populations that have been studied, where approximately 10% of women have cytologic evidence of HPV infection. If a battery of diagnostic tests for HPV infection (colposcopy or cervicography, DNA hybridization, and immunoperoxidase staining) is employed in addition to cytology, this prevalence increases to 20 to 30%. Asymptomatic penile HPV infection has been studied less extensively than cervical infection. Histologically confirmed HPV infection diagnosed clinically by the presence of warts or acetowhite epithelium has been observed in 60 to 90% of male partners of women with cervical HPV infection or cervical intraepithelial neoplasia (CIN). The significance of acetowhite penile lesions is not well understood, and diagnostic and morphologic criteria have not been established.

Although genital warts were recognized as an STD in ancient times, the medical community has accepted this mode of transmission only in the last 15 years. Congenital transmission from mother to baby, causing juvenile laryngeal papillomatosis and oral and skin condylomata, has been documented. In recent years, it has been shown that the specific HPV types that cause warts in the genital area differ from those responsible for warts on the hands and feet.

The average incubation period between HPV infection and clinical appearance of a genital wart is 3 months. Limited studies have shown that 60 to 66% of sexual partners of persons with genital warts will also develop genital warts within 3 months; however, the additional percentage of partners who will become subclinically infected is unknown (Fig. 10.5).

NATURAL HISTORY AND ASSOCIATION WITH CANCER

The natural history of genital warts and subclinical HPV infection has not been well established. Warts may persist or recur despite treatment, may regress spontaneously, or, rarely, may undergo presumed malignant transformation. Cervical HPV infection appears to have a similar spectrum of behavior, although subsequent development of malignant precursors is not a rare event. Limited studies suggest that as many as 10% of women with cervical HPV infections will develop CIN within a year.

The epidemiology of cervical and other genital cancers is consistent with a sexually transmissible infectious etiology, and HPV meets several criteria for oncogenicity. Although mounting evidence suggests a strong association between HPV and genital dysplasia and cancer, a causal role has not been established (Fig. 10.6). Papillomaviruses are known to produce tumors in animals, and certain types are capable of transforming normal cells to neoplastic cells in vitro. Integration of HPV DNA into the genome of the host cell is usually observed only in invasive carcinomas and cervical carcinoma cell lines, whereas in benign and premalignant lesions the HPV DNA is usually extrachromosomal. Certain types of HPV DNA—especially types 16, 18, and 31—have been found in all types of genital cancers and cancer precursors. However, many clinically and microscopically normal tissues harbor HPV DNA. Epidemiologic studies show that women with cytologic evidence of HPV have an increased risk of cervical dysplasia and cancer. Prospective studies are needed to show whether HPV infection actually precedes the development of dysplasia or cancer and to investigate the role of HPV infection as a cofactor rather than the sole etiologic agent.

Clinical Manifestations

The spectrum of HPV-associated conditions in the anogenital region ranges from the typical papillomas of condylomata acuminata found on the external genitalia, perineum, and vaginal, cervical, perianal, and urethral mucosa to clinically inapparent

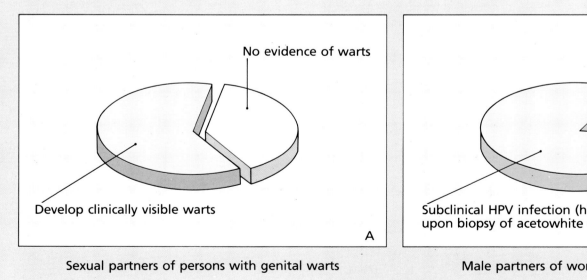

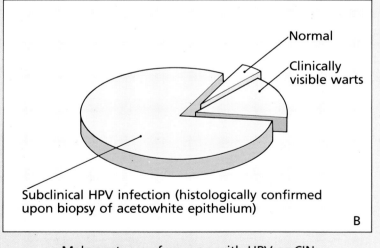

Sexual partners of persons with genital warts   **Male partners of women with HPV or CIN**

Figure 10.5 Transmission of HPV infection. Although only two-thirds of sexual partners of patients with genital warts develop genital warts within 3 months, many more may be infected subclinically. Limited studies suggest as many as 90% of partners are infected, yet only a small fraction have clinically apparent warts.

infection of the same areas. Additionally, HPV has been found in vulvar, vaginal, and penile carcinoma in situ or intraepithelial neoplasia, including bowenoid papulosis, CIN, and invasive carcinoma of the genital tract.

CONDYLOMATA ACUMINATA

These flesh-colored papillomatous pedunculated or sessile growths occur anywhere on the vulvar, penile, scrotal, perineal, or perianal skin or in the urethra (Fig. 10.7). They may be smooth but usually have fingerlike projections that cause them to have a rough surface—thus the term *condylomata acuminata* (*condylomata*, knuckles; *acuminata*, pointed) (Fig. 10.8). Single lesions usually range from 1 to 4 mm in diameter and from 2 to 15 mm in height. Multiple papules may become confluent, plaquelike, or multilobed masses (Fig. 10.9). Spread of the infection can result in an increase in the number of warts, in the size of individual warts, or both. In some cases, the size of large plaques or masses may reach several centimeters (Fig. 10.10). Condylomata may become so large as to cause deformity of normal structures. These large lesions are sometimes called

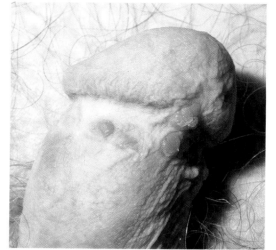

Figure 10.7 Condylomata acuminata—penile. Asymptomatic, flesh-colored papules present on the shaft of the penis.

EVIDENCE LINKING HPV WITH CIN AND CERVICAL CANCER

Epidemiology suggests a sexually transmissible infectious etiology of CIN and cervical cancer

40 to 95% of cases of CIN contain HPV DNA

80 to 90% of cases of invasive cancer contain HPV DNA

Cervical HPV increases risk of CIN and cervical cancer

Figure 10.6 Evidence linking HPV with CIN and cervical cancer.

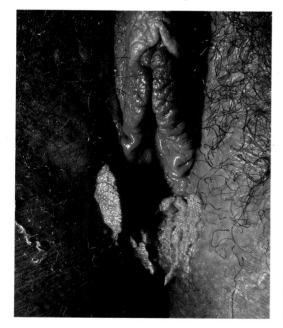

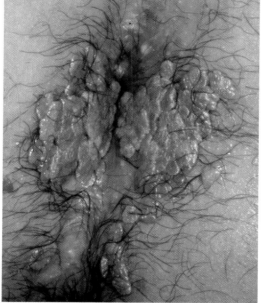

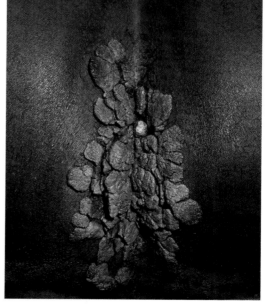

Figure 10.8 Condylomata acuminata—vulvar. The rough, corrugated surface is characteristic and papillary projections may form as seen here.

Figure 10.9 Condylomata acuminata—perianal. Both discrete and confluent masses of condylomata are present. The large size may result in irritation or other secondary symptoms.

Figure 10.10 Condylomata acuminata—perianal. Treatment of these large, recurrent warts was complicated by poor compliance with office follow-ups by the patient.

giant condylomata of Buschke and Löwenstein (Fig. 10.11). Obstruction by condylomata of the urethral meatus is not infrequent in males. In males, condylomata occur earliest near the frenulum of the penis and are most frequent on the coronal sulcus, the shaft (Fig. 10.12), and the preputial borders (Fig. 10.13). In females, earliest lesions are seen most often around the introitus and frequently on the fourchette and labia, but condylomata may be present on any part of the vulva (Fig. 10.14). In at least 20% of women, the perineum and perianal skin are also involved (Fig. 10.15). The natal cleft is another frequently missed site, especially in obese patients.

FLAT WARTS (CONDYLOMATA PLANA)

Flat warts appear on the vulva or penis as flesh-colored or hypopigmented, nearly invisible flat papules (Fig. 10.16). Application of 3 to 5% acetic acid enhances visualization of this subclinical form of infection (Figs. 10.17 and 10.18). Examination of the acetowhite areas with a colposcope or hand lens improves diagnostic accuracy and recognition of flat warts, but the specificity is unknown. Acetowhitening may occur in other conditions such as intraepithelial neoplasia, as well as in histologically unremarkable tissue (Fig. 10.19). When the vulva is extensively involved, large confluent whitened areas appear af-

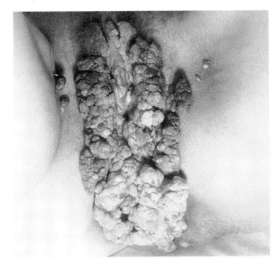

Figure 10.11 Condylomata acuminata—vulva and perineum. The clinical diagnosis was giant condylomata of Buschke and Löwenstein. Such large and confluent lesions should be carefully examined and multiple biopsies obtained to rule out underlying malignancy.

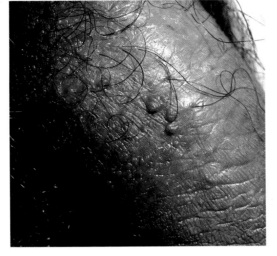

Figure 10.12 Condylomata acuminata—penile shaft. Very early lesions may be difficult to see.

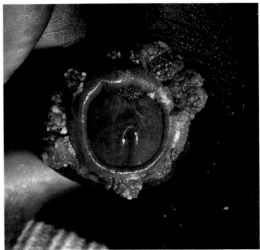

Figure 10.13 Condylomata acuminata—preputial borders. These lesions had become secondarily infected due to the occlusion of the foreskin.

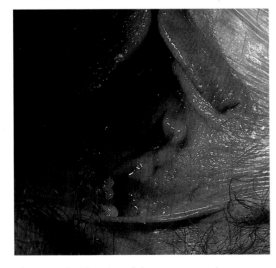

Figure 10.14 Condylomata acuminata—vulvar introitus. These small papules seen at the fourchette are nearly invisible to the examiner and asymptomatic to the patient.

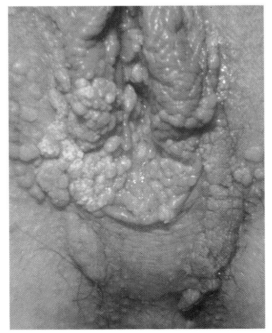

Figure 10.15 Condylomata acuminata—vulva and perineum. This patient has extensive involvement around the introitus and the labia with extension onto the perineum and perianal region.

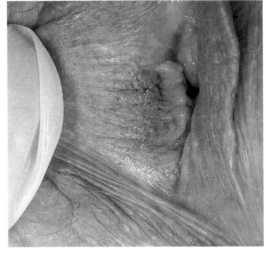

Figure 10.16 Condylomata plana—vulvar. Use of 3% acetic acid enhances visualization of these difficult-to-see flat vulvar warts on the labia minora.

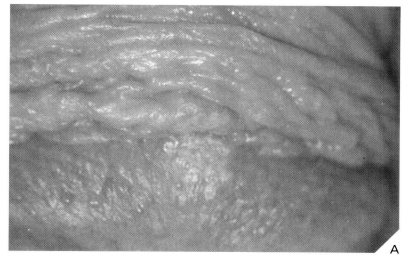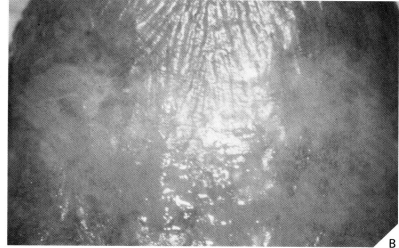

Figure 10.17 A and **B** Acetowhite penile lesions. Penile skin after application of 3 to 5% acetic acid showing areas of "acetowhitening," representing histologically confirmed subclinical HPV infection. Without use of acetic acid and a magnifying lens, these lesions were not clinically apparent.

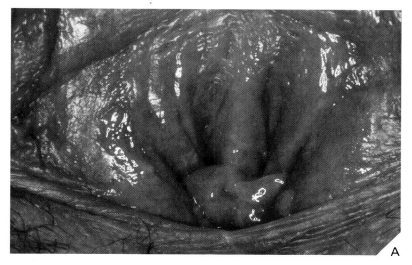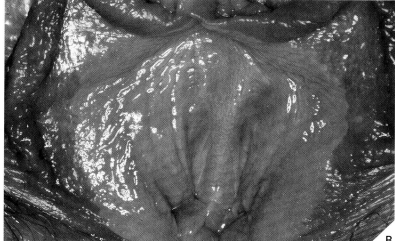

Figure 10.18 Acetowhitened vulva. **A** External vulvar skin appearing normal before application of 3 to 5% acetic acid. **B** This is the same vulvar skin after application of acetic acid. The entire area proximal to Hart's line (demarcation of keratinized and unkeratinized stratified squamous epithelium) appears "acetowhite." Acetowhitening is one sign of subclinical HPV infection; however, its specificity is not known.

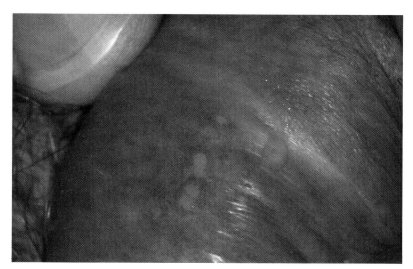

Figure 10.19 Carcinoma in situ—penis. These flat penile papules appear white after acetic acid application and biopsy showed carcinoma in situ. All lesions that are suspicious, clinically atypical, or unresponsive to initial treatment should be biopsied to rule out premalignant and malignant changes.

ter the acetic acid-soaked gauze is removed from the area. Vaginal warts are not seen as commonly as cervical or vulvar warts. They may have a spiked appearance, but also may be flat or invisible to the naked eye.

BOWENOID PAPULOSIS

A specific clinicopathologic entity termed *bowenoid papulosis* was described by Wade et al in 1979. These flat, multicentric papules, often seen in young people, histologically resemble carcinoma in situ but may be indistinguishable clinically from condylomata acuminata. In males, they are usually multiple and are erythematous, hyperpigmented, or flesh-colored papules scattered along the shaft or glans of the penis (Fig. 10.20). In females, the vulva and perineum are the sites of this typically multifocal disease (Fig. 10.21). The natural history of these lesions appears to be benign, but the disease may persist for years and in some cases spontaneously regress. The lesions are reported to be associated with HPV types 16 and 18, specific types known for their oncogenic potential. Well-documented reports of progression to invasive carcinoma, however, are very rare. These lesions may be interspersed within groups of condylomata acuminata and be indistinguishable from them. Other forms of intraepithelial neoplasia of the penis and vulva (e.g., Bowen's disease) that do not resemble condylomata are also associated with HPV, usually types 16, 18, or 31. They appear as hyperkeratotic or whitish plaques or papules that are usually visible without acetic acid. The risk of conversion to invasive carcinoma has been reported in less than half of these cases.

CERVICAL HPV INFECTIONS

Cervical HPV infections similarly may have various presentations: from invisible "flat condylomata" (subclinical infection) to "spiked," exophytic, or florid papillomata. All are associated with the presence of HPV particles (Fig. 10.22). The exophytic condylomata with a rough acuminate appearance are white, gray, or red and may be hyperkeratotic or secondarily infected and ulcerated. Flat condylomata are most common and often occur in great numbers, but they may be invisible without colposcopy along with 3 to 5% acetic acid application. Although colposcopic criteria have not been standardized, certain morphologic features such as color, margin contour, vascular pattern, and iodine staining appear to be useful in distinguishing cervical HPV infection from dysplasia or other cervical abnormalities. Cervicography is a recently developed screening tool

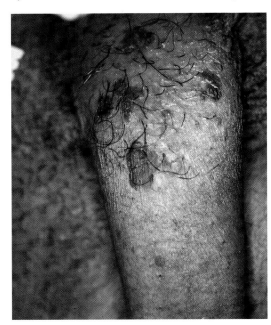

Figure 10.20 Bowenoid papulosis—penis. These large, hyperpigmented, flat papules on the shaft of the penis were asymptomatic. Biopsy to rule out carcinoma in situ is essential in such cases.

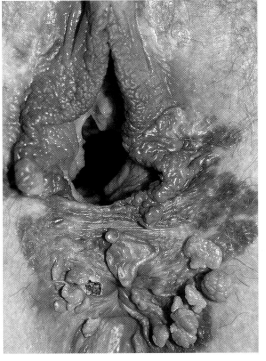

Figure 10.21 Bowenoid papulosis—vulvar and perineal. Although these lesions clinically resemble condylomata, multiple pigmented papular lesions in a young woman should raise the possibility of bowenoid papulosis, and biopsies should be obtained.

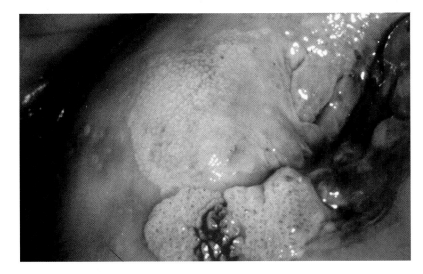

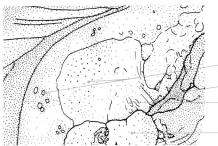

Subclinical HPV infection

Cervical os

Cervical intraepithelial neoplasia

Exophytic condyloma

Figure 10.22 Colpophotograph of cervix showing an exophytic condyloma, an area of subclinical HPV infection, and an area of high-grade CIN. Differentiation of these lesions is difficult and should be attempted only by experienced colposcopists.

that involves taking a photograph of the cervix through a special lens for subsequent interpretation (Fig. 10.23). Preliminary evaluation suggests that cervicography has a higher sensitivity than the Papanicolaou smear in the detection of HPV and CIN.

DIFFERENTIAL DIAGNOSIS

Condylomata acuminata ordinarily present a distinct and easily recognized clinical picture. However, the clinician should be familiar with some of the other common entities in the differential diagnosis. The most common of these are discussed briefly here; for a more detailed discussion the reader is referred to Chapter 12. Verrucae vulgaris—usually caused by HPV types

2, 3, and 4—may occur in or near the genital region, especially on skin of the lower abdomen, upper thigh, or buttocks (Fig. 10.24). A thickened, dry, hyperkeratotic appearance is more typical of verrucae vulgaris, but differentation of the two entities may require histopathologic examination. Treatment is similar to that for condylomata acuminata.

The umbilicated papules of molluscum contagiosum infection frequently resemble condylomata acuminata and appear in the genital region in sexually active patients (Fig. 10.25). The umbilication of the papules helps distinguish them from condylomata acuminata, but crusting or other secondary changes may obscure this helpful feature. This pox virus infection trans-

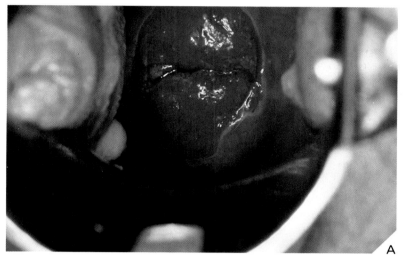
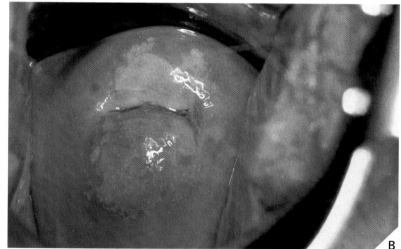

A

B

Figure 10.23 A Cervigram showing normal cervix, including the transformation zone. B Cervigram showing an area of acetowhitening with irregular borders, which is typical of subclinical HPV infec-

tion of the cervix. Cervicography may prove to be a useful adjunct to the Papanicolaou smear for cervical cancer screening.

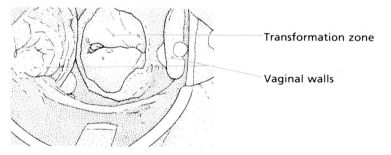

Transformation zone

Vaginal walls

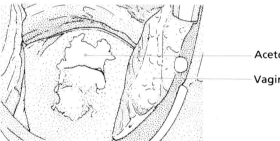

Acetowhitening

Vaginal wall

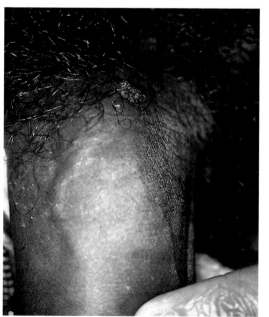

Figure 10.24
Verruca vulgaris—penis. This raised, rough papule at the base of the penis appeared similar to condylomata acuminata but proved to be verruca vulgaris on biopsy.

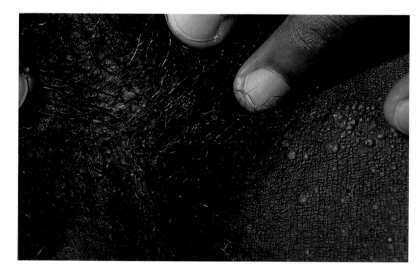

Figure 10.25 Molluscum contagiosum—inguinal. The characteristic umbilicated papules are typically asymptomatic but may become secondarily infected, crusted, or pruritic.

mitted by sexual and nonsexual routes is usually self-limited but may be progressive in immunocompromised patients. It can easily be diagnosed by its characteristic inclusions seen on cytologic or histologic examination. Treatment should be conservative.

Seborrheic keratoses are rough and usually brown or black hyperpigmented, flat, broad papules. They have a waxy texture and minute puncta on the surface. These benign tumors may be multiple and are treated only for cosmetic reasons.

Condylomata lata of secondary syphilis must always be considered when condylomata acuminata are present (Fig. 10.26). The two entities may not only look remarkably similar but may coexist, as patients with multiple sexual partners frequently are exposed to and become infected with more than one STD at a time. Condylomata lata, however, are typically more moist than condylomata acuminata and may even be ulcerated. In condylomata lata, dark-field examination almost always demonstrates spirochetes and syphilis serology is invariably reactive. Skin tags (acrochordons) and pearly penile papules may also be confused with condylomata acuminata. Hemorrhoids may look like pedunculated condylomata acuminata, but they have a smooth, rather than rough, surface. They may also bleed

and be tender; these features are rare in condylomata acuminata.

Bowen's disease of the vulva may also appear verrucous but is usually a flat, velvety, gray-white plaque with surrounding erythema that may be pruritic or otherwise symptomatic (Fig. 10.27). Ulceration is not rare. Giant condylomata of Buschke and Löwenstein, slowly growing lesions of uncertain malignant potential, resemble condylomata acuminata; in fact, HPV has been found associated with this tumor. Proper biopsies are mandatory to rule out malignancy in recalcitrant or exceptionally large and confluent condylomata.

Laboratory Tests

Diagnosis of typical condylomata acuminata is made primarily on clinical appearance aided by application of acetic acid and use of magnifying lenses. Clinical diagnoses should be confirmed by histology and cytology whenever necessary. Additional tools for the detection of viral antigens and viral DNA that are used primarily in research are immunohistochemical and hybridization techniques. These diagnostic techniques are

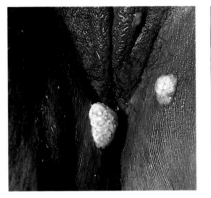

Figure 10.26 Condylomata lata—perineal and upper thigh. The rough texture of these papules mimics condylomata acuminata. Dark-field examination and serology were positive in this case of secondary syphilis.

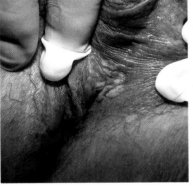

Figure 10.27 Bowen's disease of the vulva. This white plaque has well-defined borders and slight ulceration. Biopsy was diagnostic of Bowen's disease.

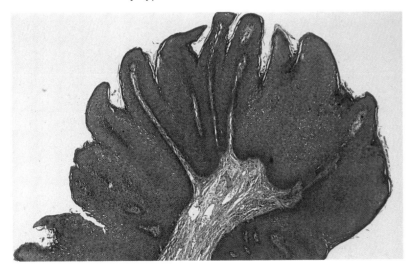

Figure 10.29 Anogenital condylomata. Histologic preparation of condyloma showing hyperkeratotic squamous epithelium with multiple papillary fronds. This appearance of condyloma is diagnostic, irrespective of anatomic site.

DIAGNOSIS OF HPV INFECTIONS AND LIMITATIONS OF VARIOUS METHODS

DIAGNOSTIC TESTS	PRACTICAL LIMITATIONS
Inspection/magnifying lens	May not detect subclinical infection
Cytology	Insensitive; sampling error
Histology	Invasive; differentiation of condylomatous atypia from CIN is difficult
Colposcopy, urethroscopy, anoscopy	Differentiation from dysplasia is difficult
Cervicography	Not well studied; not widely available
DNA hybridization	Not widely available; time-consuming and expensive
Southern blot	Fresh tissue required; most specific hybridization method
Dot blot	Fresh tissue required; specific
In situ (tissue)	Insensitive and less specific
In situ (filter)	Fresh tissue required; least specific hybridization method
Immunoperoxidase stain	Specific for antigens not present in malignant lesions; insensitive
Electron microscopy	Not practical; insensitive; time-consuming
Serology	Specific test for genital infection not available
Culture	Not available

Figure 10.28 Diagnosis of HPV infections and limitations of various methods.

particularly useful in those cases of HPV infection that are not readily visible by clinical means. Successful techniques for propagating HPV recently have been reported, but in vitro cultures are not available for routine diagnostic work. Serologic testing is not useful in diagnosis (Figure 10.28).

HISTOPATHOLOGY
Condylomata Acuminata
In anogenital condylomata, the most obvious histologic changes are papillomatosis and acanthosis of the malpighian layer. The dermal papillae are usually elongated, narrow, and branching in a pattern of a pseudoepitheliomatous hyperplasia (Fig. 10.29). The most characteristic feature, according to Lever, is the presence of "koilocytes" in the upper stratum malpighii, stratum granulosum, and stratum corneum. These are large, epithelial cells with small or large, dense, irregular, crumpled-looking nuclei (Fig. 10.30). Because cytoplasmic organelles congregate at the periphery of the cell and the remainder of the cytoplasm is clear, a "halo" in the perinuclear area can be seen. In addition, many mitotic figures and multinucleated and dyskeratotic cells may be present (Fig. 10.31). Hyperplasia of the parabasal cells may be present beneath the atypical cells. Orthokeratosis and parakeratosis are common. Chronic inflammatory cells and dilated capillaries and edema are usually present in the dermis.

Cervical Condylomata
Hyperkeratosis, acanthosis, and cellular atypia create a similar overall architectural pattern in the exophytic condylomata (Fig. 10.32). Papillomatosis is absent in the flat condylomata except for occasional small peaks of superficial epithelium. Koilocytosis seen in the upper layers of the cervical mucosa is a characteristic finding of flat cervical condylomata. A significant amount of cellular atypia may accompany these changes, thus mimicking CIN. It is often difficult to distinguish between condylomatous atypia and true CIN. In general, the former is seen in the superficial layers and the latter in the deeper layers of the epithelium. It is common to see both components together in a cervical biopsy.

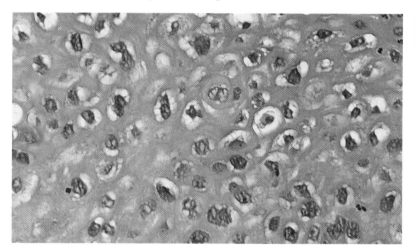

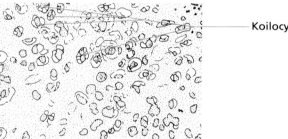

Figure 10.30 Anogenital condylomata. Histologic examination shows multiple large cells with clear cytoplasm and atypical wrinkled nuclei. These cells, called koilocytes, suggest HPV infection.

Koilocytes

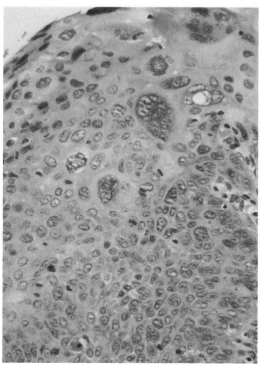

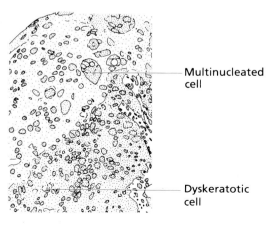

Multinucleated cell

Dyskeratotic cell

Figure 10.31 Cervical condyloma. Histologic examination of condyloma may show large, extremely atypical nuclei. These changes do not necessarily indicate malignancy. Condylomatous atypia and premalignant dysplastic changes are often difficult to distinguish by histologic examination alone.

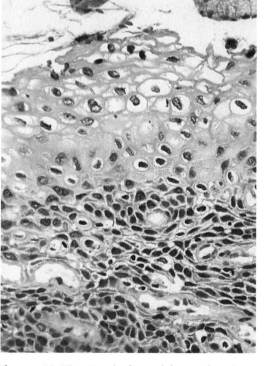

Figure 10.32 Cervical condyloma showing large, vacuolated koilocytes in the superficial layers of the mucosa.

Bowenoid Papulosis

Hyperkeratosis, parakeratosis, and psoriasiform epidermal hyperplasia with a focally prominent granular zone are accompanied by crowding of epidermal nuclei, increased mitotic figures of the upper half of the epidermis, and atypical mitotic figures (Fig. 10.33). Necrotic and large multinucleated keratinocytes may be present. Keratinocytes with hyperchromatic and pleomorphic nuclei also are characteristically present and produce a pattern of squamous cell carcinoma in situ (Fig. 10.34). Koilocytosis may be present, but is less prominent than in classic forms of condylomata. Skin adnexa are generally spared from the process, and the confluent growth pattern of the proliferating epithelium is not seen.

CYTOLOGY

The Papanicolaou smear is the most commonly used means of detecting asymptomatic cervical HPV infections, but it is relatively insensitive and subject to sampling error. Viral atypia and koilocytosis are characteristic cytologic features of cervical HPV infection. Koilocytosis is considered fairly specific for HPV infection (Fig. 10.35). Koilocytes have an irregular, hyperchromatic nucleus surrounded by a clear, cytoplasmic halo, which,

in turn, is surrounded by peripherally located dense cytoplasm. Diagnosis of HPV infection is further suggested by other cytologic findings such as dyskeratocytosis, multinucleation, anucleation, and parakeratosis. The association of these changes with HPV has been confirmed by immunoperoxidase and electron-microscopic studies of the same tissues.

DEMONSTRATION OF VIRUS

Because HPV cannot routinely be propagated in tissue culture, specific viral diagnosis requires detection of viral proteins or DNA. However, these types of tests are not yet widely available. In the absence of a "gold standard" reference test for comparison, the sensitivity and specificity of these methods have not been determined. Each test is relatively insensitive when used alone.

DNA Hybridization

Nucleic acid hybridization identifies a specific HPV DNA type by using a DNA or RNA "probe" made from a known type of HPV (Fig. 10.36). The probe is obtained by cloning the known HPV DNA in a bacteriophage, denaturing it into single strands, and then radioactively labeling it. Cellular and viral (if present)

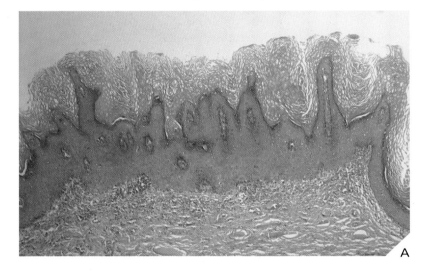

A

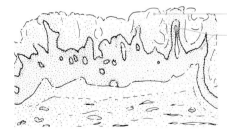

Hyperkeratosis
Papillomatosis

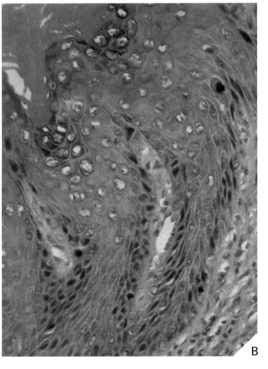

B

Figure 10.33
Bowenoid papulosis of the vulva. **A** Hyperkeratotic benign squamous epithelium with multiple papillary projections. **B** Same tissue at a higher magnification to show hyperkeratosis, papillomatosis, and reactive atypia of the squamous epithelium. The superficial layers of the epidermis show atypical cells with large, empty-looking nuclei suggesting a viral infection.

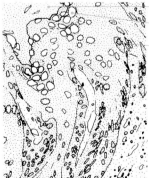

Hyperkeratosis
Vacuolated cells
Dyskeratosis

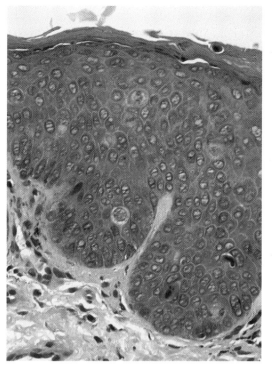

Figure 10.34 Bowenoid papulosis of the vulva. Histologic examination showing the presence of hyperchromatic nuclei, multiple mitoses, and disruption of the maturation sequence imparting a carcinoma in situ appearance to the epidermis.

Hyperkeratosis

Mitoses

Hyperchromatic nuclei

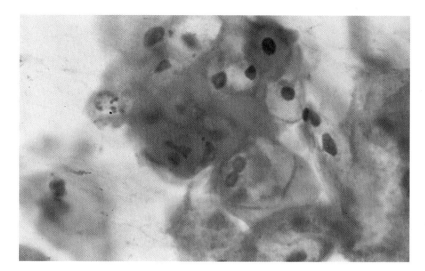

Figure 10.35 Koilocyte and superficial desquamated epithelial cells on Papanicolaou smear. The koilocyte is the cell with the perinuclear halo. It is a relatively specific yet insensitive diagnostic indicator of HPV infection.

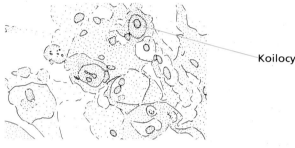

Koilocyte

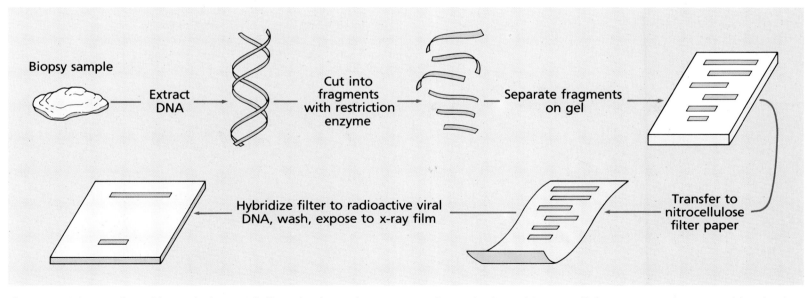

Biopsy sample → Extract DNA → Cut into fragments with restriction enzyme → Separate fragments on gel → Transfer to nitrocellulose filter paper → Hybridize filter to radioactive viral DNA, wash, expose to x-ray film

Figure 10.36 Southern blot technique. Of all methods used to detect HPV DNA, this one is the most specific. DNA from patient specimens is cleaved into small fragments and separated by size before allowing the known DNA probe to attach.

DNA is extracted from tissue specimens and denatured, then mixed with the nucleic acid probe. In Southern blot hybridization, the homologous DNA strands combine (anneal) to form radioactive double-stranded DNA, which is visualized by autoradiography (Fig. 10.37). The various methods of hybridization differ mainly in the way the DNA from the patient specimen is extracted and purified; therefore, they vary widely in sensitivity and specificity.

The "Southern blot" and "dot blot" are popular nucleic acid hybridization techniques that require extraction of DNA from fresh tissue. DNA is not extracted from cells for "in situ" methods of hybridization. Tissue in situ hybridization (TISH) employs biotinylated probes to give a colorimetric reaction and may be performed on cytologic smears or formalin-fixed and paraffin-embedded tissues (Fig. 10.38); automation may become available. Cellular detail and localization of the hybridized DNA within the architecture of the tissue are the advantages to this method, but it is less sensitive than the Southern blot method.

Filter in situ hybridization (FISH) is a new technique in which whole cells are collected on filter paper and then denatured; this method is quicker and more sensitive but less specific than the Southern blot technique.

Immunoperoxidase Stain

Immunoperoxidase staining of cells or tissues directly detects HPV capsid antigen. In this technique, commercially prepared antibodies (directed against disrupted virions) are attached to an enzyme (peroxidase) that will yield a colored reaction product. Immunoperoxidase stains may be performed on tissues (Fig. 10.39A) or cytologic smears (Fig. 10.39B); however, this method is even less sensitive than routine cytologic examination. Because only viruses that are actively proliferating produce capsid antigens, tissues that stain positively are considered infectious. The likelihood of detecting capsid antigen decreases with increasing severity of dysplasia, and immunoperoxidase stains are invariably negative in genital cancers that contain HPV DNA.

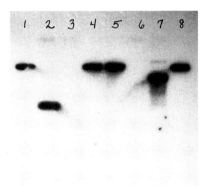
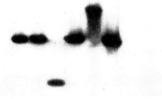

Figure 10.37 Southern blot hybridization of DNA fragments from patient specimens on nitrocellulose filter paper. Migration patterns of DNA in the numbered lanes are compared with known standards ("fingerprints") of specific types of HPV DNA. The intensity of the black spot roughly indicates the amount of DNA present.

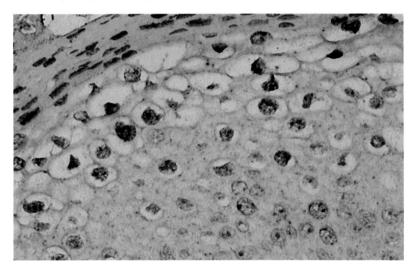

Figure 10.38 Tissue in situ hybridization of biotinylated HPV type 11 DNA to formalin-fixed, paraffin-embedded vulvar condyloma. Dark brown-black signal over nuclei indicates presence of HPV DNA. Signal is strongest at surface in koilocytic cells and decreases toward basal layer. However, many nonkoilocytes also demonstrate positive hybridization indicating infection.

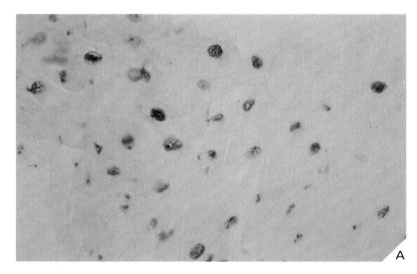

A

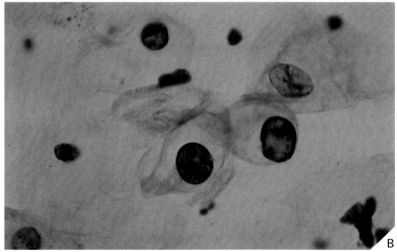

B

Figure 10.39 Immunoperoxidase stain. **A** Tissue and **B** cytologic smear containing HPV identified by the immunoperoxidase method, which stains the intranuclear capsid antigen brown. Capsid antigen is generally found only in the superficial layers of tissue. Presence of capsid antigen indicates infectiousness.

SEROLOGY

Currently, serologic diagnosis is not feasible since antibodies to genital types of HPV cannot reliably be distinguished from those produced in response to nongenital warts.

ELECTRON MICROSCOPY

Electron microscopy is extremely time-consuming and insensitive compared with other diagnostic methods. Genital wart tissues contain only 1/10,000 as many virions as common skin warts; therefore, electron microscopy is not a practical procedure for diagnosis.

Treatment

Treatment of genital warts may be frustrating since it often requires multiple office visits and recurrence is quite common. HPV has been recovered from seemingly uninvolved margins of surgical resection of condylomata, perhaps accounting for some clinical recurrences of the lesion. Recurrence results from failure to completely eradicate all HPV-containing epithelial cells or from reinfection by infected sexual partners. Local treatment entails application of antimetabolites or caustic agents (e.g., podophyllin, trichloroacetic acid, or 5-fluorouracil), cryotherapy, electrodesiccation, or surgical removal. Patients with internal (intraurethral, rectal, cervical, vaginal) warts should be referred to appropriate specialists for treatment. All women with warts should have a Papanicolaou smear to rule out coexistent CIN. Although laser surgery is being used commonly, its efficacy compared with that of other methods has not been established. A serious drawback of laser therapy could be the destruction of the lesion without any histologic evaluation to rule out malignancy. When condylomata are large, confluent, necrotic, and rapidly growing, and the patient is old or immunoincompetent, the lesion should be properly biopsied before being treated by laser or any other locally destructive therapy. These patients should also be carefully followed. Intralesional and intramuscular injection of interferon has limited efficacy and significant adverse side-effects. Current research studies are investigating local use of 5-fluorouracil cream to suppress recurrences after eradication with other methods. The necessity for treatment of all persons with subclinical infection has not been established.

Treatment of bowenoid papulosis or other clinical forms of genital intraepithelial neoplasia should be referred to dermatologists or gynecologists familiar with these entities. Superficial destruction or excision is frequently curative. Because of reports of spontaneous remission, low malignant potential, and the possibility of surrounding latent infection, extensive or mutilating surgical procedures are not recommended, but close follow-up with biopsies is mandatory.

Picture credits for this chapter are as follows: Fig. 10.15 courtesy of Woodruff JD, Parmley TH: Atlas of Gynecologic Pathology. New York, Gower Medical Publishing, 1988; Fig. 10.16 courtesy of Marilynne McKay, MD; Figs. 10.17 and 10.19 courtesy of Michael Campion, MD; Figs. 10.18, 10.22, and 10.23A courtesy of Richard Reid, MD; Figs. 10.20 and 10.24 courtesy of Heidi Watts, PA-C; Fig. 10.21 courtesy of D.R. Popkin, MD; Fig. 10.23B courtesy of National Testing Laboratories Inc.; Figs. 10.29 to 10.31 and 10.34 courtesy of J. Michael Hall, DDS; Fig. 10.38 courtesy of Beth Unger, MD; Fig. 10.39B courtesy of Nancy Kiviat, MD.

BIBLIOGRAPHY

Beckmann AM, Myerson D, Daling JR, et al: Detection and localization of human papillomavirus DNA in human genital condylomas by in situ hybridization with biotinylated probes. J Med Virol 16:265, 1985.

Bonfiglio TA, Stoler MH: Human papillomavirus and cancer of the uterine cervix. Human Pathol 19:621, 1988.

Ferenczy A, Mitao M, Nagai N, et al: Latent papillomavirus and recurring genital warts. N Engl J Med 313:784, 1985.

Gissmann L, de Villiers EM, zur Hausen H: Analysis of human genital warts (condylomata acuminata) and other genital tumors for human papillomavirus type 6 DNA. Int J Cancer 29:143, 1982.

Gross G, Hagedorn M, Ikenberg, H, et al: Bowenoid papulosis. Arch Dermatol 121:858, 1985.

Grubb G: Human papillomavirus and cervical neoplasia: Epidemiological considerations. Int J Epidemiol 15:1, 1986.

Guijon FB, Paraskeras M, Brunham R, et al: The association of sexually transmitted diseases with cervical intraepithelial neoplasia: A case-control study. Am J Obstet Gynecol 151:185, 1985.

Howley PM: On human papillomaviruses, editorial. N Engl J Med 315:1089, 1986.

Jenson AB, Kurman RJ, Lancaster WD: Human Papillomavirus, in Belshe RB (ed): Textbook of Human Virology. Littleton, Mass, PSG Publishing Company, Inc, 1984, pp 951–968.

Lever WF, Schaumberg-Lever G: Histopathology of the skin, ed 6. Philadelphia, J.B. Lippincott Company, 1983.

Mitchell H, Drake M, Medley G, et al: Prospective evaluation of risk of cervical cancer after cytologic evidence of human papillomavirus infection. Lancet 573, 1986.

Oriel JD: Genital warts, in Holmes KK, Mardh PA, Sparling PF, Wiesner PJ (eds): Sexually Transmitted Diseases. New York, McGraw-Hill Book Co, 1984, pp 496–507.

Reid R, Greenberg M, Jenson AB, et al: Sexually transmitted papillomaviral infections: I. The anatomic distribution and pathologic grade of neoplastic lesions associated with different viral tpes. Am J Obstet Gynecol 156:212, 1987.

Reid R, Scalzi P: Genital warts and cervical cancer: VII. An improved colposcopic index for differentiating benign papillomaviral infection from high-grade cervical intraepithelial neoplasia. Am J Obstet Gynecol 153:611, 1985.

Reid R, Stanhope CR, Herschman BR, et al: Genital warts and cervical cancer: I. Evidence of an association between subclinical papillomavirus infection and cervical malignancy. Cancer 50:377, 1982.

Reid R (ed): Obstet Gynecol Clin N Am vol 14, June 1987 (entire issue).

Rush-Presbyterian-St. Luke's Medical Center, Chicago, and Sinai Hospital of Detroit: Human Papillomavirus and Squamous Carcinoma. Second International Conference. Chicago, October 27–29, 1986, pp 1–90.

Southern EM: Detection of specific sequences among DNA fragments separated by gel electrophoresis. J Mol Biol 98:503, 1975.

Spitzer M, et al: Comparative utility of repeat Papanicolaou smears, cervicography and colposcopy in the evaluation of atypical pap smears. Obstet Gynecol 69:731, 1987.

Wade TR, Kopf AW, Ackerman AB, et al: Bowenoid papulosis of the genitalia. Arch Dermatol 115:306, 1979.

Infestations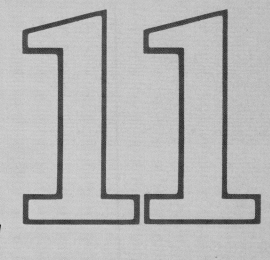

J. G. LONG

Introduction

Scabies and pubic lice are parasitic insects that live on or within the skin. The dermatidides that they produce are generally considered to be STDs, although they are also spread by nonsexual activity involving skin-to-skin contact. Sexual acquisition can often be assumed when the patient is a young adult with multiple sexual partners. Among young children, however, most cases do not imply sexual exposure.

SCABIES

Scabies is a pruritic dermatosis caused by the mite *Sarcoptes scabiei*. This condition, recognized for centuries as the "seven-year itch," was associated with the mite as early as 1654. The causal relationship between the mite and the rash was much debated and not generally accepted until this century.

The female mite is primarily responsible for the rash and is the form most frequently recovered from infested patients (Figs. 11.1 and 11.2). The adult female measures approximately 400 × 300 μm and is translucent, barely perceptible to the naked eye. Transverse grooves cover the body, and small denticles form a variable pattern on the dorsal surface. Although there is no distinct head, large, protruding jaws identify the anterior end (Fig. 11.3). Four pairs of legs are found in adult mites. In the female, the most posterior of these ends in long tendrils, while in the male the pair ends in suckers.

On the skin surface, the female can walk 2.5 cm/min, moving from the neck to the wrist within a few hours. Upon selecting a suitable site, the fertilized female digs into the skin to the stratum granulosum, where she lays her eggs and feeds on cellular material (Fig. 11.4). Each day, she extends the burrow by 0.5 to 5 mm and lays two to three eggs. Under optimal conditions, the mite will continue to burrow and lay eggs for a month or more, never returning to the skin surface. After three to four days, the eggs hatch into larvae, which resemble the adults but have only three pairs of legs. The larvae leave the burrow but may penetrate the skin to feed. After three days, the larvae molt to produce nymphs. After three more days, the larvae molt again to produce either a second nymphal stage or an adult (Fig. 11.5).

If all eggs survived to adulthood, an infestation could produce one million mites within 2 months. In fact, less than 10% of eggs survive to reach adulthood. Scratching, bathing, and immunologic reaction all contribute to their poor survival. The

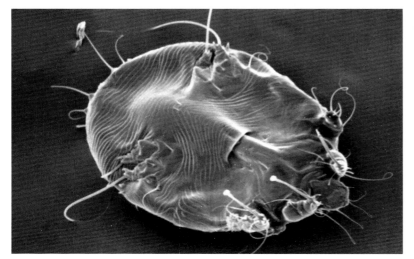

Figure 11.1 Scanning electron micrograph of the ventral surface of a female *S. scabiei* (original magnification × 300). A central bulge overlies the ovary, which contains a large egg.

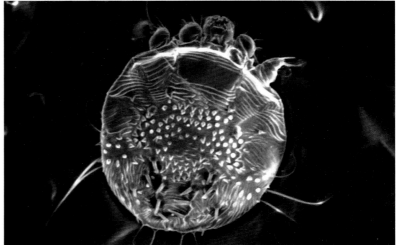

Figure 11.2 Scanning electron micrograph of *S. scabiei* showing the dorsal surface (original magnification × 200). Multiple small denticles are present except in a central bare area. Attempts to correlate the size of this bare area with biologic variants of the mite have had limited success.

Figure 11.3 Scanning electron micrograph of the jaw parts of *S. scabiei* (original magnification × 1000). These powerful jaws penetrate the skin and disrupt cells, producing a nutrient fluid on which the mite feeds.

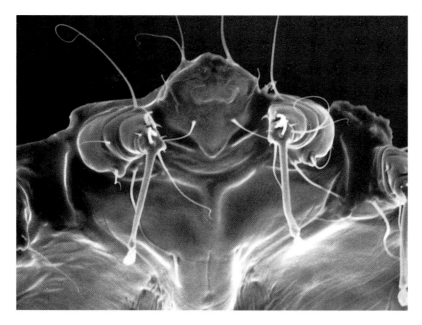

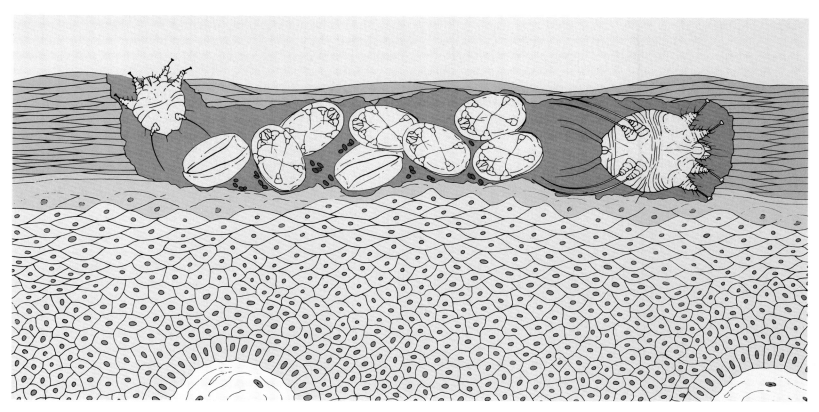

Figure 11.4 The burrow of *S. scabiei.* As the female mite advances through the stratum corneum, she leaves a trail of eggs and scybala behind. When the eggs hatch, the larval forms emerge onto the skin surface.

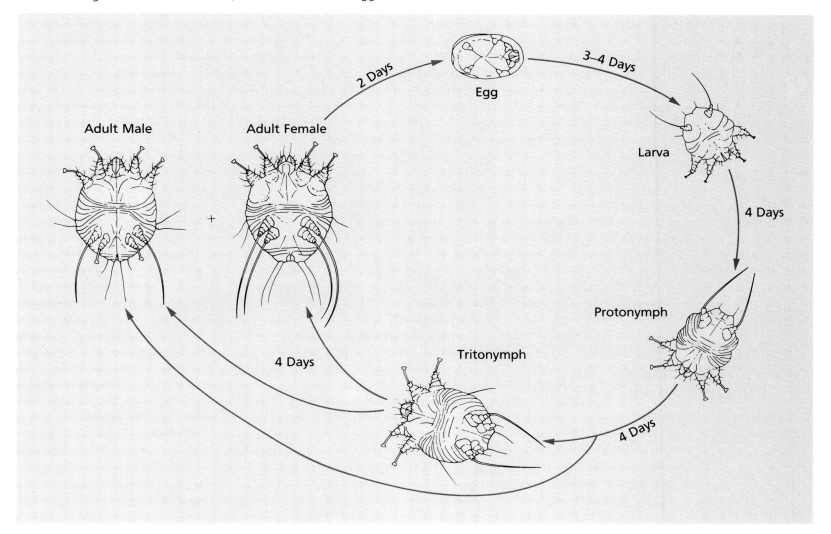

Figure 11.5 The life cycle of *S. scabiei.* Females complete the cycle from egg to egg in 19 days, with fertilization occurring on day 15. Males are mature after only 10 days.

average patient with scabies is infested with 11 mites, but half have no more than five (Fig. 11.6).

The clinical manifestations of scabies primarily reflect the host's immunologic response to the invading parasite. Under experimental conditions, mites placed on volunteers initially produce only minor erythema and no symptoms, even though burrows containing mites are present. It is not until a month after infestation that the characteristic pruritus and rash appear. However, volunteers who have been previously infested with the mite will develop symptoms within a day of exposure. The number of mites infesting a patient reaches a peak at about 3 months and then begins to decline. It is not known whether the immune system can eventually clear the infestation if treatment is withheld. Under experimental conditions, it is more difficult to establish infestation in individuals with prior exposure to scabies. This suggests that there is an immunologic defense against reinfestation.

Several types of immunologic responses to the scabies mite have been studied, but investigations have been hampered by an inability to cultivate the mite in sufficient quantities to extract and purify specific antigens. The predominant response involves the cellular branch of the host's immune system. Histopathologic examination of the skin lesion shows a perivascular infiltrate—predominantly lymphocytes, histiocytes, and eosinophils (Fig. 11.7). Patients with impaired cellular immunity have fewer symptoms, but can develop a more severe infes-

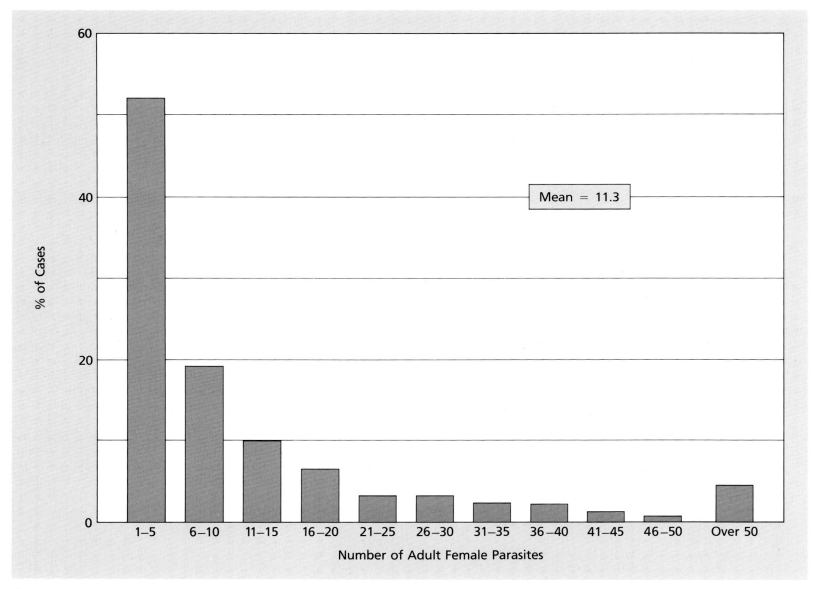

Figure 11.6 The number of adult female mites recovered from a large series of carefully examined patients.

tation known as *crusted scabies*. Circulating immune complexes, vasculitis, and IgE-mediated reactions have also been associated with scabies.

Specific physical characteristics and local immunologic properties of skin at different sites may explain the mite's predilection for certain areas. The mite remains somewhat insulated from the full force of the host's immunologic response by burrowing only to the stratum granulosum, well away from the dermis.

Epidemiology

Scabies is known throughout the world. In underdeveloped countries, it is most prevalent among young children and adolescents, while in developed nations it is more uniformly distributed across age groups. The attack rate appears to be the same for males and females. Decreased susceptibility among blacks has been suggested; however, African blacks are commonly infested, which does not support the idea of genetic immunity.

Although scabies is an STD, it is transmitted by skin-to-skin contact rather than specific sexual activity. Scabies differs from other STDs in that it is not especially prevalent among young adults or homosexual men. The occurrence of scabies in infants and children further supports the view that nonsexual skin contact is an important mode of transmission. Most transmission occurs within families, although outbreaks have been observed in hospitals and nursing homes. Schools and fomites have not been shown to play an important role in the spread of scabies. Mites are immobilized by cold and killed by brief exposure to heat, so they seldom survive long away from the host. However, in a warm, moist environment they can survive for two to three days, suggesting at least the potential for in-direct transmission. Fomites may be more important in institutional outbreaks, particularly when cases with large mite burdens occur.

It has been widely accepted that epidemics of scabies occur in 30-year cycles consisting of 15 years of high prevalence followed by 15 years of relatively few cases. Neither changes in population immunity nor a cyclical change in the mite has been found to explain this cycle. Recently, this phenomenon has been reevaluated, and the apparent cycles may be more properly attributed to the great social upheavals caused by world wars. The scabies mite infests 40 different mammalian hosts, the largest number for any permanent parasite. Although the mites that infest different hosts are morphologically indistinguishable, there appear to be biologic differences that limit interspecies spread. Transmission to humans from domestic animals is recognized, especially from dogs.

Clinical Manifestations

A patient's clinical history may offer important clues to the diagnosis of scabies. The typical patient seeks medical advice between 2 and 4 weeks after the onset of itching. The pruritus is usually most intense at night, especially upon first undressing and going to bed. Some patients itch only at night. Warmth intensifies the discomfort, and antipruritics may offer little relief. The rash typically begins on the hands and then spreads to the wrists, elbows, and other parts of the body. The presence of a pruritic rash on the hands and trunk is very suggestive of scabies, as is a report that other family members are also itching.

A variety of skin lesions may result from scabies infestation (Fig. 11.8). Typical lesions of scabies are usually found on the flexor surfaces of wrists, elbows, anterior axillary folds, areola

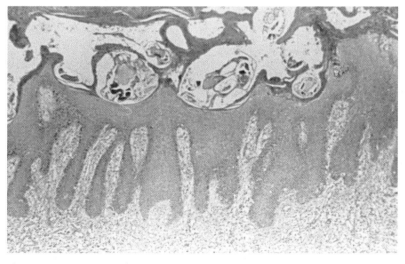

Figure 11.7 Histology of a burrow and the inflammatory response of skin to scabies infestation. Typically, a superficial and deep perivascular infiltrate of lymphocytes, histiocytes, and eosinophils is present. When tissue sections do not reveal the mite, the pathologic pattern may be mistaken for a drug eruption, erythema multiforme, or malignant lymphoma.

SKIN MANIFESTATIONS OF SCABIES

COMMON	UNUSUAL
Papules	Scaling crusts
Burrows	Urticaria
Excoriations	Vasculitis
Nodules	Attenuated or exaggerated lesions
Vesicles	
Pyoderma	
Eczema	

Figure 11.8 Skin manifestations of scabies.

in women, belt line, lower portion of buttocks and upper thighs, and the male genitalia (Fig. 11.9). The back is conspicuously free of lesions except in infants and the debilitated.

In contrast to adults, infants often show heavy infestation of the palms, soles, head, neck, face, and back (Fig. 11.10). The individual papules and burrows maintain their characteristic appearances. Infants may refuse feedings and fail to grow because of scabies infestation. Secondary bacterial infection is common.

Several specific types of skin lesions may be present in a single patient. The classically described burrow, although pathognomonic for the disease, is increasingly difficult to find. The burrow consists of a gray, dirty-appearing, 2-to-15-mm wavy line, usually seen on the wrist, interdigital web, or the side of a finger (Fig. 11.11). A tiny vesicle containing the mite may occasionally be seen at one end of the burrow (Fig. 11.12). The more typical lesion is a small, erythematous papule with surrounding erythema (Fig. 11.13). Lesions are usually sparse, but in some areas may become nearly confluent. These lesions are caused by larvae and nymphs that do not burrow.

In patients who bathe frequently, the manifestations of scabies may be subtle, with only a few lesions and rare burrows (Fig. 11.14). Bathing undoubtedly destroys many developing mites, thus limiting the number that reach maturity. Despite the paucity of characteristic lesions, the distribution and symmetry of the dermatitis provide a clue to diagnosis. In cases in

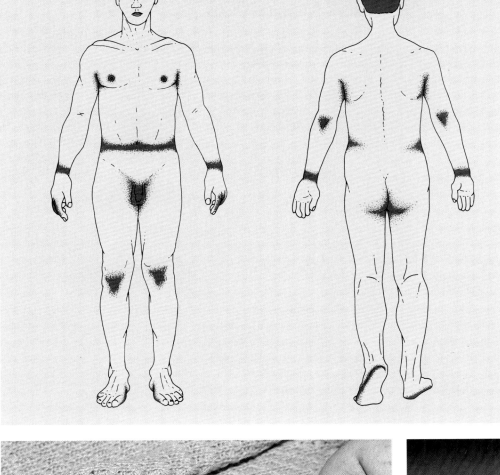

Figure 11.9 Distribution of skin lesions of *S. scabiei* infestation. Unshaded areas are rarely affected in healthy adults.

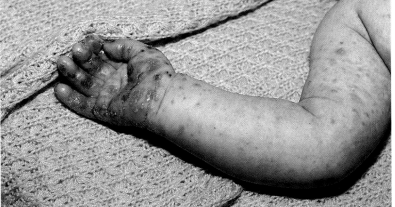

Figure 11.10 Scabies of the palm with secondary pyoderma in an infant. Lesions on the palms, soles, head, neck, and back are rare except in infants and debilitated adults.

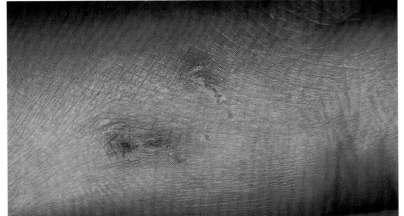

Figure 11.11 Burrow of *S. scabiei* on the side of a finger. Upper lesion shows the pathognomonic dirty-appearing wavy line extending out from an erythematous papule. In the lower lesion, the burrow has been nearly obliterated by excoriation.

which only a single body site is involved, the recognition of an infested contact may be the key to diagnosis.

Excoriation, denudation, eczematization, and subsequent infection may alter the appearance of scabies lesions so that they resemble chronic eczema or pyoderma (Fig. 11.15A). Infection, usually caused by *Staphylococcus aureus* or *Streptococcus pyogenes*, can produce local complications, including impetigo,

ecthyma, furunculosis, and cellulitis or more serious systemic disease such as bacteremia and internal abscesses. Eczematous changes induced by scratching may be exacerbated by the irritant or drying effect of topical antipruritic and antiscabietic medications. Scratching may also cause trauma to superficial blood vessels, resulting in petechial or ecchymotic lesions (Fig. 11.15B).

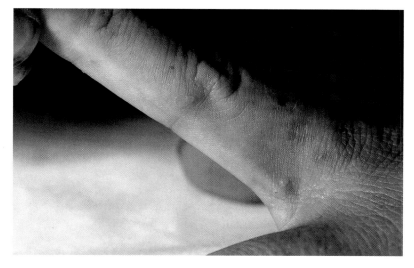

Figure 11.12 Vesicular scabietic lesions on the lateral surface of a finger and interdigital web.

Figure 11.13 Multiple larval papules on the abdomen. Such papules, which may be clustered or widely scattered, occur when immature mites penetrate the skin. These papules greatly outnumber burrows, which are formed only by the adult female mites.

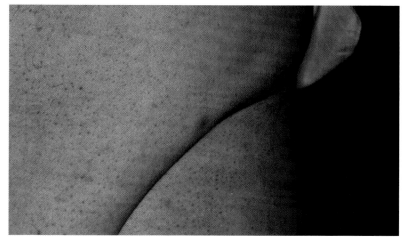

Figure 11.14 Scabies in the clean. Frequent bathing kills immature mites and limits the severity of the infestation. This man had only a few pruritic papules such as this isolated lesion on the lower abdomen.

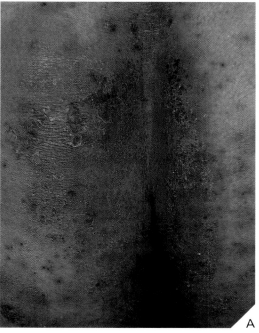

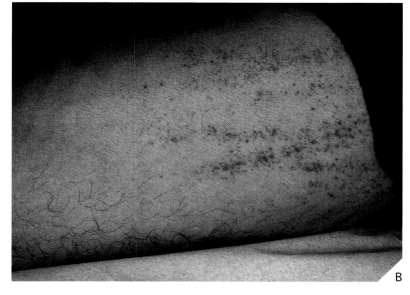

Figure 11.15 Excoriated lesions. **A** Eczematization may result from repeated excoriation or from the irritating effect of topical medications. A scaling, pruritic rash on the buttocks is a common manifestation of scabies. **B** Petechiae and ecchymoses may also be caused by excoriation. These rows of petechiae resulted from capillary breakage during vigorous scratching.

A

B

Manifestations of scabies may be altered by the presence of any other chronic or acute dermatosis. Scabies is frequently associated with other STDs. The diagnosis of scabies in sexually active individuals indicates a need to examine for other STDs.

NODULAR SCABIES

Firm, reddish-brown *nodules* may appear on covered parts of the body (Figs. 11.16 and 11.17). Most commonly found on the male genitalia, including the glans penis, shaft, and scrotum, they are also frequently seen on elbows and in the anterior axillary folds. These nodules may persist long after treatment and probably represent an immunologic reaction to the dead mite. Viable organisms are seldom found in nodules. Both clinically and histologically, nodular scabies may be confused with lymphoma and histiocytosis X.

URTICARIAL REACTIONS

A systemic allergic reaction to mite antigens may result in urticaria (Fig. 11.18). Such a response is not common, but when

it occurs it may completely overshadow the small number of scabies lesions. The urticaria resolves within a few days of antiscabietic therapy.

VASCULITIS

Although vasculitis is often present histologically, *vasculitic lesions* are not common. It is possible that some lesions that appear to be ulcerated due to excoriation or superinfection may actually be the result of a localized vasculitis (Fig. 11.19).

CRUSTED SCABIES

Crusted scabies is characterized by lesions, resembling psoriasis, whose thick scales contain large numbers of mites (Fig. 11.20). Pruritus is minimal. The disease is usually seen in immunologically incompetent or physically debilitated patients. It has also been associated with the use of topical fluorinated steroids. Months are required for the generalized lesions of crusted scabies to develop. An impaired immune response or inability to scratch allows the mite to multiply unchecked. The

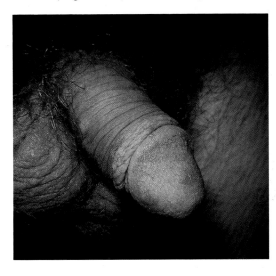

Figure 11.16
Nodular lesions of scabies on the male genitalia. Nodules generally occur on covered parts of the body. In this patient, erythematous, indurated lesions are present on the glans, penile shaft, and scrotum.

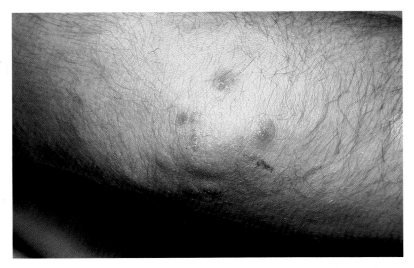

Figure 11.17 Nodular scabies on the extensor surface of the elbow. Such lesions may persist long after antiscabietic therapy. Their clinical and histologic appearances have caused them to be mistaken for neoplasms.

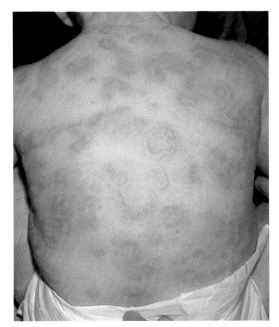

Figure 11.18
Urticaria associated with scabies. This child had multiple wheals over the face, trunk, and extremities. Typical scabietic burrows on the palms and soles were initially overlooked. The urticaria disappeared 48 hours after treatment with lindane lotion.

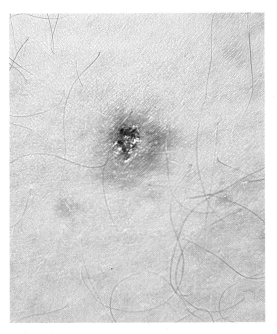

Figure 11.19 Lesion with necrotic center suggestive of vasculitis. Histologic evidence of localized vascular inflammation is frequently present on biopsy, but a generalized vasculitic reaction is rare.

shedding of tremendous numbers of mites causes this form of scabies to be extremely contagious.

SCABIES INCOGNITO
Topical application of steroids may markedly attenuate symptoms as well as reduce the number of lesions and alter their distribution. Such a presentation has been labeled *scabies incognito* (Fig. 11.21). Potent fluorinated steroids have also been associated with crusted scabies.

SCABIES AND AIDS
Patients with AIDS may have an atypical or exaggerated cutaneous response to many infections, including scabies infes-

tation (Fig. 11.22). The absence of burrows, an unusual distribution of lesions, and the scaling or crusted character of the dermatitis often delay diagnosrs. Repeated treatments are required to eradicate the infestation, probably because of the large mite burden.

Laboratory Tests
An attempt should be made to confirm the diagnosis of scabies in all suspected cases. A number of techniques have been used to demonstrate the mite, its burrow, eggs, or scybala (feces), any one of which is diagnostic. Although a positive diagnosis can probably be made in almost all cases if one searches with

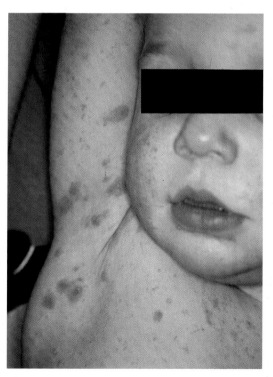

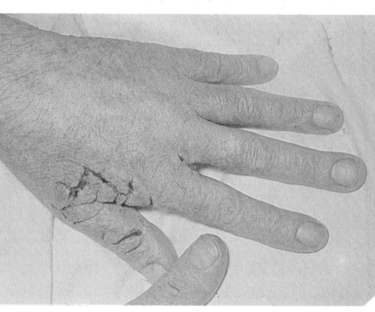

Figure 11.20
Crusted scabies. Thick, scaling lesions resembling psoriasis are the hallmark of crusted scabies. Affected patients are often debilitated or suffer from immunologic impairment. The exfoliated scales, which contain numerous mites, readily transmit the infestation. **A** Extensive crusted lesions of the abdominal wall. **B** Involvement of the hand in the same patient.

Figure 11.21
Scabies incognito. Atypical lesions in a child treated with topical steroids. Steroids may either exacerbate or reduce the cutaneous response to infestation.

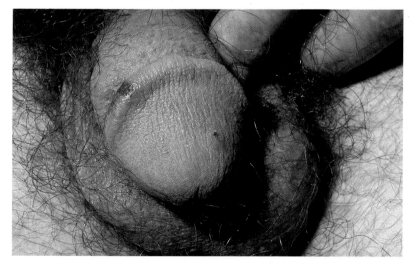

Figure 11.22 Cutaneous lesions of scabies in a patient with AIDS. As with steroid therapy, the clinical manifestations of scabies may be either diminished or exaggerated in patients with AIDS.

sufficient diligence, the success rates of various techniques are reported to range from 30 to 90%. Success with any technique increases with the skill and experience of the examiner.

SKIN SCRAPING

Preparation of a skin scraping is probably the most frequently used test for the scabies mite (Fig. 11.23). First the patient should be examined carefully in good light using a magnifying lens to select a burrow or papule that has not been excoriated. Lesions on the finger webs, wrists, or elbows are most likely to yield a positive diagnosis. Place a drop of mineral oil on the lesion and use a small disposable scalpel to scrape gently across the surface until the topmost layer of skin is removed. No bleeding should occur. Gently collect the mineral oil con-

taining the flecks of skin onto the scalpel blade and transfer it to a glass microscope slide. Add a cover slip and examine under low magnification.

Visualization of any adult or larval mite forms, eggs, or scybala is diagnostic of scabies (Fig. 11.24). Some clinicians prefer to omit the mineral oil and transfer the dry skin scrapings to a slide containing a drop of 10% KOH. Although this may help to disperse the cellular material for easier examination, it will destroy the fecal pellets that in some specimens are the only clues to the diagnosis.

EPIDERMAL SHAVE BIOPSY

This technique offers improved sensitivity and may be less likely to cause injury in an uncooperative patient (Fig. 11.25). Lift the

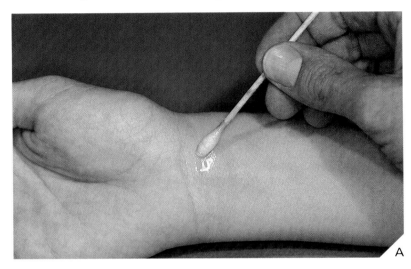

A

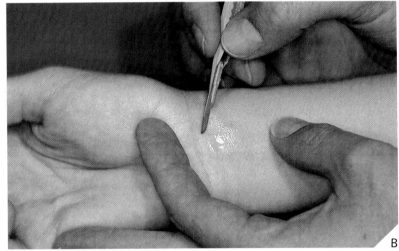

B

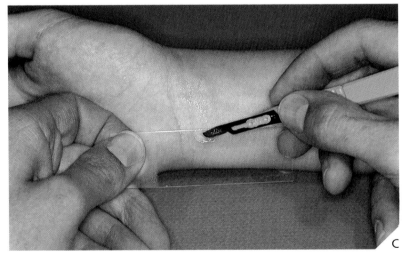

C

Figure 11.23 Preparation of a skin scraping. **A** Select an unexcoriated burrow or papule, preferably on the hand or wrist. Cover the lesion with a thin layer of mineral oil. **B** Hold a sterile scalpel perpendicular to the skin. Gently scrape the lesion until the superficial skin is removed. Collect the mineral oil containing skin particles and mites onto the scalpel blade. **C** Transfer the mineral oil to a microscope slide and cover with a glass cover slip. Add another drop of oil if necessary to eliminate any air bubbles. Examine under a microscope with a low-power objective.

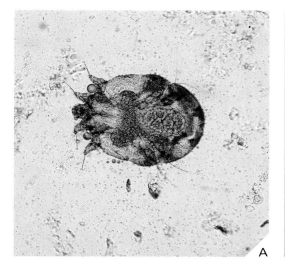
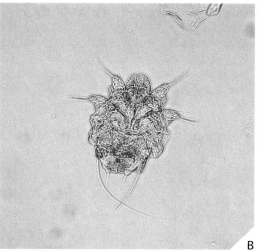
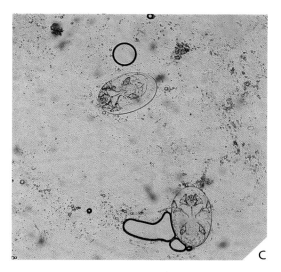

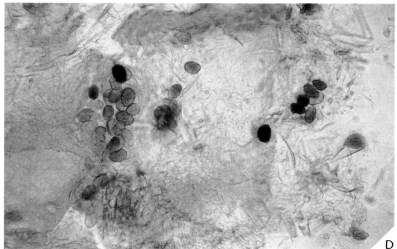

Figure 11.24 Positive skin scrapings. Any of the following are diagnostic of scabies infestation: **A** Adult female mite. **B** Larval stage of mite, which has only two hind legs. **C** Eggs. **D** Feces.

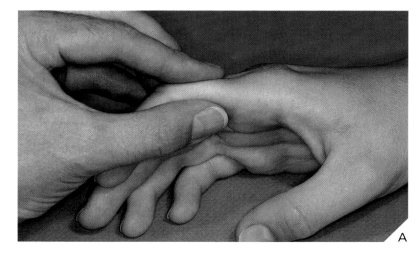
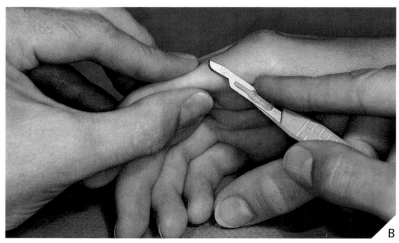

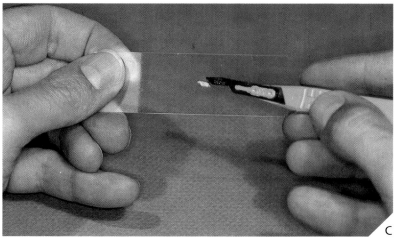

Figure 11.25 Preparation of a shave biopsy. **A** Select a lesion and hold it firmly between the thumb and index finger so that it is slightly elevated above the surrounding skin. **B** Hold a sterile scalpel with its blade parallel to the skin surface. Use a fine sawing motion to carefully shave off the outer layer of skin. **C** Use the scalpel blade to transfer the shaving to a microscope slide. Place a drop of oil over the specimen, then add a cover slip. Examine under a microscope using a scanning objective.

selected lesion between the thumb and index finger. Gently shave off the outer layer of skin with a sterile scalpel. Use a fine sawing movement while holding the scalpel blade tangential to the skin surface. Transfer the shaving to a microscope slide, add a drop of mineral oil and cover slip, and then examine under the microscope for mites, eggs, or scybala (Fig. 11.26).

CURETTAGE

Use a small cutting curette to scrape the epidermal layer off of a selected papule or burrow. This technique is particularly useful for infants or other uncooperative patients for whom the use of a scalpel might be hazardous. Place the scrapings on a slide with oil or KOH and examine.

BURROW INK TEST

Use a fountain pen to cover a papule with ink, then clean off the ink with alcohol (Fig. 11.27). A positive result is seen when the ink penetrates the papule, revealing a dark, zigzag line running across and away from the papule (Fig. 11.28). A positive ink test is specific for scabies; however, a shave biopsy on a positive lesion will demonstrate the actual mite. Topical tetracycline may be used instead of ink and washed off with alcohol after five minutes. A Wood's light will reveal burrows as areas of linear yellow-green fluorescence.

SEWING NEEDLE

An intact burrow must be present with the mite visible as either a dark point in Caucasian skin or a white point in blacks. Using a needle or pin, perforate the burrow at this point and move the needle from side to side, holding it parallel to the skin. The mite will attach itself to the needle and can be transferred to a slide for examination.

GLUE STRIPPING

Place a drop of methacrylate glue on a glass slide and push down firmly over an intact lesion. Allow the glue to set, then strip the slide off of the lesion briskly. Repeat the process two more times to obtain deeper organisms, then examine microscopically.

CELLOPHANE TAPE

Prepare the lesion by cleaning with ether, then apply a short length of clear cellophane tape. Briskly strip the tape from the skin and affix to a microscope slide. Repeat this several times for each lesion, using a new piece of tape each time.

PUNCH BIOPSY

If none of the above techniques are successful, a small 2-mm punch biopsy from an unexcoriated lesion may reveal the mite.

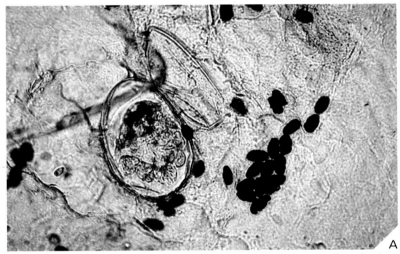

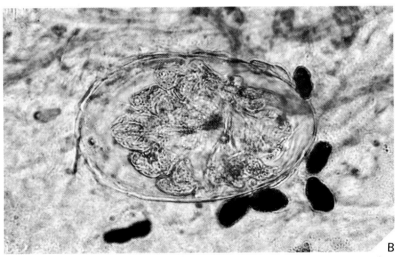

Figure 11.26 Positive shave biopsies. **A** Two eggs, one hatched and one containing a developing nymph, are visible within the skin shaving. Multiple small, dark fecal particles surround the eggs (original magnification × 50). **B** Egg and scabyla under higher magnification. The egg contains a larva that is nearly ready to emerge (original magnification × 100).

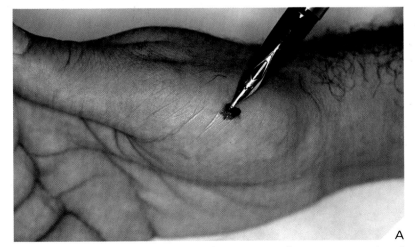

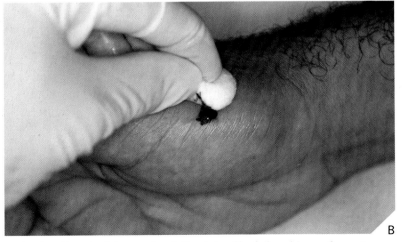

Figure 11.27 Burrow ink test technique. **A** Select an unexcoriated burrow or papule for the test. Cover the lesion with water-soluble ink from a fountain pen. **B** After five minutes, use an alcohol-soaked cotton ball to wash all the ink off of the skin surface. Examine the lesion for evidence of ink remaining within the scabies burrow.

Instruct the laboratory to make serial sections, all of which should be closely studied for evidence of the mite (see Fig. 11.7).

Treatment

Decisions in scabies therapy center on the choice of drug and on selection of contacts for prophylaxis. Because scabies may not become symptomatic until one month following infestation, it is essential to treat contacts prophylactically in order to prevent reexposure. In general, all household and sexual contacts should be treated. Decisions on whether to treat other contacts should be based on the degree of skin-to-skin contact they have with the patient. Three drugs are commonly used to treat scabies: lindane, crotamiton, and sulfur (Fig. 11.29).

Lindane (gamma benzene hexachloride) in a 1% lotion is the most frequently used scabicide. After the patient bathes, lindane is applied to the entire body from the neck down. Twelve hours later, it is washed off. A second treatment is not necessary unless there is evidence of treatment failure or reinfestation. Because lindane is toxic to the central nervous system and approximately 10% of the drug is absorbed through the skin, it should be used cautiously. To avoid overuse, only the amount actually needed (about 1 oz for an adult) should be prescribed. Lindane should not be used by young children, pregnant women, or patients with neurologic disorders because of the potential for toxicity.

Crotamiton, an effective scabicide with minimal toxicity, is suitable for use in small children and pregnant women. It is applied nightly for two nights, then washed off 48 hours after the last application. Crotamiton is more likely than lindane to require a second course of therapy.

Sulfur as 6% precipitated sulfur in petrolatum is an ancient therapy that remains effective although seldom used because of its disagreeable odor and staining. It is applied nightly for three nights then washed off 24 hours after the last application.

Upon completing the regimen of topical therapy, the patient should wash all clothes and bed linen used within the preceding two to three days. Usually, pruritus begins to resolve within two days of therapy, but may not be completely resolved for several weeks. It is important that the patient know what to expect because overuse of scabicides or other topical medications may lead to an irritant dermatitis that can be confused with treatment failure. Cases of apparent resistance to lindane and crotamiton are rare and may be due to improper use or reinfestation.

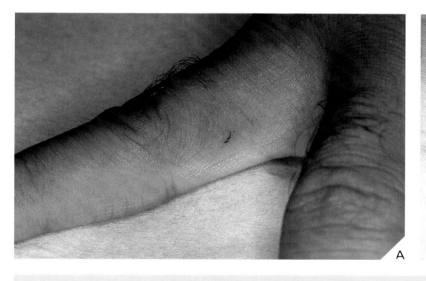

A

B

Figure 11.28 Positive burrow ink test. **A** An ink-filled burrow on the side of a finger is clearly visible after washing ink from the surface of the lesion. **B** A close-up view demonstrates the scabies burrow tracking across skin lines. The ink helps to define the morphology and limits of the burrow.

Figure 11.29   Treatment of scabies.

TREATMENT OF SCABIES

LINDANE 1% LOTION OR CREAM

Apply a thin layer to entire body from the neck down and allow to dry. Wash off completely after 8 to 12 hours. One application is usually curative.

CROTAMITON 10% CREAM

After bathing, massage cream into skin from neck down. Apply again after 24 hours. Wash off medication 48 hours after second application.

PRECIPITABLE SULFUR 6% IN PETROLATUM

Apply nightly from the neck down for three nights. Wash off medication thoroughly 24 hours after final application. (May stain clothing.)

PHTHIRUS PUBIS

Phthirus pubis, the crab louse, is one of the three members of the order Anoplura that infests man. The other two are *Pediculus humanus capitis*, the head louse, and *Pediculus humanus corporus*, the body louse (Fig. 11.30). Only P. *pubis* is primarily sexually transmitted. The insect's short, broad body and large, clawlike legs bear a remarkable resemblance to a crab, thus accounting for its common name (Fig. 11.31). The head, conical and pointed anteriorly, contains stylets that can pierce human skin, enabling the louse to suck blood from its host. Three pairs of legs extend from the anterior abdomen. The first is long and thin, while the second and third have thick claws specially suited for grasping hairs (Fig. 11.32). Four sets of small, conical appendages ending in bristles arise from the posterior abdomen.

The life cycle of P. *pubis* includes five stages from egg to adult. The eggs, called nits, are encased in a cement substance and firmly affixed to the hair shaft. Each nit has a convex cap containing air pores through which the first nymphal stage emerges after six to nine days (Fig. 11.33). Nymphs resemble adults ex-cept for their smaller size and sexual immaturity. A tough, chitinous exoskeleton restricts the nymph's growth so that a series of three molts is necessary to reach adulthood, a process requiring 2 to 3 weeks. Adults mate frequently, and the female begins to lay eggs shortly after fertilization, producing 20 to 30 eggs during her 3-week adult life.

Crab lice are found mainly in the pubic area, but may spread to the buttocks, legs, axillae, beard, scalp, and eyebrows. Their preference for certain sites is probably related to hair spacing: the 2-mm spaces between pubic hairs match the span of the louse's hind legs, with which it grasps hairs. Pubic lice are usually sedentary, moving only a few millimeters per day. They seldom travel far from the initial area of infestation unless transferred to a new site by the host. To feed, the crab grasps hairs with its clawlike legs and pierces the skin to obtain blood from a capillary. It often remains attached and feeds intermittently for hours before moving to a new site. P. *pubis* feeds exclusively on human blood and can survive less than 24 hours away from a human host.

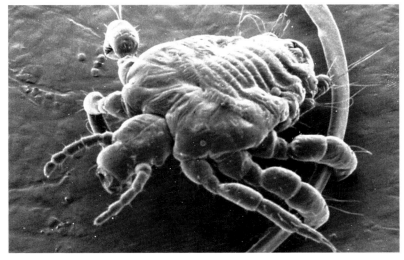

Pediculus humanus corporis
Magnification ×20

Pediculus humanus capitis
Magnification ×20

Phthirus pubis
Magnification ×20

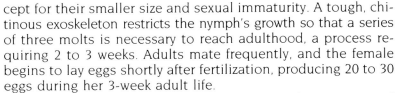

Figure 11.30 Lice that infest humans. The crablike appearance of *P. pubis* makes it easy to distinguish from the head louse (*Pediculus humanus capitis*) and body louse (*Pediculus humanus corporus*). *P. pubis* may be found outside the pubic area, so diagnosis must be based upon the appearance of the louse rather than its site of infestation.

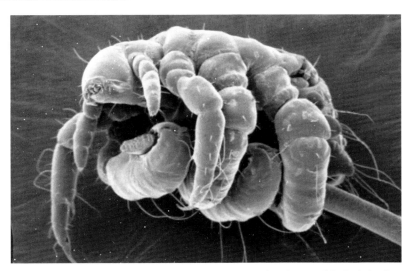

Figure 11.31 Scanning electron micrograph of *P. pubis* (original magnification ×50).

Figure 11.32 Scanning electron micrograph of *P. pubis* (original magnification ×100). Clawlike legs encircling a pubic hair produce a firm grip that can be difficult to dislodge.

Epidemiology

P. *pubis* spreads predominantly through intimate sexual contact. Transmission via nonsexual contact or fomites may occur occasionally, but is unusual.

Because P. *pubis* infestation is not reportable in the United States, limited epidemiologic information is available. Many believe that the incidence of infestation has increased markedly during the past two decades, paralleling increases in other STDs during a period of changing sexual behavior. Most available epidemiologic information comes from STD clinics. However, such data certainly underestimate cases because the availability of effective nonprescription therapy makes it unnecessary to consult a physician for this disease.

Among new patients seen in one clinic in England, the prevalence of crabs increased from 0.8% in 1954 to 3.2% in 1968. Patients with crabs were generally similar to those with other STDs. Males were more likely to be infested than females except among 15 to 19 year olds. Nearly half of the patients with crabs also had another STD. In 1986 in DeKalb County (Atlanta), Georgia, 3% of patients attending a public STD clinic were infested with crabs.

Clinical Manifestations

Patients who present to a physician with P. *pubis* infestation usually have seen lice or are complaining of severe pruritus in the pubic area. Excoriations and secondary infection are common findings in symptomatic patients. Ten or fewer adult lice are usually present at diagnosis.

In an STD clinic, half of infested patients are asymptomatic. The diagnosis is often made during examination for an unrelated problem. Occasionally the only complaint is the presence of multiple rust-colored spots on the patient's underclothes, resulting from bleeding at sites of bites or from excrement from the louse after a blood meal (Fig. 11.34). Most patients do not notice pruritus until one month after exposure to an infested partner. This incubation period is probably related to development of the host's immunologic response and growth of the lice population to a size sufficient to cause discomfort.

An uncommon manifestation of P. *pubis* infestation is the macula caerulea, an asymptomatic bluish-gray macule that does not blanch under pressure. This lesion represents the bite of the louse and a resultant small hemorrhage into the skin. More commonly seen are small, punctate, red lesions near hair follicles that mark the sites of recent bites (Fig. 11.35). These lesions, when inflamed and excoriated, resemble folliculitis.

Laboratory Tests

P. *pubis* infestation diagnosis is usually straightforward and requires finding only one of the crablike insects on the patient. The search is aided by good lighting and a magnifying lens. Their yellow-gray color makes the lice difficult to see on Caucasian skin, but after a blood meal they have a more visible

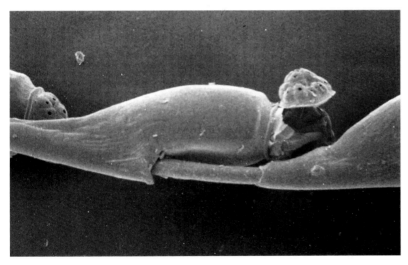

Figure 11.33 Scanning electron micrograph of an egg, or nit, with nymphal stage of *P. pubis* preparing to emerge. The cap containing air pores is pushed off during this process (original magnification × 100).

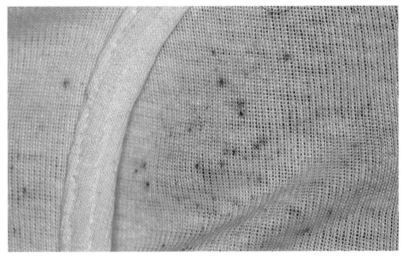

Figure 11.34 Rust-colored spots on underclothing may result from bleeding at sites of bites or from excrement from the louse after a blood meal. In patients without symptoms, these spots may be the first clue to the presence of infestation.

Figure 11.35 Bite marks of *P. pubis*. These punctate lesions with surrounding erythema are typical of the tiny papules that arise at sites of crab louse bites.

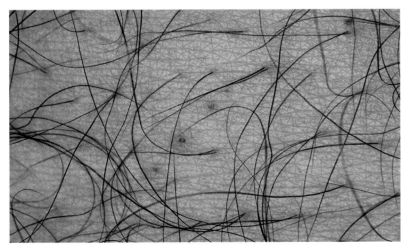

rust color (Fig. 11.36). Occasionally the lice are found only in extrapubic areas such as the axilla, extremities, buttocks, scalp, or eyelashes (Fig. 11.37). Demonstration of adults, nymphs, or nits is sufficient for diagnosis. Nits are usually easiest to find, but may be confused with hair casts or scales of skin from seborrhea (Fig. 11.38). Nits may be distinguished from the latter by microscopy and by their firm adherence to the hair shaft. Unless removed with a special fine-tooth comb, nits will remain attached to the hair after therapy and move outward as the hair grows. If treatment failure or reinfestation is suspected, only those eggs close to the base of the hair shaft should be considered significant. Empty egg casings do not indicate active infestation, but can be distinguished from viable eggs only by microscopic examination (Fig. 11.39).

Treatment

Lindane and synergized pyrethrins are the drugs of choice for treatment of P. pubis infestations and are equally effective (Fig. 11.40). Lindane is available as a lotion, cream, or shampoo.

The cream and lotion require a 12-hour application for complete killing of lice and ova, but the shampoo is effective in only four minutes. The use of lindane in small children, pregnant women, and patients with extensive dermatologic or neurologic disorders should be avoided. However, if used correctly, the brief exposure to the shampoo presents a very limited opportunity for absorption of the drug.

Pyrethrins synergized with piperonyl butoxide are available without prescription in lotion and shampoo forms. The infested hair must be covered with the lotion or lathered with the shampoo for ten minutes, then washed with water. Toxicity is not a problem with this drug, which may be used safely during pregnancy.

With either drug, it is important to instruct the patient in the proper use of the medication. In most cases, treatment of the pubic and perianal hair is sufficient, although other sites should be inspected and treated if necessary. In individuals with much body hair, medication should be applied to the lower abdomen, thighs, and buttocks regardless of whether or not lice are found in these areas.

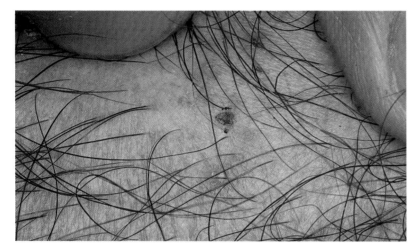

Figure 11.36 *P. pubis* feeding on its host. To obtain a meal of human blood, the crab louse uses its clawlike legs to grasp a hair on either side, then penetrates the host's skin with its mouth. Firmly anchored in this position, the louse may feed for hours. During feeding, the body takes on a red-brown color more easily seen against Caucasian skin.

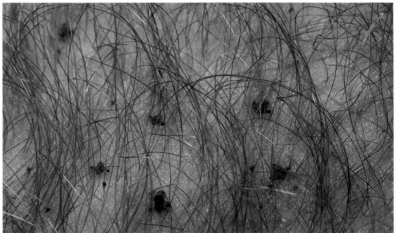

Figure 11.37 Extrapubic infestation. *P. pubis* may infest almost any area in hirsute individuals. This cluster of lice was present on the buttock of a patient whose pubic hair was not infested.

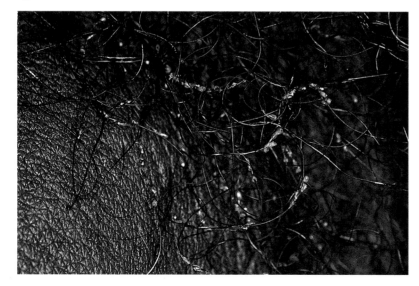

Figure 11.38 Pubic hair with multiple nits. Hairs such as these with numerous nits are easily recognized as a sign of *P. pubis* infestation. When only a few nits are present, a careful search with a magnifying lens may be necessary to establish the diagnosis.

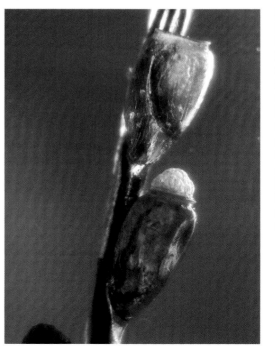

Figure 11.39 Photomicrograph of two nits on a hair shaft. The upper egg is empty, but the lower one still contains a developing nymph. Empty nits may be a sign of past rather than current infestation. After therapy, unhatched nits at the base of hairs indicate treatment failure or reinfestation.

After treatment, any clothing and bed linen used during the preceding 24 hours should be washed. Because the louse survives for less than a day away from the host, it is not necessary to treat furniture and other potential fomites with insecticide. In cases in which the eyelashes are involved, petrolatum applied to the lashes twice a day for eight days is safe and effective. If nits remain after this treatment, they may be removed with forceps.

Sexual contacts should be examined and treated prophylactically; household contacts should be treated only if actually infested. Patients infested with P. *pubis* should be examined for other STDs.

Resistance of P. *pubis* to insecticides has not yet been reported. Most cases of treatment failure can be attributed to incorrect use of medication, failure to medicate all infested body sites, or reexposure to an untreated partner. Persistent pruritus does not warrant additional therapy in the absence of active infestation. Repeated treatments with lindane may exacerbate the itching by causing a skin irritation. Delusions of parasitosis are not uncommon after successful therapy and frequently result in the overuse of medications.

Picture credits for this chapter are as follows: Figs. 11.1–11.3 and 11.31–11.33 courtesy of Patricianne Hurd, PhD, John Pietrahita, and Danny Blankenship, Fernbank Science Center, DeKalb County Board of Education; Fig. 11.5 adapted from Orkin M, Maibach HI (eds.): Cutaneous Infestations and Insect Bites. *New York, Marcel Dekker, 1985. Fig. 11.6 adapted from Johnson CG, Mellanby K: The parasitology of human scabies.* Parasitology *34:286, 1942, courtesy of Cambridge University Press; Fig. 11.7 courtesy of S.D. Glazer, MD; Figs. 11.17 and 11.20 courtesy of du Vivier A. McKee PH:* Atlas of Clinical Dermatology. *London, Gower Medical Publishing Ltd., 1986; Fig. 11.18 courtesy of Chapel TA: Scabies presenting as urticaria.* JAMA *246:1441, 1981 with permission, © 1981 American Medical Association; Fig. 11.21 courtesy of Heidi Watts; Figs. 11.22 and 11.24A and C courtesy of Adele Moreland, MD; Fig. 11.28B courtesy of David Woodley, MD.*

BIBLIOGRAPHY

Ackerman AB: Crabs—The resurgence of *Phthirus pubis*. NEJM 278:950, 1968.

Burkhart CG: Scabies: An epidemiologic reassessment. *Ann Intern Med* 98:498, 1983.

Chapel TA, Krugel L, Chapel J, Segal A: Scabies presenting as urticaria. JAMA 246:1440, 1981.

Dahl MV: The immunology of scabies. *Ann Allergy* 51:560, 1983.

Estes SA, Kummel B, Arlian L: Experimental canine scabies in humans. J Am Acad Dermatol 9:397, 1983.

Fernandez N, Torres A, Ackerman B: Pathologic findings in human scabies. *Arch Dermatol* 113:320, 1977.

Fisher I, Morton RS: *Phthirus pubis* infestation. Br J Vener Dis 46:326, 1970.

Johnson CG, Mellanby K: The parasitology of human scabies. *Parasitology* 34:285, 1942.

Martin WE, Wheeler CE Jr: Diagnosis of human scabies by epidermal shave biopsy. J Am Acad Dermatol 1:335, 1979.

Orkin M, Maibach HI: Modern aspects of scabies. *Curr Probl Dermatol* 13:109, 1985.

Orkin M, Maibach HI (eds.): *Cutaneous Infestations and Insect Bites.* New York, Marcel Dekker, 1985.

Parish LC, Nuttig WB, Schwartzman RM (eds.): *Cutaneous Infestations of Man and Animal.* New York, Praeger, 1983.

Sadick N, Kaplan MH, Pahwa SG, Sarngadharan MG: Unusual features of scabies complicating human T-lymphotropic virus type III infection. J Am Acad Dermatol 15:482, 1986.

Woodley D, Saurat JH: The burrow ink test and the scabies mite. J Am Acad Dermatol 4:715, 1981.

Figure 11.40   Treatment of *P. pubis* infestation.

TREATMENT OF *PHTHIRUS PUBIS* INFESTATION

LINDANE 1% SHAMPOO

Apply shampoo to pubic hair and any other infested areas (except eyelashes). Add water to produce a thick lather, then wash off after four minutes. If the 1% cream or lotion is used, it should be washed off after 12-hours.

PYRETHRIN WITH PIPERONYL BUTOXIDE

Lotion, gel, and shampoo preparations are available without prescription. Apply medication to thoroughly cover infested hair (except eyelashes). Wash off after 10 minutes.

PETROLATUM

Use only for infestation of the eyelashes. Apply twice daily for eight days. Any nits remaining after treatment can be physically removed.

Nonvenereal Genital Dermatoses

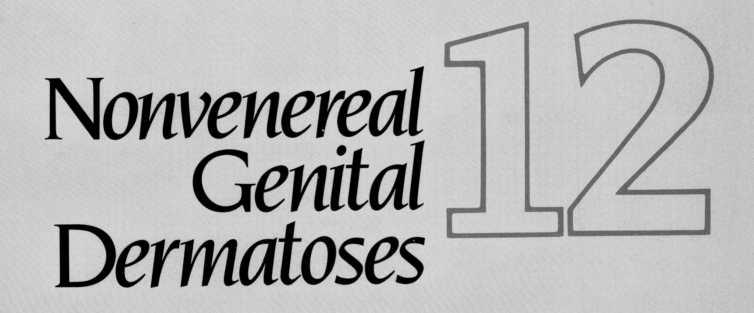

12

M. McKAY, A.A. MORELAND

Introduction

Skin changes (cutaneous disorders) of the genital skin may be assumed either by patient or physician to be of a sexually transmitted nature because of their location. This chapter will review common cutaneous disorders of the genitalia that are not sexually transmitted but that may be seen in a venereal disease clinic or be mistaken for an STD.

Although it is traditional to classify and discuss infectious diseases and conditions with respect to etiology, this approach has significant shortcomings when applied to cutaneous disorders. A 3-mm papule, for example, can be a congenital nevus, a benign or malignant neoplasm, or the result of infection with a bacteria, a virus, or a fungus. Since the skin lesion itself is the usual starting point for the development of a differential diagnosis, the traditional dermatologic approach is to seek out a so-called "primary lesion," one that recreates the pathophysiology of the disease process. This usually implies a search for a fresh, fully developed lesion, rather than for one that has dried, crusted, been scratched, or become secondarily infected. In addition to describing the morphology of the primary pro-cess, observation of the distribution and configuration of the lesions on the skin helps to identify the disorder, as it may be one of many dermatoses that are more easily identified by finding similar lesions on other areas of the body.

With these principles in mind and for the purpose of this discussion, the nonvenereal genital dermatoses will be grouped into seven different morphologic categories. Six of these are defined by the primary lesion, such as pustules, pigmentary disorders, and dermatitis. The seventh category, erosions and ulcers, deals with the so-called "minus" lesions, wherein the original morphology has been altered by the loss of superficial epidermis (erosion) or of the entire skin surface itself (ulcer). This latter category may be difficult to assess, for normal morphologic clues to differential diagnosis frequently are absent.

Dermatitis/Eczema

The term *dermatitis* simply means inflammation of the skin. The Greek root *eczema*, which means "boiling over or out," is remarkably descriptive of the oozing, wet appearance of dermatitic

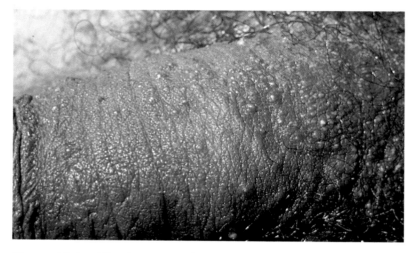

Figure 12.1 Allergic contact dermatitis of the penis due to spermicidal jelly. Note the typical appearance of microvesicles on the glans penis. This patient complained of pruritus and rash developing approximately two days after use of the product.

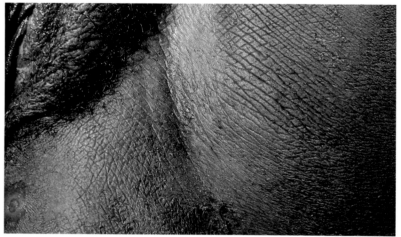

Figure 12.2 Lichenification of intertriginous skin as a result of chronic rubbing and scratching.

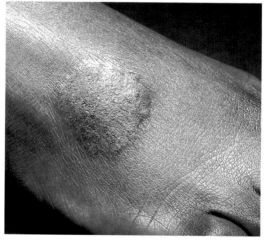

Figure 12.3 Lichen simplex chronicus on the foot. The hallmark of this diagnosis is the leathery appearance of the skin.

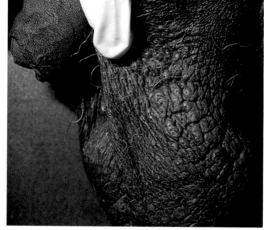

Figure 12.4 Lichen simplex chronicus of the scrotum. The accentuation of normal skin markings is shown clearly. The inguinal area is hyperpigmented—a milder sign of continuous rubbing.

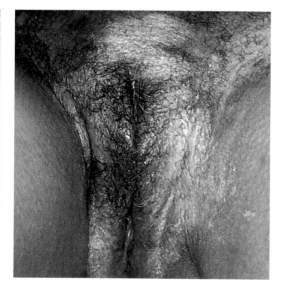

Figure 12.5 Vulvar lichen simplex chronicus. The extensiveness of the area involved suggests that pruritus has been present for several months or more. The skin is lichenified, scaly, and in some areas hyperpigmented.

skin. Eczemas characteristically are pruritic. The patient complains of itching, and scratch marks (excoriations) may be seen on the skin surface. Dermatitis typically changes its appearance over time. The first sign simply may be an erythema, which is followed by a pebbly appearance to the skin surface that rapidly evolves into small blisters which may ooze and crust (Fig. 12.1). As dermatitis evolves, the skin becomes thickened, leathery, and often scaly, with increased skin markings. These findings are the hallmark of *lichenification* (Fig. 12.2) and are even more important than scaling in making this diagnosis. The patient's rubbing or scratching of the initial condition will increase the likelihood of lichenification, which persists long after the original insult has been removed. Acute dermatitis, then, is seen as a plaque that is erythematous, edematous, and oozing; chronic dermatitis is a plaque that may be purplish, hyperpigmented, and lichenified. In the latter case, the patient is said to have *lichen simplex chronicus*, a descriptive term that indicates only that the patient has a plaque of thickened skin that has been rubbed or scratched. Any area of the body may be involved (Fig. 12.3), but genital skin is a common area of involvement (Figs. 12.4 and 12.5). Some underlying skin conditions, such as atopic dermatitis, may make it more likely that the patient will develop areas of lichen simplex chronicus. In other cases, the skin reaction is due to something that has come in contact with the epidermis. The offending substance may be an irritant such as urine or a true allergen. Neomycin and benzocaine are relatively common allergens found in nonprescription topical medications. These medications may be self-prescribed by patients or prescribed by physicians to treat both pruritus and any type of irritation, abrasion, or ulcer.

Papulosquamous Disorders

The papulosquamous dermatoses, as the name implies, are characterized by papules and plaques that typically have a scaly surface. While a plaque of lichen simplex chronicus might fit this description, it should be noted that lichenification is *secondary* to rubbing and scratching of the affected skin. The papulosquamous dermatoses, on the other hand, begin with a scaly papule as the *primary* lesion. Of all dermatologic disorders, probably the most commonly encountered are those in the papulosquamous category, and it is important for the clinician to develop a logical approach to the differential diagnosis of these problems (Fig. 12.6).

Figure 12.6 Differential diagnosis of common papulosquamous dermatoses.

DIFFERENTIAL DIAGNOSIS OF COMMON PAPULOSQUAMOUS DERMATOSES

CONDITION	ERYTHEMA	SKIN CHANGES THICKENING	PRURITUS	ASSOCIATED LESIONS
Psoriasis	+ +	+ + +	+/−	Red plaques with silvery scale on knees, elbows, scalp. Nail pitting.
Seborrheic dermatitis	+ +	+	+	Scaling/erythema on eyebrows, nasolabial folds, hairline, occasionally on axillae.
Dermatophyte (tinea cruris)	+ +	Raised border	+ +	Annular plaque with central clearing and peripheral scale. KOH shows hyphae.
Candidiasis	+ +	Edema	+ + +	Acute erythema, edema, peeling, satellite pustules. Gram stain shows budding yeast.
Lichen simplex chronicus	+ +	+ + +	+ + +	May be limited to vulva; other common sites are ankle, nape of neck, arm.
Chronic dermatitis (contact or irritant)	+ + +	+ +	+ +	Often eczematous and oozing. May involve congruent areas, eyelids. May generalize.
Lichen planus	Violaceous	+ +	+ +	Purple polygonal papules and plaques, especially on wrists and legs. Lacy white pattern on buccal mucosa.
Lichen sclerosus and mixed dystrophy	+	−	+/−	Usually limited to vulva, anus ("keyhole" pattern). White, nonscaly. Dermis thick, epidermis atrophic.

The acute onset of a pruritic annular lesion anywhere on the body, especially in intertriginous areas, should raise the suspicion of a *dermatophyte* (Fig. 12.7) infection. Scraping a bit of scale from the border of a lesion and examining it under 10 to 20% potassium hydroxide (KOH) solution will allow the visualization of fungal hyphae (Fig. 12.8). Dermatophyte infections are more common in men than in women, but the latter are more likely to develop candidal infections, usually as a result of spread from the vagina (see section on pustular disorders). Griseofulvin is effective only for dermatophytes and nystatin only for *Candida*, but the imidazole antifungals are effective treatment for both dermatophyte and candidal infections. Annular lesions also may occur in secondary syphilis, but syphilis

only rarely itches, and no hyphae can be seen on KOH and, of course, the serology is positive.

Psoriasis is another commonly encountered papulosquamous disorder with a distinct familial association, even though many patients are unaware of family members with psoriasis. Typically seen as thick, red plaques with adherent white scales, psoriasis occurs most commonly on the arms (Fig. 12.9), knees, elbows, trunk, and sacrum, as well as the scalp. Genital lesions, however, are apt to have little if any scale, and may be seen simply as persistent intertriginous erythema (Figs. 12.10 and 12.11). Scaly plaques may be seen on the penis and scrotum as well as on the pubic area, and in some cases may closely resemble the papulosquamous form of secondary syphilis (see Fig. 1.34B,

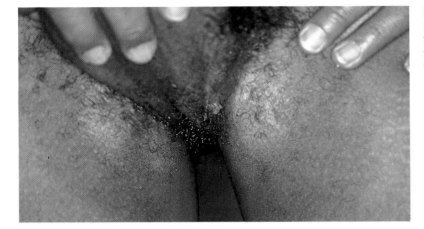

Figure 12.7 Tinea cruris. Erythema and scaling associated with pruritus are typical features of a dermatophyte infection. Scrapings for potassium hydroxide (KOH) and fungal cultures should be taken from the leading edge of the involved skin, even though scaling there may be minimal.

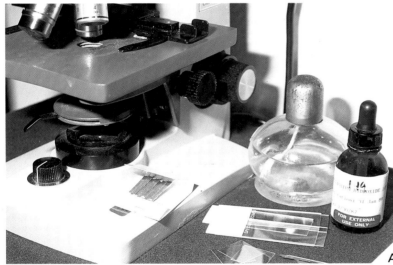

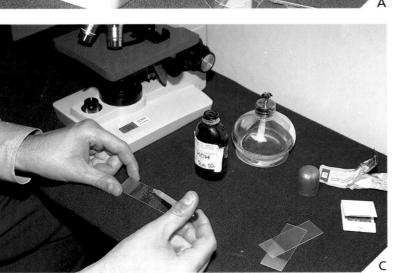

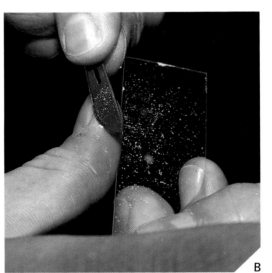

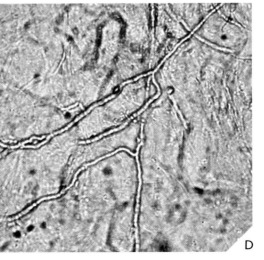

Figure 12.8 **A** Equipment needed for KOH examination. Curved scalpel blades, glass microscope slides, 10 to 20% KOH, glass coverslips, heat source, and microscope are shown. **B** A curved scalpel blade allows gentle scraping of the skin with minimal trauma. The scale should be collected directly onto a glass slide and the coverslip applied. **C** KOH applied by dropper to the edge of the covered specimen allows it to penetrate under the coverslip by capillary action. The slide is *gently* warmed, *without* boiling, to allow clearing of the specimen. The alcohol lamp produces a cleaner flame than do matches. **D** Microscopic view of branched hyphae among cleared keratinocytes as they appear in a positive KOH preparation.

Chapter 1), with minimal involvement of the rest of the body. Fingernail pitting may lead one to suspect the diagnosis of psoriasis in a persistent genital papulosquamous disorder. A mild topical corticosteroid (hydrocortisone 1%) generally is effective in treating genital psoriasis. The use of strong fluorinated steroids on genital skin may lead to the development of striae, which are permanent and unsightly.

Seborrheic dermatitis usually is seen as scaling in the hairy areas of the body, with a more or less prominent erythematous and papular component. Most commonly diagnosed in the scalp as "dandruff," seborrheic dermatitis also affects the eyebrows, nasolabial folds (Fig. 12.12), axillae, central chest, and genital region. Women usually experience only mild erythema and scaling on the mons pubis (Fig. 12.13), but men may have ery-

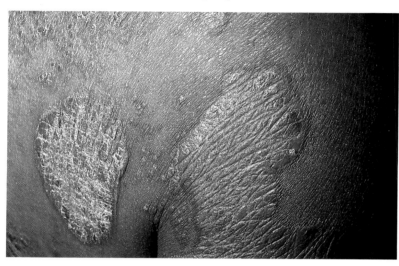

Figure 12.9   Psoriasis. Thick reddish plaques with an adherent thick white scale are typical on nongenital skin such as the arms, elbows, knees, and scalp.

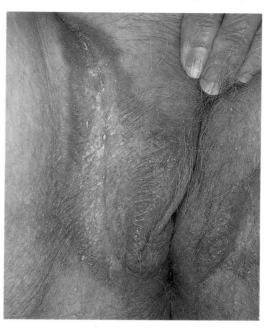

Figure 12.10
Psoriasis of the vulva. The typical thick scale seen here is sometimes absent when psoriasis occurs on the genital skin, leaving erythematous patches and plaques with a more macerated and moist scale, or with no scale at all.

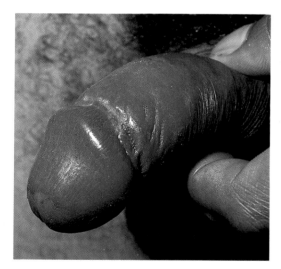

Figure 12.11
Psoriasis of the penis. The typical intense erythema of psoriatic plaques, but with complete lack of scale, is seen in this largely intertriginous plaque of psoriasis under the foreskin.

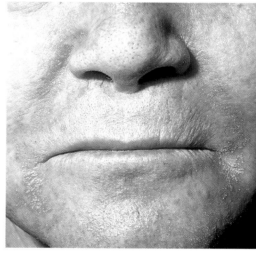

Figure 12.12
Typical seborrheic dermatitis in the nasolabial crease. Erythema with mild scaling is seen.

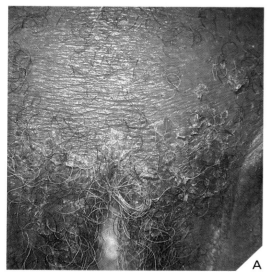

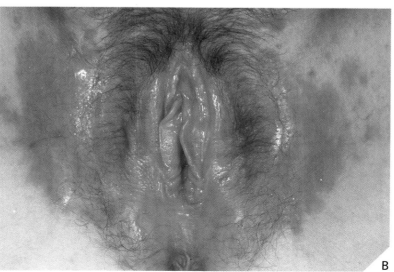

Figure 12.13   A and B Seborrheic dermatitis of the vulva may present as pruritus of the vulva or mons. The skin appears red or slightly pigmented, and thick "dandruff" scales may be seen.

A

B

thematous plaques on the penis (Fig. 12.14) that are difficult to differentiate from psoriasis or secondary syphilis (see Fig. 1.35A, Chapter 1). Treatment with mild corticosteroids is effective in this condition, as well.

Lichen planus (classically described as purple, pruritic, polygonal papules and plaques) is not as scaly as are the above disorders. The typical areas of involvement are the flexor surfaces of the wrists, the trunk (Fig. 12.15), and the anterior shins. An examination of the tongue (Fig. 12.16) or buccal mucosa (Fig. 12.17) may show a lacy white pattern and sometimes erosions difficult to distinguish from *Candida* or thrush. This lacy white pattern also may be seen on genital mucosal surfaces, but violaceous papules with or without scale (Fig. 12.18) also may be seen. Treatment of lichen planus is symptomatic, with corticosteroids and, if necessary, antipruritic agents.

Lichen sclerosus and the so-called "mixed dystrophies" (see below) may be responsible for thickened, scaly plaques appearing on the genitalia. Although these disorders are not always pruritic, itching may occur primarily or may be secondary to medications that have been applied to the affected area. A biopsy may be necessary to differentiate lichenified dermatitis from a primarily papulosquamous disorder.

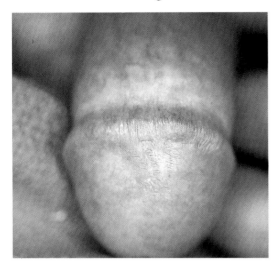

Figure 12.14 Seborrheic dermatitis on the penis. Erythematous changes are sometimes difficult to differentiate from psoriasis, and may resolve with a mottled hypopigmentation.

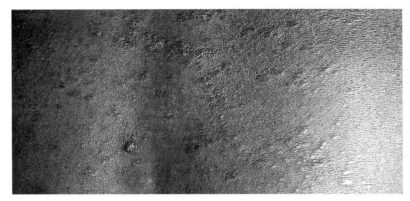

Figure 12.15 Lichen planus on the trunk. Typical violaceous flat-topped papules are seen, some with angular borders and adherent scale in the form of "Wickham's striae."

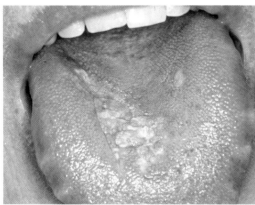

Figure 12.16 Oral lichen planus of the tongue. Whitish plaques are seen centrally.

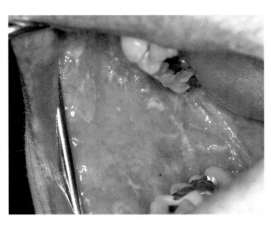

Figure 12.17 Oral lichen planus. Thin whitish linear streaks or Wickham's striae are seen on the buccal mucosa. This is not symptomatic unless it is erosive.

Figure 12.18 Penile lichen planus. **A** Flesh-colored papules of lichen planus have a lacy white surface and assume an annular configuration. **B** These papules on the glans are scalier and more extensive than those in the previous example.

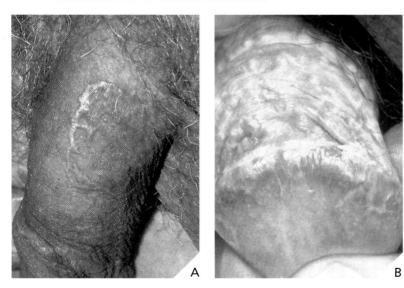

A   B

Pigmentary Disorders

HYPERPIGMENTATION

A black macule on the genitalia is an obvious lesion of concern, for it is important to rule out *malignant melanoma* as a diagnostic possibility. Typically, however, a melanoma (Fig. 12.19) is a single lesion with an irregular "notched" border with variable hyperpigmentation, which also may show areas of depigmentation within the larger macule. This malignant change should be distinguished from that of *freckle* or *lentigo* (Fig. 12.20)—benign macules having regular borders and smooth pigmentation. Diffuse hyperpigmentation as a result of chronic inflammation, *post-inflammatory hyperpigmentation*, also can occur as multiple ma-

cules, giving a "spotty" appearance to genital skin, especially around the vaginal introitus (Fig. 12.21).

Another form of diffuse hyperpigmentation, but with a thickened velvety appearance to the skin, is that of *acanthosis nigricans*. This pigmentary change may be seen around the neck (Fig. 12.22), genitalia, (Fig. 12.23), and the axillae of genetically predisposed obese individuals or in some patients with endocrine abnormalities. This "benign" or pseudoacanthosis nigricans cannot be distinguished clinically or histologically from the form that is associated with internal malignancy, usually a gastric adenocarcinoma. Thus a thorough evaluation for malignancy should be made in patients who present with new-onset

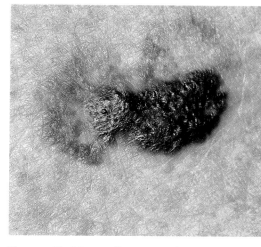

Figure 12.19 Malignant melanoma. Note the asymmetry, irregular contours, and variable pigmentation that are the hallmarks of this malignancy.

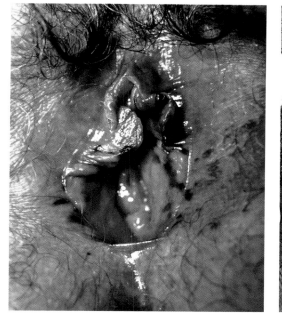

Figure 12.20 Lentigines of the vulva. Multiple dark macules or freckles on the labia minora and vaginal introitus may appear as a result of previous inflammation, but single lesions should be evaluated carefully to rule out the possibility of malignant melanoma.

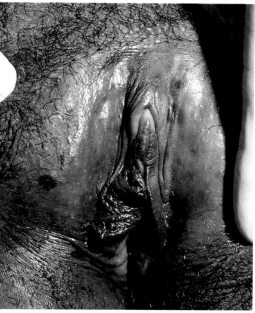

Figure 12.21 Post-inflammatory hyperpigmentation of the vulva. The spotty hyperpigmentation on the right labium majora and left labium minora is seen in association with a more diffuse hypopigmentation around the clitoris and the lower introitus.

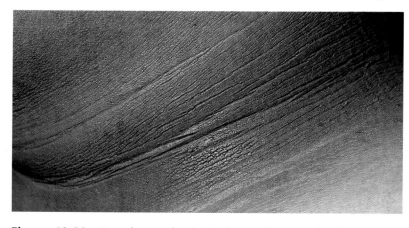

Figure 12.22 Pseudoacanthosis nigricans of the neck. The finely papillated surface of the skin gives it a velvety appearance. This feature, in combination with hyperpigmentation, is the cardinal sign of acanthosis nigricans of any etiology.

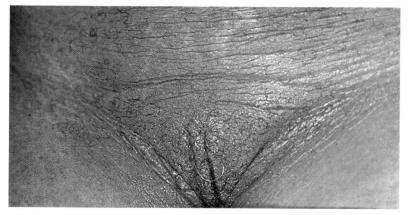

Figure 12.23 Acanthosis nigricans of the vulva. This patient, who has extensive involvement of all intertriginous skin and of the hands and mouth, was found to have gastric adenocarcinoma—the most common cancer associated with this disorder. The acute onset of thick, velvety intertriginous plaques, hyperpigmented or not, should prompt a thorough evaluation for internal malignancy.

acanthosis nigricans. Unfortunately, the malignancy may be well established by the time the cutaneous changes are seen.

HYPOPIGMENTATION

By far the most common color change on the genitalia is the loss of pigment in the form of *vitiligo*. This pigment loss is quite remarkable in persons with dark complexions and may be overlooked entirely in fair-skinned people. Characteristically symmetric in distribution, it may be seen as white patches on the glans penis (Fig. 12.24) or as a "keyhole" pattern around the vagina (Fig. 12.25) and anus. When it occurs on other areas of the body, it also is often periorificial, around the mouth, eyes (Fig. 12.26), and nares. Vitiligo also may develop distally over the fingers and toes, again, in a typically symmetric pattern. Asymmetric vitiligo is unusual but does occur, often in a dermatomal distribution. Some vitiligo patients have autoimmune thyroid disorders or diabetes, but many have no systemic abnormalities. Treatment should be directed to a dermatologist, but spontaneous repigmentation has been known to occur. Post-inflammatory hypopigmentation may be seen after an episode of primary or secondary syphilis (Fig. 12.27), any form of genital ulcer, a dermatophyte infection, or chronic intertrigo (Figs. 12.28 and 12.29).

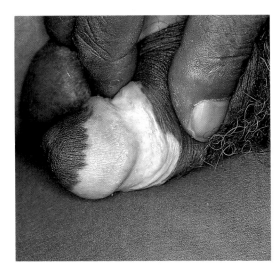

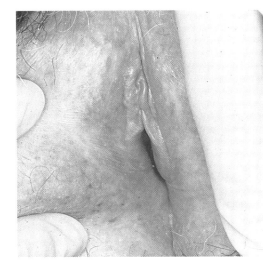

Figure 12.24 Vitiligo of the glans penis. This is a relatively common condition, which, although asymptomatic, may be a source of great anxiety for the patient.

Figure 12.25 Vitiligo of the vulva. This photograph shows the typical symmetric loss of pigmentation from the periorificial skin. Notice that the epidermis is quite normal in appearance. There is no sign of the atrophy usually associated with lichen sclerosus, which also may be hypopigmented.

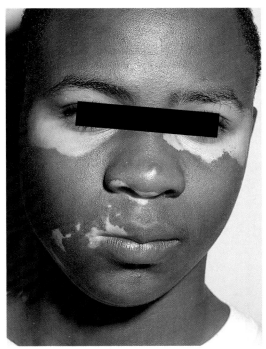

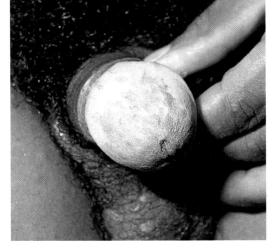

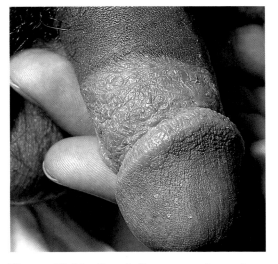

Figure 12.26 Periorificial facial vitiligo. The patchy symmetric loss of pigmentation in vitiligo may be localized to one area of the body or it may involve many sites. In this patient, the vitiligo was confined to the face and extremities.

Figure 12.27 Post-inflammatory hypopigmentation and hyperpigmentation of the penis. A syphilitic chancre may have been the cause of the spotty pigmentation of the glans that appeared months prior to the development of a generalized papular eruption. This generalized eruption, visible on the penis, scrotum, and legs, proved to be a manifestation of secondary syphilis.

Figure 12.28 Post-inflammatory hypopigmentation of the foreskin and corona of the penis. Seborrheic dermatitis caused the pigment changes in this patient, who visited the STD clinic for this problem.

Atrophy

Itching or burning may be the presenting symptom in *lichen sclerosus* (*lichen sclerosus et atrophicus*). Occurring more commonly on female genitalia, this condition is seen clinically as depigmentation of the skin (Fig. 12.30). The atrophic epidermis shows fine "cigarette paper" wrinkling, while the sclerotic or thickened dermis obscures normal capillary filling, giving a white appearance to the skin. Severe cases may result in complete resorption of the labia minora, and vulvar adhesions are not uncommon. The etiology of this condition is unknown, and occasionally it may be seen in young girls, in some cases resolving at puberty. Symptoms vary in such cases of lichen sclerosus, ranging from the patient's complete unawareness of the problem to severe itching and burning. The thinned epidermis is extremely friable, and petechiae or purpura may be seen as a result of scratching. When seen in the male, lichen sclerosus may cause the glans penis to have an extremely white, scarred-down appearance known as *balanitis xerotica obliterans* (Fig. 12.31). As with lichen sclerosus in the female, balanitis xerotica may respond to topical treatment with glucocorticoids or androgens (testosterone).

In some cases, lichen sclerosus may develop discrete areas of thickened hyperkeratotic stratum corneum. When these changes are seen in conjunction with the more typical atrophic ones, this is known as a *mixed dystrophy* (Fig. 12.32) and should be evaluated carefully for the presence of neoplasm. Several biopsies should be taken from different areas of thickened dystrophic skin to rule out the possibility of vulvar intraepithelial neoplasia (VIN).

Atrophic vaginitis may be seen in the postmenopausal woman, though cutaneous changes may consist only of mild thinning and loss of subcutaneous substance.

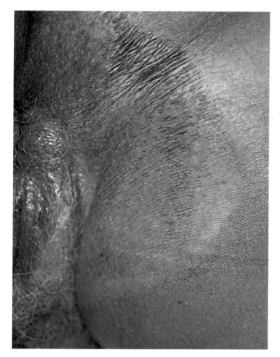

Figure 12.29 Post-inflammatory hypopigmentation and hyperpigmentation of chronic intertrigo. Pigment variations may be seen as inflammatory cutaneous conditions flare and resolve.

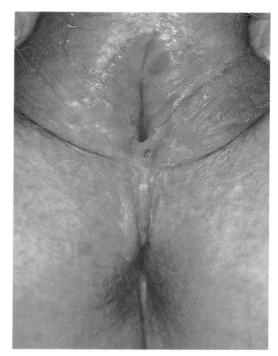

Figure 12.30 Lichen sclerosus of the vulva. Thinning and atrophy of epidermal skin are seen with loss of architecture of the labia minora, including adhesion formation at the posterior introitus. Note the presence of erosions and petechiae secondary to mild trauma of the fragile skin.

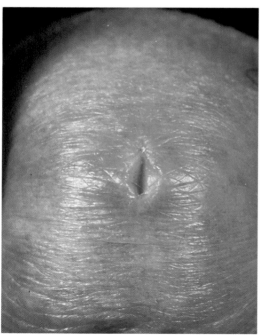

Figure 12.31 Balanitis xerotica obliterans. Lichen sclerosus on the glans penis exhibits white atrophic patches similar to those seen on the vulva. Meatal stenosis may occur.

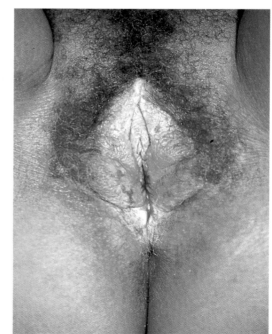

Figure 12.32 Mixed dystrophy of the vulva. This nomenclature describes hypertrophic, white thickened areas of vulvar skin in association with lichen sclerosus. This patient has biopsy-proven lichen sclerosus with areas of cutaneous hyperplasia. There was no evidence of malignancy.

Pustules

Most physicians regard the presence of pustules on the skin as prima facie evidence of infection. In most cases this is true, and infection certainly should be ruled out when pus-containing papules are seen. There are, however, certain cutaneous conditions that are characterized by the presence of aggregates of white cells that are sterile to culture for bacteria, fungi, or a virus. In the following section, we will discuss the pustular conditions of the genitalia (Fig. 12.33).

Figure 12.33 **A** Infectious pustular conditions occurring on the genitalia. **B** Noninfectious pustular conditions occurring on the genitalia.

INFECTIOUS PUSTULAR CONDITIONS OCCURRING ON THE GENITALIA

CONDITION	FINDINGS	TREATMENT
Candida	Most common, itches and burns.	Clotrimazole, miconazole.
	Intense erythema; often edema, satellite lesions.	Nystatin vaginal suppositories. Oral ketoconazole in resistant cases— short course.
Tinea	Serpiginous "active" border, itchy, relatively unusual in women.	Oral griseofulvin. Topical imidazoles.
Impetigo	Usually secondary to pruritic dermatitis, excoriations, secondary bacterial colonization.	Topical antibacterial scrubs. Erythromycin or dicloxacillin.
Folliculitis	Pustules at base of hairs (rule out gram-negative infection if patient is on antibiotics).	Erythromycin or dicloxacillin unless gram-negative; then according to sensitivities.
Furunculosis "boils"	Painful, deep-seated nodules may be topped by pustules; may suppurate; recurrent lesions may indicate transmission by close contact.	Early treatment with erythromycin or dicloxacillin may abort early lesions and prevent suppuration.
Herpes simplex	WBCs in old intact vesicles may cause lesions to look pustular.	Acyclovir or topical antibiotics in mild cases.
Syphilis	Scattered scaly pustules may be seen in secondary syphilis.	Penicillin: see treatment schedule in Chapter 1.

A

NONINFECTIOUS PUSTULAR CONDITIONS OCCURRING ON THE GENITALIA

CONDITION	FINDINGS	TREATMENT
Pseudofolliculitis	Ingrown hairs indicate mechanical trauma.	Stop shaving.
Acneiform rashes	Withdrawal of potent topical steroids; contact with oils, hydrocarbons.	Wean off with hydrocortisones. Eliminate work-related industrial exposure.
Hidradenitis suppurativa	Chronic acneiform condition with sinus tracts and scarring.	Minocin, 100 mg *po* daily. Surgical excision of affected area.
Pustular psoriasis and/or Reiter's	Often associated with arthritis; usually a previous history of disease.	Methotrexate therapy. Dermatology consult.
Pemphigus	Chronic familial form (Hailey-Hailey) or acquired (pemphigus vulgaris).	Antibiotics and oral corticosteroids. Dermatology consult.

While the presence of pus generally implies infection, this finding is not specific. Just as there are nonpyogenic infections, there are certain pustular skin conditions not at all associated with infectious organisms. Gram stains of pustule contents should be examined for bacteria and gram-positive budding yeast forms; KOH of the pustule roof may reveal fungal hyphae; and bacterial cultures should be done on material from cleaned, intact lesions. If lesion morphology suggests herpes, Tzanck smears and viral cultures should also be performed; dark-field examination should be done if syphilis is suspected.

B

INFECTIOUS PUSTULES

One of the most common causes of genital pustules, especially with inflammation, is cutaneous *candidiasis* or *monilia* (Fig. 12.34). Skin lesions generally are seen in conjunction with a candidal vaginitis in the female (Fig. 12.35). Males may also harbor the organism (*Candida albicans*), in the inguinal or gluteal folds, on the scrotum, and, especially if uncircumcised, on the penis (Fig. 12.36). Factors predisposing to cutaneous candidiasis include immunosuppression, diabetes mellitus, and the administration of systemic antibiotics. While candidal pseudohyphae sometimes may be seen on KOH examination of material from superficial intertriginous erosions, the better diagnostic tests for this organism are a Gram or PAS stain of material from a pustule. The typical budding yeast forms are gram-positive and somewhat larger than lymphocytes (Fig. 12.37).

Acute inflammatory *tinea* infections may have a vesiculopustular scaly border (Fig. 12.38). KOH of a blister or pustule roof will demonstrate fungal hyphae. In the presence of a chronic intertrigo, foci of dermatophyte infections may remain deep in follicles, which can occasionally become nodular (Majocchi's granuloma). The diagnosis of fungal folliculitis should be considered when the patient fails to respond to systemic antibiotics.

Discrete, scattered pustules in hairy areas of the body generally are caused by *Staphylococcus*—"Bockhart's impetigo." Since many cutaneous staphylococci are penicillinase producers, treatment should be with erythromycin or with penicillinase-resistant penicillins such as dicloxacillin.

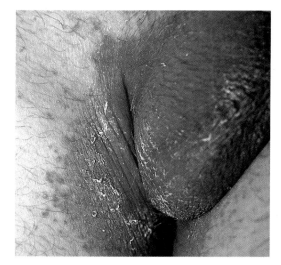

Figure 12.34 *Candida* infection showing the intense inflammation with satellite pustules. Note that the pustules are superficial and not located at the base of hairs.

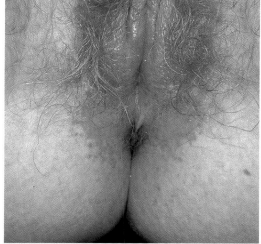

Figure 12.35 *Candida* vulvovaginitis. Intense erythema and edema appear around the introitus, perineum, and perianal areas. The discrete erythematous macules at the active borders are resolving pustules.

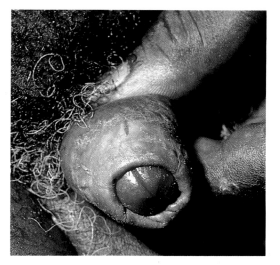

Figure 12.36 *Candida* balanitis showing edema and erythema with satellite pustules. This is seen most commonly in uncircumcised males. *Candida* should be considered a sexually transmissible disease, and treatment with imidazole creams may facilitate satisfactory topical treatment of both partners.

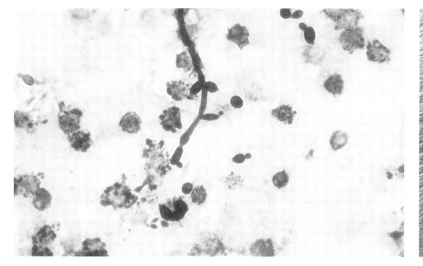

Figure 12.37 PAS stain of budding yeast and pseudohyphae seen in *Candida albicans*.

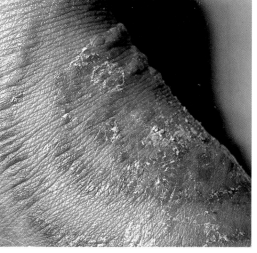

Figure 12.38 Tinea corporis showing vesicles and pustules at the active advancing edge of a typical scaly plaque.

In susceptible individuals, folliculitis may develop into a larger cutaneous abscess called a *carbuncle* or a *furuncle* (Fig. 12.39). Typically caused by *Staphylococcus*, early lesions will respond to systemic antibiotics. Most later lesions benefit from application of warm compresses until spontaneous rupture of the abscess occurs, but fully developed walled-off abscesses may require incision and drainage. Recurrent furunculosis does not necessarily imply that a patient has an immune deficiency. Phage-typing of staphylococci has been used to identify cluster groups of patients who pass the infection back and forth, usually in a close-living or sexually active situation. Pustules also may be seen in mixed bacterial *impetigo* (Fig. 12.40), an extremely common skin infection that may be the result of secondary bacterial colonization of a preexisting dermatitis.

While the umbilicated papules of *molluscum contagiosum* (Fig. 12.41) are not actually pustules, the initial appearance of these lesions may mislead the patient and physician. Since usually they are pale or flesh-colored, they can give the appearance of pustules; however, they actually are rather sturdy papules, which may persist for many weeks. The central dell or umbilication is characteristic of the viral etiology of these lesions, which are caused by a pox virus. Therapy is directed toward destruction of the lesion, with curettage or blistering agents applied to the lesions.

NONINFECTIOUS PUSTULES

In most clinical situations, the presence of pus implies infection, and it is entirely appropriate to obtain bacterial, fungal,

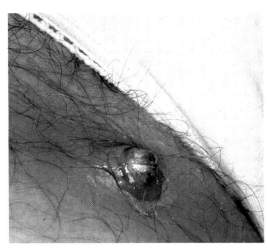

Figure 12.39 Carbuncle on the upper thigh. A thick crust with surrounding erythema and tenderness is characteristic.

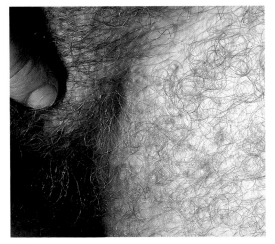

Figure 12.40 Impetigo. Pustules, pus-filled bullae, crusts, and erosions all present in this superficial bacterial skin infection, which may be localized to the groin in sexually active patients.

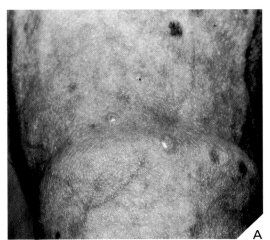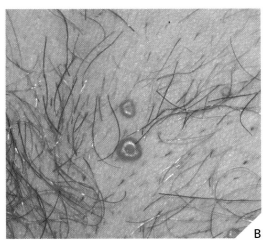

A B

Figure 12.41 A and B Molluscum contagiosum. Flesh-colored papules of molluscum may be distinguished by their umbilicated centers. The papules contain a white cheesy substance, which may be stained for the presence of viral inclusion bodies.

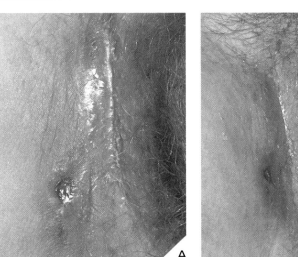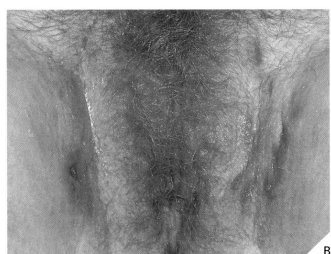

A B

Figure 12.42 A and B Hidradenitis suppurativa of the vulva. Indolent painful pustules and nodules are associated with this chronic disorder. Sinuses and scars result.

and/or viral cultures in this setting. There are certain dermatologic conditions, however, in which pustules or the accumulation of white cells in the epidermis is initiated by stimuli other than bacterial infection.

While bacterial superinfection can play an important part in *hidradenitis suppurativa* (Fig. 12.42), the mechanism of this severe acneiform eruption in the groin and/or axillae is related to occlusion of hair follicles and retention of follicular contents, resulting in an inflammatory process that includes hair follicles and sweat glands. Secondary bacterial infection is common. The presence of multiple papules, pustules, cysts, and sinus tracts is the cutaneous constellation common to cystic acne, hidradenitis, and dissecting folliculitis of the scalp, which may occur together. In some chronic cases, keloid formation may be the most prominent feature of a "burned-out" case of hidradenitis. Antibiotic therapy can be helpful in acute flares of this disease, and resistance to tetracycline or erythromycin should raise the suspicion of superinfection·with gram-negative organisms. Surgical excision and grafting remains the treatment of choice for recalcitrant cases, although the vitamin A analogs (e.g., isotretinoin) have shown some promise in the treatment of this distressing condition.

Pustular psoriasis (Fig. 12.43) may begin as groups of sterile pustules in intertriginous areas, which rapidly enlarge and spread across the trunk and extremities in waves that coalesce, forming "lakes" of pus in the superficial epidermis. This severe form of psoriasis is associated with high fevers and malaise. It occurs primarily in patients already diagnosed with psoriasis and is seen sometimes as a result of systemic steroid therapy. Acute episodes may be difficult to manage, and generally respond best to systemic therapy with antimetabolites such as methotrexate or with the vitamin A analog etretinate (RO 10-9359).

Reiter's disease is an uncommon condition in which urethritis and arthritis may be associated with psoriasis-like lesions on the skin, including an inflammatory condition of the penis known as *circinate balanitis*. The urethritis and involvement of genital mucosa make the STD clinic a likely setting in which to diagnose this disease. The circinate balanitis (Fig. 12.44) may appear as nonscaly erythematous plaques, or the eruption may be more pustular, crusted, and scaly. On nongenital skin, it is very similar in appearance to pustular psoriasis (Fig. 12.45). Arthritis also is a typical feature, and conjunctivitis also may be seen. Patients with Reiter's disease usually have histocompatibility antigen HLA-B27, with a high risk of developing ankylosing spondylitis. A link to infections such as *Chlamydia* has been postulated. Fortunately, skin lesions often respond to low-potency topical corticosteroids. The arthritis may be more difficult to treat and can be disabling.

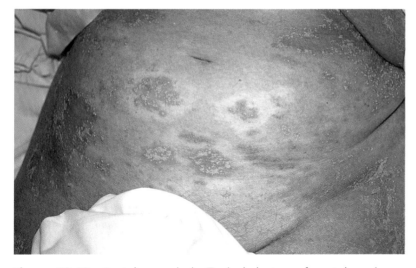

Figure 12.43 Pustular psoriasis. Typical clusters of pustules arise in intertriginous areas and spread outward, forming "lakes" of pus at the periphery of the eruption. Patients are febrile and ill, although the pustules are sterile. This form of psoriasis is relatively rare but may be precipitated by systemic corticosteroid therapy.

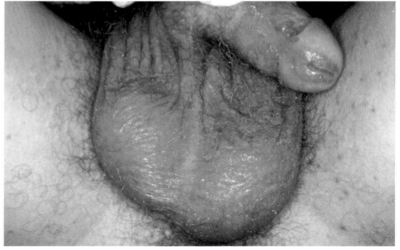

Figure 12.44 Reiter's disease of the penis. The typical erythema and scale are seen producing the psoriasis-like picture of circinate balanitis. This disorder is associated with HLA-B27, and symptoms of arthritis are extremely common.

Figure 12.45 Reiter's disease. Scaly papules cover the instep and heel. Palmar and plantar involvement is termed *keratoderma blennorrhagica*.

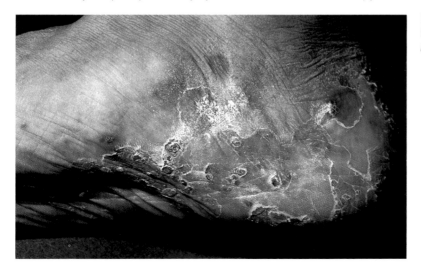

Benign familial pemphigus (*Hailey-Hailey disease*) presents as pustules and erosions in intertriginous areas (Fig. 12.46), but this inherited disorder can easily become superinfected with *Candida* or bacteria, which may obscure the initial diagnosis. The familial occurrence and chronicity, as well as a typical histologic picture, make diagnosis relatively easy, although the varied spectrum of lesions from hyperkeratotic papules to erosions may mislead the clinician who looks for fluid-filled vesicles in this so-called "bullous disease."

Nodules and Tumors

Epidermoid cysts are firm, yellow, subcutaneous nodules that may occur singly or, in some cases, prolifically over the vulva or scrotum (Fig. 12.47). Treatment usually is sought when the cysts rupture or become secondarily infected. Although cutaneous crusting and erosion may be present over the cyst, the nodular nature of the lesion is unlike other sexually transmitted genital ulcers, which are more superficial. Antistaphylococcal antibiotics and *sitz* baths usually resolve the secondary infection,

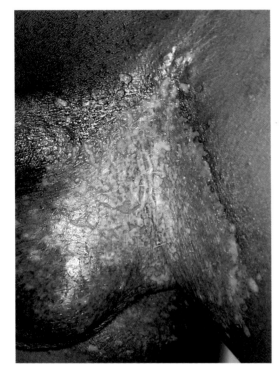

Figure 12.46 Erosive lesions of benign familial pemphigus (Hailey-Hailey disease) on the scrotum and groin. Traumatic loss of the blister roof in an intertriginous area may cause an otherwise typical bullous disease to appear as multiple erosions.

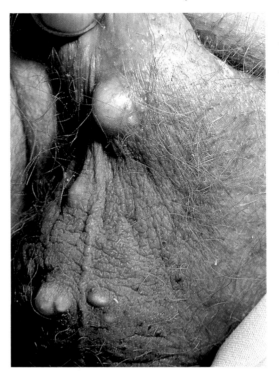

Figure 12.47 Epidermoid cysts of the scrotum. Generally asymptomatic, these lesions occasionally may rupture and cause discomfort to the patient. These lesions should be differentiated from steatocystoma multiplex, which contain a gel-like material rather than the thick, yellow, sebaceous substance typical of the epidermoid cyst.

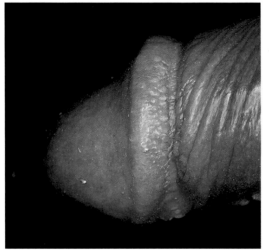

Figure 12.48 "Pearly penile papules." A normal variant, these tiny papules are sometimes mistaken for condylomata.

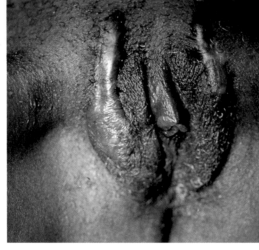

Figure 12.49 Vulvar keloids. Thickened, linear nodular scars are present on both labia majora. Inciting factors in susceptible individuals include any inflammation or infectious or traumatic insult to skin.

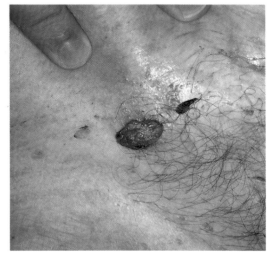

Figure 12.50 Seborrheic keratosis. This thickened, warty lesion has a typical "stuck-on" appearance. Similar lesions may be found elsewhere on the trunk.

and, if necessary, the cyst may later be removed. In most cases, the patient is aware of the diagnosis, although with multiple lesions one also should consider the possibility of *steatocystoma multiplex*. The latter cysts extrude a clear to yellowish gel-like material when punctured, and often appear on the face, neck, upper trunk, and axillae as well. This condition is a hereditary disorder, primarily of cosmetic concern.

Pearly penile papules (Fig. 12.48) are 1-to-2-mm pink papules that occur in one or two orderly rows along the corona of the glans penis. They frequently are mistaken for condylomata acuminata, but their consistency in size and regular distribution help to establish the diagnosis. Histologically, the papules are angiofibromas. No treatment is indicated for this condition.

Fox-Fordyce disease is characterized by aggregations of tiny 1-to-2-mm papules in the groin or axilla. This hereditary condition affects the apocrine sweat ducts and is much more common in women than in men. The most common complaint is severe pruritus, which may respond to systemic estrogen therapy.

Keloids (Fig. 12.49) are irregular, often linear, firm nodules, seen most often in patients with recurrent episodes of folliculitis or hidradenitis. They should be differentiated from epidermoid cysts, for often they will respond to intralesional steroid therapy, and excision may worsen the condition.

Seborrheic keratoses are elevated "stuck-on" growths that may be pigmented or flesh-colored, which most often appear on the trunk (Fig. 12.50) but may occur on the genitalia. These warty growths are quite benign, and similar lesions usually are found elsewhere on the body. They require removal only if they occur in areas where friction of clothing causes irritation. In intertriginous areas, seborrheic keratoses or even simple *acrochordons* (skin tags) may, with time, become pedunculated and prominent (Fig. 12.51). When one of these lesions becomes twisted on its stalk the entire lesion may infarct, becoming black and alarming the patient.

Hyperkeratotic or ulcerated lesions that are asymmetrically located on the genitalia should be evaluated carefully for the possibility of *squamous cell carcinoma* (Figs. 12.52 and 12.53). The lesions may be asymptomatic, and patients may be unaware of them or deny the chronicity of the problem. Biopsy is recommended for suspicious lesions, and multiple biopsies should be taken of all suspicious areas. In some forms of squamous cell carcinoma, such as Bowen's disease of the vulva and bowenoid papulosis, the presence of certain human papillomaviruses (HPV 16 and 18) has been reported (see Chapter 10). Evaluation of the patient with a suspicious lesion should include palpation of regional lymph nodes. It may be appropriate to refer the patient directly to a specialist for evaluation and biopsy, although physicians should be aware that apprehension may make the patient reluctant to seek appropriate and timely consultative care. For this reason it may be expeditious to per-

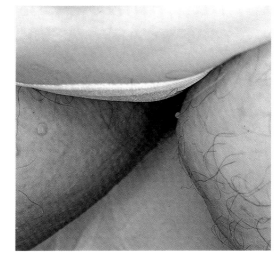

Figure 12.51 Acrochordons. "Skin tags" often are found in intertriginous areas. They usually are asymptomatic unless traumatized.

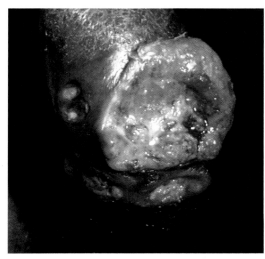

Figure 12.52 Squamous cell carcinoma of the penis. This large chronic ulcer had been present for over a year. Patients may delay consultation with a physician because they are afraid that a malignancy will be diagnosed.

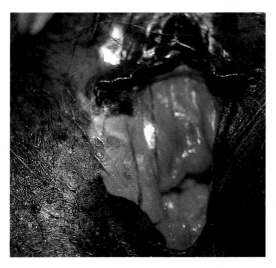

Figure 12.53 Carcinoma in situ of the vulva. Note the asymmetric, rough, whitish, eroded, thickened appearance of this malignancy on the labium.

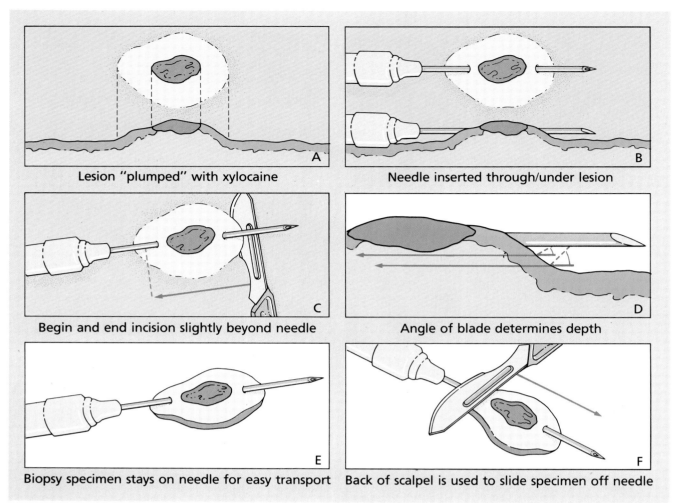

Figure 12.54
Needle shave technique for skin biopsy.

A Lesion "plumped" with xylocaine

B Needle inserted through/under lesion

C Begin and end incision slightly beyond needle

D Angle of blade determines depth

E Biopsy specimen stays on needle for easy transport

F Back of scalpel is used to slide specimen off needle

A Using a small (27-to-30-gauge) needle, a wheal is formed under and around the lesion with local anesthetic (generally less than 1 cc of 1% xylocaine with epinephrine). For the biopsy, a half-inch 25-gauge needle is preferable, as a 30-gauge needle tends to bend when lifting up on the skin. Placing the needle on a syringe provides a "handle" for better control.

B The orientation of needle insertion is not critical, but a good guide might be the direction of what is to be the long axis of the biopsy. The needle is inserted just proximal to the lesion, advanced just under it, and exited just distal to it.

C The scalpel blade (#15 is small and manageable) should also be mounted on a handle for good control. The long axis of the scalpel and the needle are maintained at approximate right angles to one another, and the blade is inserted *under* the point of the needle, with the back of the blade actually touching the distal needle shaft. The biopsy incision is begun slightly distal to the exit point of the needle, and is directed toward the hub for maximum control.

D The angle of the blade should be determined before beginning the incision—a shallow angle for a superficial incision and a wider angle for a deeper specimen. The blade angle (depth of cut) should be maintained as consistently as possible, as the scalpel is drawn toward the hub of the syringe. Running the blade along the undersurface of the needle should be avoided as the incision will be too shallow and tissue immobilization will be lost as the specimen shifts off the needle. "Scooping" with the blade also should be avoided since the incision will then be wider and deeper than necessary, and wound edges will be ragged.

E The incision is begun and ended slightly *beyond* the needle entrance and exit. The skin is lifted *gently* with the needle, as the blade slices underneath; the specimen on the needle should not "pop" free as the biopsy is completed. The biopsy specimen should smoothly come free of the surrounding skin, impaled neatly on the needle for ease of handling. The biopsy specimen may be left on the needle and set aside briefly until bleeding is stopped or it may be placed directly into fixative.

F To remove the biopsy specimen from the needle, use the *back* of the scalpel blade to slide the specimen off into the bottle of fixative.

form a biopsy on the first visit so that the correct diagnosis may be made (Fig. 12.54).

Erosions and Ulcers

An erosion is defined as the loss of epidermis, while an ulcer extends through the epidermis into the dermis. The lack of a primary lesion makes evaluation of erosions and ulcers extremely difficult for most physicians, and biopsies rarely are helpful unless taken from the edge of a fresh lesion. Infectious ulcers have been covered in other chapters, so this discussion will be limtied to noninfectious genital erosions and ulcers.

BULLOUS DISEASES

The fragility of a blister roof in an intertriginous area makes erosions the most common presentation of the bullous diseases, which classically appear as blisters elsewhere on the skin. Erythema multiforme (EM) typically appears as "target" or "bull's-eye" lesions on the extremities (Fig. 12.55). Involvement of the oral mucosa (Fig. 12.56), palms, soles, and glans penis (Fig. 12.57) is seen most often in the bullous form called the Stevens-Johnson syndrome. EM often is associated with ingestion of drugs or a preceding herpes simplex virus (HSV) infection; however, other infections such as mycoplasma, pneumonia, or other viral or bacterial infections may be associated with the occurrence of this disorder. Recurrent episodes are not uncommon and may be limited to mucous membranes such as the mouth and genitalia. It is important to inquire of the patient whether or not there has been an episode of HSV preceding the outbreak of EM, for control of HSV recurrences with acyclovir may lead to control of EM as well.

As mentioned previously in the section on pustular dermatoses, *benign familial pemphigus* is most commonly seen as localized erosions in the groin. *Pemphigus vulgaris*, however, also may present with similar ulcers or erosions. Chronic pemphigus may even result in somewhat heaped-up, friable papules (*pemphigus vegetans*.)

ULCERATIVE DERMATOSES

Ulcerative forms of dermatoses may occur when a dermatologic condition makes the skin exceptionally fragile and easily traumatized. When these conditions occur on the genitalia, their presentation may be obscured by their erosive appearance.

Seen most commonly on the glans penis or hands, the *fixed drug eruption* (Fig. 12.58) has been linked with tetracycline therapy, phenolphthalein found in certain laxatives, and several other drugs (Fig. 12.59). Typically appearing as a hyperpigmented round macule on the skin, acute lesions may be eczematous, bullous, or erosive in appearance. The appearance of genital lesions in a patient who is being treated with tetracycline for an STD may cause that patient to believe that he or she is experiencing a relapse of the disease or has another STD (see Chapter 1, Differential Diagnosis).

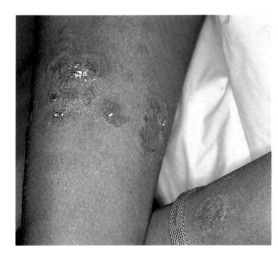

Figure 12.55
Erythema multiforme (EM) on the arms. The concentric shape ("target" lesions) and presence of bullae are helpful clues to the recognition of this skin disorder, in which many different morphologic types of lesions may be present.

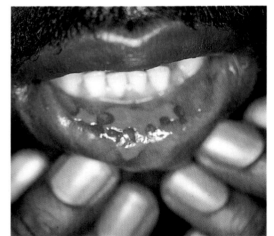

Figure 12.56
Oral erythema multiforme (Stevens-Johnson syndrome). This patient's lips exhibit painful erosions and crusting. On the palms and soles were multiple tender erythematous plaques.

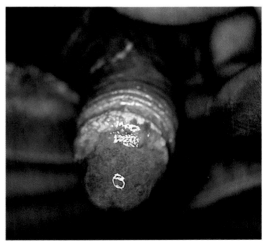

Figure 12.57 Penile erosion in erythema multiforme. These painful shallow erosions developed after a herpesvirus infection of the mouth—a relatively common association.

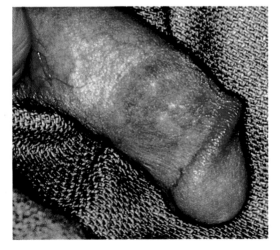

Figure 12.58 Fixed drug eruption of the penis. Lesions may appear elsewhere on the body as hyperpigmented round macules or bullae that flare with readministration of the offending drug.

DRUGS COMMONLY CAUSING FIXED DRUG ERUPTIONS

Barbiturates

Chlordiazepoxide

Dapsone

Oxyphenbutazone

Phenolphthalein

Quinine and derivatives

Sulfonamides

Tetracycline

Figure 12.59 Drugs commonly causing fixed drug eruptions.

Lichen planus was discussed under its most typical presentation as a papulosquamous disorder, but ulcerative forms of this disorder do occur on mucous membranes (Fig. 12.60) and can be extremely difficult to manage. Vulvovaginal erosions may be extensive, and their chronicity may cause the physician to consider the possibility of malignancy. Superinfection with *Candida* also may occur in this disorder, and should be considered and treated, if present. Treatment for ulcerative lichen planus generally is symptomatic, and topical steroids may be necessary.

Lichen sclerosus was discussed under the category of atrophy, but the extreme friability of the epidermis in this condition makes the presence of erosions, petechiae, and purpura a common occurrence. The patient should be examined carefully for the typical white atrophic epidermis occurring symmetrically around the rectum and perineum in this condition.

Cutaneous trauma is an often overlooked source of genital ulceration. A relatively innocuous dermatitis on the genitalia may be extremely pruritic and bothersome, and may result in the patient's traumatizing the skin during bouts of itching and scratching. *Erosions* can be deep and severe (Fig. 12.61), and secondary infection may make evaluation difficult. Questioning the patient about his underlying symptoms frequently will evoke an admission of intractable pruritus, and therapy should be directed toward alleviation of symptoms. Trauma induced by the patient's sexual partner also should be considered, especially with oral sex. *Human bites* (Fig. 12.62) are notoriously infectious, and cultures may be necessary to determine appropriate broad-spectrum antibiotic therapy. The presence of symmetric bruises or cuts encircling the penis should lead the physician to suspect cutaneous trauma as a likely etiology; this becomes especially important in the evaluation of children for possible sexual abuse.

SYSTEMIC DISEASES

Systemic diseases also may lead to secondary genital ulcers. *Behçet's disease* is a multisystem disorder that may present with skin involvement in a majority of cases. In the full-blown syndrome, oral and genital ulcerations are present (Fig. 12.63), as well as a pustular eruption, which may involve the genitals. A

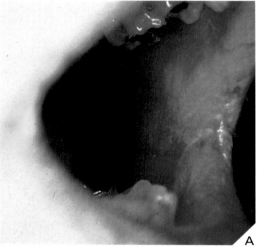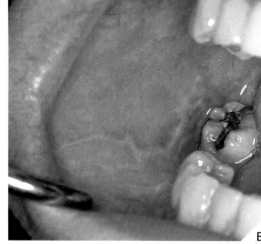

Figure 12.60 Erosive lichen planus on the oral mucous membrane. **A** The lips and buccal mucosa are seen. **B** The buccal mucosa is seen.

A

B

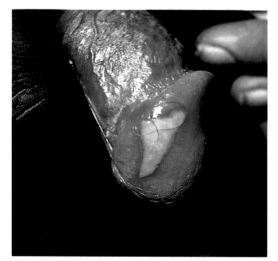

Figure 12.61 Traumatic ulcer of the penis. The sharply angled borders of this lesion are a clue to its traumatic rather than infectious etiology.

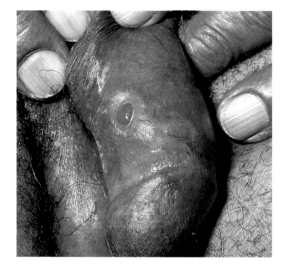

Figure 12.62 Ulcers secondary to human bite of the penile shaft. Secondary infection is a common sequela of human bite wounds and cultures may be necessary for appropriate antibiotic therapy.

spectrum of ocular involvement includes conjunctivitis, photophobia, uveitis, and optic neuritis. Central nervous system changes are variable and can be severe, thus frequently dominating the clinical picture. Fever, arthralgias, and cardiac or pulmonary involvement also may be present. The mucosal ulcerations are nonspecific, and more common causes should be excluded before a diagnosis of Behçet's is made on the basis of oral and genital ulcers alone.

Pyoderma gangrenosum (Fig. 12.64) is a shaggy, painful, "dirty"-appearing ulcer with a bluish overhanging border. The name reflects the exceptionally infectious appearance of this actually noninfectious ulcer. It is seen most commonly in patients with inflammatory bowel disease, but also may be seen in conjunction with multiple myeloma or other hematologic or immunologic disorders.

Although pyoderma gangrenosum may be seen with gastrointestinal disease, cutaneous Crohn's disease classically presents as long "knife-cut" ulcers along the intertriginous groin folds.

Flares of these cutaneous lesions often parallel the course of the GI disease, and control of one often will lead to control of the other.

Asymmetric ulcers on the genitalia that do not heal with appropriate therapy should be biopsied to rule out carcinoma. Biopsies should be multiple and taken from the thickest part of lesions and the edge of ulcers. Squamous cell carcinoma was discussed in detail under nodules and tumors. Extramammary Paget's disease may have a remarkably eczematous appearance on first examination. Hallmarks of this diagnosis are its chronicity, asymmetry, and lack of response to topical therapy.

Picture credits for this chapter are as follows: Figs. 12.16, 12.17, and 12.60 courtesy of Emory University School of Dentistry; Figs. 12.56 and 12.57 courtesy of Heidi Watts; Figs. 12.13B, 12.18, 12.31, 12.41, and 12.42 courtesy du Vivier A: Atlas of Clinical Dermatology. New York, Gower Medical Publishing, 1986.

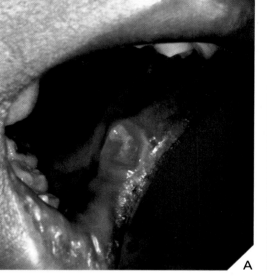
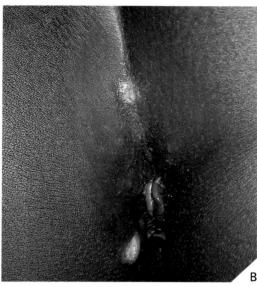

A

B

Figure 12.63 A and B Behcet's disease. Nonspecific painful recurrent ulcers of the oral and genital mucosa were the presenting complaints in this young woman in whom Behcet's disease was diagnosed.

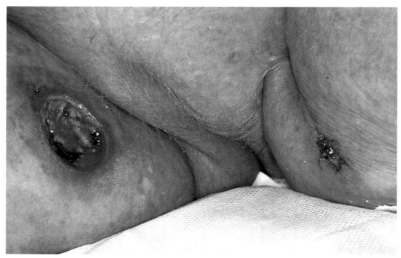

Figure 12.64 Pyoderma gangrenosum. Multiple deep necrotic ulcers with dusky overhanging margins are characteristic of pyoderma gangrenosum. These lesions may be seen in patients with various systemic diseases.

BIBLIOGRAPHY

Ackerman AB, Kornberg R: Pearly penile papules—acral angiofibromas. *Arch Derm* 108:673, 1973.

Betterle C, Caretto A, DeZio A, et al: Incidence and significance of organ-specific autoimmune disorders (clinical, latent, or only autoantibodies) in patients with vitiligo. *Dermatologica* 171:419, 1985.

Brewerton DA, Nicholls A, Oates JK, et al: Reiter's disease and HL-A 27. *Lancet* 996, 1973.

Fischer A: *Contact Dermatitis*, ed 3. Philadelphia, Lea and Febiger, 1986, 195–198 and 220–227.

Fitzpatrick B, Eisen A, Wolff K, et al: *Dermatology in General Medicine*, ed. 3. New York, McGraw-Hill, 1987.

Friedrich EG Jr: *Vulvar Disease*, ed 2. Philadelphia, WB Saunders Co., 1983.

Hall J, Moreland A, Cox J, et al: Oral acanthosis nigricans: Report of a case and comparison of oral and cutaneous pathology. *Am J Dermatopathol* 10:68, 1988.

Landthaler M, Braun-Falco O, Richter K, et al: Malignant melanomas of the vulva. *Dtsch Med Wochenschr* 110:789, 1985.

Lemak MA, Duvic M, Bean SF: Oral acyclovir for the prevention of herpes-associated erythema multiforme. *J Am Acad Derm* 15:50, 1986.

Lyell A, Gordon A, Dide H, et al: Mycoplasma and erythema multiforme. *Lancet* ii:1116, 1967.

Nethercott JR, Choi BC: Erythema multiforme (Stevens-Johnson syndrome)—Chart review of 123 hospitalized patients. *Dermatologica* 171:383, 1985.

Powell FC, Schroeter AL, Su WPD, et al: Pyoderma gangrenosum: A review of 86 patients. *Q J Med* 55:173, 1985.

Reyman L, Milano A, Demopoulos R, et al: Metastatic vulvar ulceration in Crohn's disease. *Am J Gastro* 81:46, 1986.

Rook A, Wilkinson DS, Ebling FJG, et al: *Textbook of Dermatology*, ed 4. Boston, Blackwell Scientific Publications Inc., 1986.

Sehgal VH, Gangwani OP: Genital fixed drug eruptions. *Genitourin Med* 62:56, 1986.

Sheagren JN: Staphylococcal infections of the skin and skin structures. *Cutis* 36:2, 1985.

Slaney G, Muller S, Clay J, et al: Crohn's disease involving the penis. *Gut* 27:329, 1986.

Strauss WB, Maibach HI: Bacterial interference, treatment of recurrent furunculosis JAMA 208:861, 1969.

Tokoro Y, Seto T, Abe Y, et al: Skin lesions in Behçet's disease. *Int J Derm* 16:227, 1977.

Wolska H, Jablonska S, Langner A, et al: Etretinate therapy in generalized pustular psoriasis (Zumbusch type). *Dermatologica* 171:297, 1985.

Laboratory Evaluation of Victims of Sexual Abuse for Sexually Transmitted Diseases

1

J.S. KNAPP, S.A. MORSE

Introduction

Sexual abuse is defined as "the involvement of dependent, developmentally immature children and adolescents in sexual activities that they do not fully comprehend, to which they are unable to give informed consent, or that violate the social taboos of family roles."

Sexual abuse of children is not a new phenomenon. It is increasingly recognized as one of the most common forms of child abuse. As recently as 1976, sexual abuse was regarded as an uncommon problem; fewer than 2,000 cases were reported nationwide. It is now readily recognized to be widespread in all socioeconomic groups in the United States. A recent survey of childhood abuse among 3,132 adults indicated an overall prevalence rate of 5%; 3.8% of male respondents and 6.8% of female respondents gave positive histories of sexual abuse during their childhood.

Sexually transmitted diseases represent some of the most potentially serious sequellae of sexual abuse. Therefore, evidence of STDs should routinely be sought in children with a history of sexual abuse. Children who are reported to have been sexually abused or who have physical findings suggestive of sexual abuse should be screened for a variety of STDs. Children with a history of sexual abuse have prevalence rates of gonorrhea ranging from 5% to 28%, depending on the prevalence of this disease in the community (Fig. A1.1). The high prevalence of this and other STDs in the sexually abused population make screening for STD pathogens essential. Conversely, evidence of an STD in a prepubertal child should raise the suspicion of sexual abuse and should prompt screening for other STDs. Evidence of an STD may be noted during any evaluation of childhood complaints. These complaints, including vulvovaginitis and anogenital lesions, should prompt an evaluation that includes, but is not limited to, screening for clinically compatible STDs.

Incidence

National data for nonreportable STDs such as chlamydia, herpes, and genital herpes in pediatric age groups are not available. The trend of occurrence of these diseases in children can be extrapolated only from the trends in reportable STDs and from local studies. Figure A1.2 shows that the number of reported cases of gonorrhea per 100,000 population has increased substantially since 1966, especially in the 10 to 14 year olds and in females. In most studies, girls predominate as victims of sexual abuse.

Laboratory Evaluation

Because the identification of an STD agent from a child is indicative of possible sexual abuse, it is important that these agents be correctly identified for several reasons: (1) to provide appropriate therapy to victims infected with sexually transmitted pathogens and to prevent complications that may arise from these infections; (2) to initiate appropriate investigations of sexual abuse when a sexually transmitted pathogen is identified in a child; and (3) to culture individuals who have had contact with the child, at appropriate intervals, to detect sexually transmitted pathogens that would indicate those persons who should be considered as suspects in the investigation.

Fig. A1.1 Prevalence of sexually transmitted diseases in children with a history of sexual abuse. Not every child was examined for the presence of each of these infections.

PREVALENCE OF SEXUALLY TRANSMITTED DISEASES IN CHILDREN WITH A HISTORY OF SEXUAL ABUSE

INFECTION	PREVALENCE (%)
Gonorrhea	5–28
Chlamydia	4–8
Syphilis	0–1.5
Genital warts	0.7–1.5
Genital herpes	0.5
Trichomoniasis	1–4

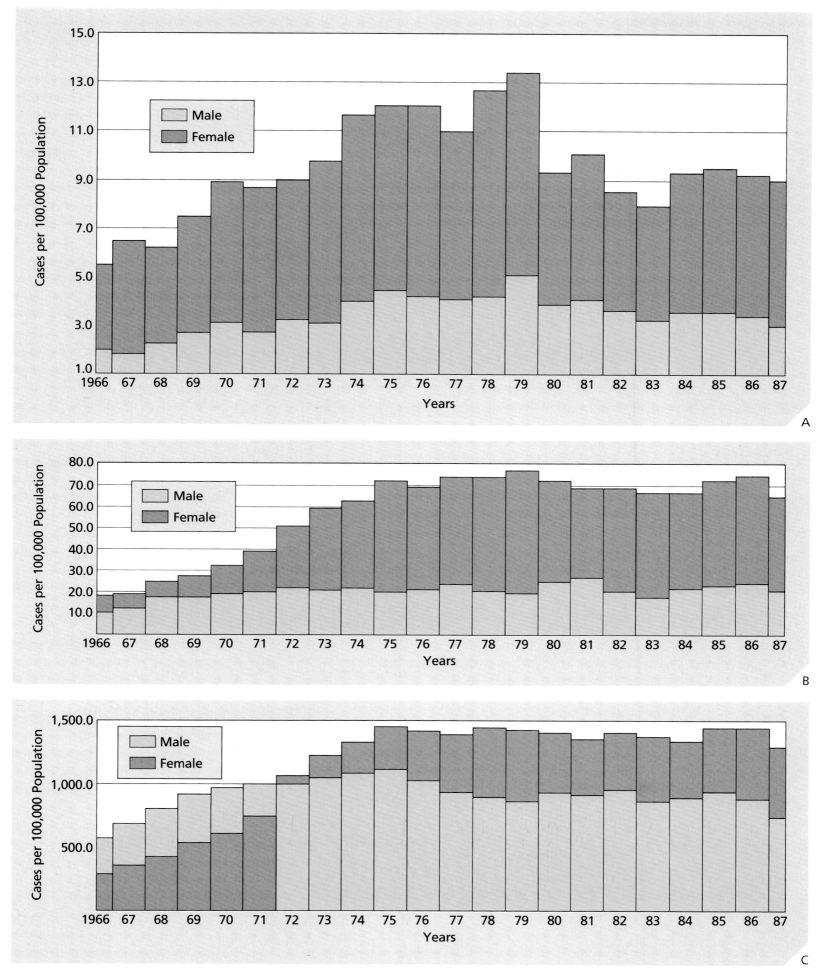

Fig. A1.2 Prevalence of gonorrhea in pediatric-age patients in the United States, 1966–1987. **A** 0 to 9 years. **B** 10 to 14 years. **C** 15 to 19 years.

In cases of suspected sexual abuse, children should be screened for the STD agents listed in Fig. A1.3. Culture is the only acceptable method for isolating many of these agents. After isolation they must be identified with confirmatory tests. It is not sufficient to diagnose an infection clinically or to identify its etiologic agent with presumptive criteria that may be acceptable when identifying the same agent in a sexually active patient population in which it is generally assumed that patients are at high risk for STDs. The confirmatory tests that may be appropriately used to identify STD agents in patients at low risk for STDs are given in earlier chapters.

Several problems may arise during the identification of STD agents in patients at low risk for these infections. The laboratory techniques for identifying some of the agents listed in Fig. A1.3, especially the viral agents and *Chlamydia trachomatis*, may not be routinely available; it may be necessary to send specimens to other laboratories. Specimens for culture must be transported by methods that have been shown to preserve the viability of the agents; if specimens cannot be transported appropriately, isolation of the agents should not be attempted. Direct tests should not be used to identify these agents in specimens from low-risk patients. Of the STDs listed in Fig. A1.3, *C. trachomatis* and *Neisseria gonorrhoeae* are probably the most prevalent in sexually abused children due to their overall prevalence in the general population. Specimens for these agents will most frequently be taken when evaluating sexual abuse victims.

CHLAMYDIA

When *C. trachomatis* strains are isolated, they may be identified with *C. trachomatis*-specific monoclonal antibody reagents. It is important that the confirmatory tests used be able to differentiate between *C. trachomatis* and *Chlamydia pneumoniae* because strains of the latter species are now being shown to be associated with respiratory infections that are not sexually transmitted. A negative culture for *C. trachomatis* followed by a positive culture 2 to 3 weeks later would not be proof of a recent infection because of the relative insensitivity of the culture method; seroconversion detected by serologic tests performed at the same time as the cultures would provide evidence of a recently acquired infection. A temptation may be, however, to use the rapid detection tests such as direct fluorescent assays (DFAs) and enzyme immunoassays (EIAs) that have recently been developed to detect chlamydia antigens in patient specimens. These tests are not acceptable for diagnosing *C. trachomatis* infections in low-risk patients. Rapid tests for detecting *C. trachomatis* in adults at high risk for chlamydia infections are not as sensitive as the cell culture method. The positive predictive value of the rapid tests for detecting *C. trachomatis* in low-risk patients is very much lower than that in high-risk patients due to the prevalence of disease in the former group of patients (see Appendix 2, Selection and Evaluation of Tests and Quality Control).

GONORRHEA

The problems associated with identifying *N. gonorrhoeae* strains in low-risk patients differ from those associated with other STD agents. The gonococcus is easily isolated and there are many confirmatory tests that can be used. In hospital laboratories where specimens for sexual abuse victims are most frequently cultured, patients are considered to be at low risk for gonorrhea and laboratorians usually identify isolates with confirmatory tests. Because of economic considerations, however, hospital laboratories may choose only one confirmatory test to identify an isolate; additional confirmatory tests may not be performed

unless an isolate from a child is being identified or the result obtained with one test is equivocal. This problem is compounded by the fact that, frequently, physicians do not provide laboratories with sufficient information, such as the age of the patient, to indicate that the specimen is from a child and that the laboratorians should interpret the results from at least two confirmatory procedures before the isolate is identified as N. *gonorrhoeae*. When physicians, in turn, receive laboratory reports identifying isolates from children as N. *gonorrhoeae*, they may immediately initiate investigations of sexual abuse without questioning the identification of an isolate. In fact, in some states in the United States, physicians who do not report suspected cases of child abuse within 48 hours of becoming aware of evidence to support such allegations may be liable for criminal prosecution.

In the past, isolates from children have been misidentified as N. *gonorrhoeae* for a number of reasons. In some instances, incorrect diagnoses of gonorrhea may have been made when (1) gram-negative diplococci have been observed in stained smears of throat or ocular specimens; (2) gram-negative, oxidase-positive diplococci have been found to be β-lactamase-positive; and (3) isolates were misidentified as N. *gonorrhoeae* because a confirmatory test gave a false-positive result. In addition, it has been assumed that β-lactamase-positive isolates were strains of N. *gonorrhoeae* because laboratorians were apparently ignorant of the fact that many strains of *Branhamella catarrhalis* also produce β-lactamase. Finally, *Neisseria lactamica* strains have been identified as N. *gonorrhoeae* in the Phadebact Gonococcus test that may not have been misidentified had the ONPG test been performed to distinguish them from gonococci, as recommended by the product's manufacturer.

In many of the incorrect diagnoses described above, health care professionals had no suspicions that the children were sexually abused until a diagnosis of gonorrhea was made. Incorrect diagnoses such as these affect not only the victims but also family members and friends who are often cultured and similarly diagnosed based on the same errors; children may be removed from their families and persons falsely accused of sexual assault.

Recently, many rapid confirmatory tests for N. *gonorrhoeae* have been developed. Gonococcal isolates may be identified in a matter of hours after isolation with one of the tests discussed in Chapter 5 (Gonorrhea). The reliability of the identifications of isolates made with these tests must be questioned under certain circumstances. In several instances, tests have not been performed according to the manufacturer's instructions. Products that were intended only for the identification of strains isolated on gonococcal selective medium have been used to identify strains isolated on nonselective media. In another instance, the result of an enzyme substrate test was interpreted as if the test was a rapid carbohydrate test. Often, required Gram stains have not been performed prior to identifying isolates; yeasts were misidentified as N. *gonorrhoeae* because they have a positive oxidase reaction and reactions identical to those of the gonococcus in rapid tests. Laboratorians *must* read the package inserts that are provided and use products in accordance with the manufacturer's instructions.

Other problems with rapid tests must be considered even when the tests are performed properly; they may go unnoticed if only one confirmatory test is used. Some isolates of N. *gonorrhoeae* may fail to produce acid from glucose in some of the rapid carbohydrate tests, whereas nongonococcal isolates (*Kingella denitrificans*, *Neisseria cinerea*) may give weak positive reactions that lead to their being misidentified as N. *gonorrhoeae* (Fig. A1.4). Similarly, some commensal *Neisseria* spp. have iden-

LABORATORY TESTS RECOMMENDED FOR THE IDENTIFICATION OF SEXUALLY TRANSMITTED AGENTS IN CHILDREN WHO ARE VICTIMS OF SUSPECTED SEXUAL ABUSE

DISEASE OR SYNDROME	RECOMMENDED TESTS	REFER TO CHAPTER
Gonorrhea	Culture; confirm the identity by tests based on two different principles	5
Syphilis	Nontreponemal test results confirmed by treponemal test; dark-field examination of material from lesions when present	1
Herpes	Culture; confirmation by typing to identify HSV I and HSV II	2
Chlamydia	Culture	6
Vaginitis (Trichomonas vaginalis)	Gram stain and wet mount of discharge; culture recommended	9
Genital warts	Viral typing and biopsy	10

Fig. A1.3 Laboratory tests recommended for the identification of sexually transmitted agents in children who are victims of suspected sexual abuse.

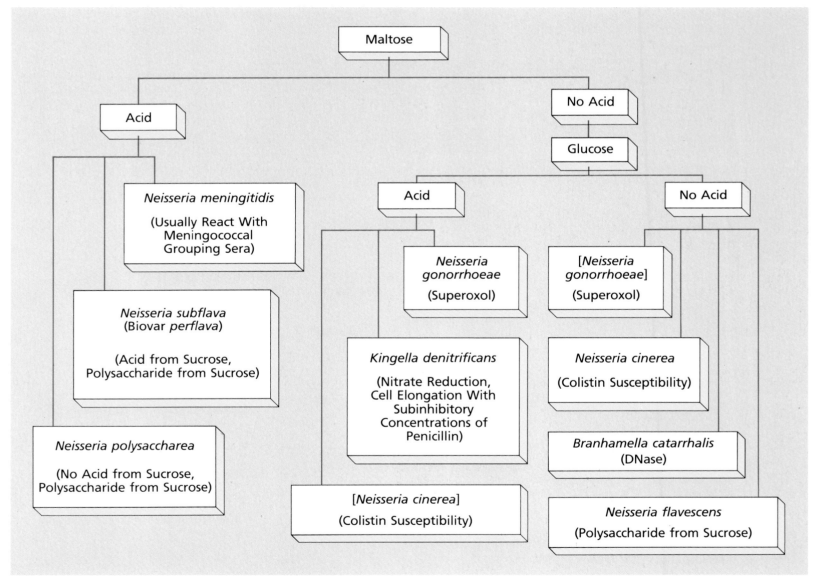

Fig. A1.4 Supplemental tests used to distinguish strains of *Neisseria gonorrhea* from other *Neisseria* and related species that may give equivocal reactions in acid production tests.

tical reactions to the gonococcus in enzyme substrate tests (Fig. A1.5). Although serologic reagents containing antibodies specific for the gonococcus have been developed, some gonococcal strains may fail to react with them, and strains of some nonpathogenic Neisseria and related species may give weak reactions that must be interpreted as positive by the manufacturer's criteria, even if they are false-positive reactions. The problems described above may occur even if the specimens are cultured correctly and the isolates are identified with tests according to the manufacturer's directions and interpreted according to the stated limitations.

Problems that may occur even if gonococcal isolation and identification procedures are performed correctly may be compounded by the fact that some nonpathogenic Neisseria spp., B. catarrhalis, and K. denitrificans are able to grow on gonococcal selective media. Colistin-sensitive strains of N. cinerea have been isolated on selective media. Also, it is often difficult, if not impossible, to differentiate between colonies of these species on selective and nonselective media such as chocolate agar (see Fig. 5.33). Specimens from children may be inoculated onto gonococcal selective media when sexual abuse is suspected. However, when sexual abuse is not initially suspected, specimens—particularly those from throats—usually will be inoculated onto nonselective media. All Neisseria and related species will grow on nonselective media; thus close attention must be paid to identification procedures. The colistin-susceptibility test performed either by disk diffusion or by testing the ability of the isolate to grow on gonococcal selective media will be useful in detecting colistin-resistant isolates that may have been isolated on nonselective medium; these isolates, which may include N. gonorrhoeae, should be identified.

Several questions must be asked, however, when such an STD agent is identified in a specimen from any site. Was the STD agent isolated? What tests were used to identify the agent? What problems are known to be associated with these tests that might result in isolates being misidentified? If the tests used to identify the isolate were not appropriate, what addi-

tional tests must be used to confirm the identity of an isolate?

The best advice that can be given at this time is that specimens from children should be cultured on gonococcal selective media, that isolates be tested in at least two tests based on different scientific principles, and that the manufacturer's limitations for the use and interpretation of rapid confirmatory tests be followed. It is important that laboratorians be aware of, and take into account, all potential problems associated with confirmatory tests when identifying isolates from low-risk patients. If in doubt, ask. Strains can be submitted to reference laboratories for confirmation.

At this time, gonorrhea cannot be diagnosed with a serologic test that detects antibodies in a person's serum.

Recent advances in gonococcal research have resulted in the development of systems for typing gonococcal isolates; these are auxotyping and serotyping. Auxotyping is a method by which the nutritional requirements of gonococcal isolates are determined. In this method, the requirement of an isolate for an amino acid such as proline is determined by testing the ability of the isolate to grow on a defined medium lacking proline. Gonococcal isolates are serotyped in coagglutination tests with a panel of monoclonal antibody reagents; gonococcal serovars are defined by the pattern of reactions of an isolate with the reagents.

An auxotype/serovar (A/S) classification has been devised to describe gonococcal isolates. The A/S classification system has been used to characterize isolates from victims and their accused assailants. If the isolates belong to the same A/S class, this would provide evidence that would support the allegations against an accused assailant. However, it must be noted that other adults who had access to the child may also be infected with the same strain and, thus, it is important that all such adults be cultured to include all infected persons as possible suspects. If the isolates from a suspect and victim do not belong to the same A/S class, it might be assumed that the suspect is not the perpetrator. However, it is possible that persons may be infected with multiple strains of N. gonorrhoeae. Urethral in-

DIFFERENTIAL TESTS USED TO DIFFERENTIATE BETWEEN *NEISSERIA GONORRHOEAE* AND RELATED SPECIES THAT GIVE SIMILAR REACTIONS IN RAPID ENZYME SUBSTRATE TESTS

ENZYME PRODUCED	SPECIES	SUPPLEMENTAL DIFFERENTIAL TESTS
Hydroxyprolylaminopeptidase only	N. gonorrhoeae K. denitrificans N. cinerea N. subflava (biovar perflava)	Superoxol Nitrate reduction Colistin susceptibility Acid from sucrose, polysaccharide from sucrose
γ-Glutamylaminopeptidase	N. meningitidis N. subflava (biovar perflava) N. polysacchrea	Serogroup Acid from sucrose, polysaccharide from sucrose No acid from sucrose, polysaccharide from sucrose
β-Galactosidase	N. lactamica	
No reaction	B. catarrhalis	

Fig. A1.5 Differential tests used to differentiate between *Neisseria gonorrhoeae* and related species that give similar reactions in rapid enzyme substrate tests.

fections with multiple strains are rarely detected in heterosexual men but occur frequently in women. It is possible that, because only a few colonies may be selected from a culture, a strain identical with that isolated from the victim may not be detected in an adult who is concomitantly coinfected with another strain. The strain identical to that isolated from the victim also may not be isolated if it grows at a slower rate than a coinfecting strain. Therefore, it may be difficult to assess gonococcal culture and typing results.

It has been suggested that the prevalence of a particular strain (A/S class) is important when assessing the probability that an infected suspect is guilty; that is, the suspect is more likely to be guilty if the strain with which he is infected is rarely isolated in the community. The prevalence of an individual A/S class in a community is of little significance. The important fact in evaluating the value of the strain-typing data as evidence in a case is dependent upon its isolation from any adult who had private access to the child within the time period during which the infection was acquired. For this reason, it is important that all adults who had private access to the child be cultured to determine if they are infected with the same strain. It is also important that the child and all adults with private access to the child be cultured at appropriate intervals after the alleged incident to ensure that their infections are sufficiently developed to obtain an inoculum that will be detectable by culture. The results of cultures from one adult cannot be extrapolated to account for culture outcome for a sexual partner; all adults should be cultured. Thus, if one person is culture negative, it cannot be assumed that his or her sexual partner is culture negative. Negative culture results may be obtained from one person if the infection is at a predetectable stage, whereas a positive culture may be obtained from a sexual partner. Such culture results may be particularly important because some strains of N. *gonorrhoeae* have a propensity to cause asymptomatic infections.

OTHER SEXUALLY TRANSMITTED DISEASES
Among the other STDs, herpes simplex virus isolates may be typed and assigned to either HSV type I or HSV type II. Sexually transmitted herpesvirus strains usually belong to HSV II,

whereas strains associated with nonsexually transmitted "cold sores" belong to HSV I. The correlation, however, between strain type and mode of transmission is not exclusive. In adults, HSV type I strains have been transmitted sexually and HSV type II strains have been transmitted nonsexually. Except in exceptional circumstances, the transmission of HSV II strains to children would normally be interpreted as occurring by sexual transmission. Thus typing data for HSV isolates must be interpreted in the context of all other evidence before they are used in the prosecution of a suspect.

Vaginosis may also occur as a result of sexual assault. The etiology of vaginosis is complex and not fully understood at this time. Among the etiologic agents associated with vaginosis, *Trichomonas vaginalis* is clearly recognized as a sexually transmitted pathogen. T. *vaginalis* cells may be detected in wet mounts of a vaginal discharge; however, culture is considered to be a more sensitive method for detecting this organism. Because the vagina has a normal flora (Fig. A1.6), it may be difficult to evaluate organisms isolated from this site as evidence of sexual assault. Several organisms—*Mycoplasma hominis*, *Ureaplasma urealyticum*, *Gardnerella vaginalis*, and *Candida albicans*—that may be sexually transmitted between adults have been isolated from the normal flora of sexually nonactive children.

G. *vaginalis* is also associated with bacterial vaginosis. Strains of this species have been biotyped; the procedures are not widely available at this time. Some reports have suggested that G. *vaginalis*-like organisms also may be normal flora in the vagina of children; thus it is doubtful that the isolation of G. *vaginalis* should be used as evidence of sexual abuse.

OTHER CONSIDERATIONS
A factor that also must be considered when assessing the significance of culture results in investigations of sexual abuse is antimicrobial use. If an assailant has taken antimicrobial agents to treat a sexually transmitted, or unrelated, infection, cultures for sexually transmitted pathogens may be negative.

Culture- and strain-typing data is circumstantial evidence of sexual abuse and must be interpreted in the light both of the considerations stated above and the physical evidence of abuse. STD infections in children less than 1 year of age may not result

NORMAL OR NONPATHOGENIC VAGINAL FLORA IN CHILDREN

Fig. A1.6 Normal or nonpathogenic vaginal flora in children.

AEROBES AND FACULTATIVE ANAEROBES

Diphtheroids	*Klebsiella* spp.
Staphylococcus epidermidis	Group B streptococci
α-Hemolytic streptococci	Group D streptococci
Nonhemolytic streptococci	*Staphylococcus aureus*
Lactobacilli (newborn and postmenarcheal)	*Pseudomonas* spp.
Escherichia coli	*Proteus* spp.

ANAEROBES

Bacteroides spp.
Peptococcus spp.
Peptostreptococcus spp.

MODELS OF NONSEXUAL TRANSMISSION OF SEXUALLY TRANSMITTED AGENTS

AGENT	MATERNAL TRANSMISSION (INTRAUTERINE/ PERINATAL)	NONSEXUAL HUMAN TRANSMISSION*	FOMITE TRANSMISSION†
Neisseria gonorrhoeae	Well documented	Not documented	Not documented
Chlamydia trachomatis	Well documented	Not documented	Not documented
Treponema pallidum	Well documented	Well documented	Not documented
Haemophilus ducreyi	Not documented	Not documented	Not documented
Calymmatobacterium granulomatis	Documented	Well documented	Not documented
Mycoplasma hominis	Well documented	Not documented	Not documented
Ureaplasma urealyticum	Well documented	Not documented	Not documented
Herpes simplex virus (HSV)	Well documented	Documented HSV1	Not documented
Papillomavirus	Well documented	Not documented	Not documented
Hepatitis B virus	Well documented	Well documented	Not documented
Human immunodeficiency virus	Well documented	Well documented	Not documented

*Includes skin–skin, skin–mucous membrane, autoinoculation, and transmission via contaminated blood.
†Excludes laboratory accidents.

Fig. A1.7   Models of nonsexual transmission of sexually transmitted agents.

MANAGEMENT OF CHILDREN WITH SUSPECTED OR CONFIRMED HISTORY OF SEXUAL ABUSE. GUIDELINES FOR DETECTION OF SEXUALLY TRANSMITTED DISEASES

I. **LABORATORY TESTS**

   A. Mandatory immediate tests
      1. Gram stain of any discharge from genitals, urethra, or anus for intracellular gram-negative diplococci.
      2. Neisseria gonorrhoeae cultures from vagina, urethra, anus, and throat; confirm positive cultures with sugar utilization tests and fluorescent antibody or coagglutination tests.
      3. Chlamydia trachomatis cultures (pharynx, vagina, and rectum).
      4. Syphilis serology.
      5. Pregnancy test in postmenarcheal girls.
      6. Wet preparations for trichomonads and clue cells.
      7. Test for presence of semen.
      8. Examine for venereal warts.

   B. Mandatory follow-up tests
      1. Test of cure 3–7 days following treatment of proven N. gonorrhoeae infection.
      2. Repeat syphilis serology, if recent assault suspected, in 1 month.

   C. Recommended follow-up tests
      1. N. gonorrhoeae cultures.
      2. Syphilis serology.
      3. C. trachomatis cultures (if available).
      4. Herpes simplex virus cultures, if suspicious lesion appears.
      5. Repeat pregnancy test, if appropriate.

II. **TREATMENT OF STD**

   A. Treat gonorrhea on the basis of positive Gram stain or cultures.
   B. No prophylaxis when assailant unknown.
   C. Epidemiologic treatment indicated if assailant suspected to have disease.

III. **GENERAL MANAGEMENT**

   A. Report to appropriate legal and child protective services.
   B. Follow-up by social worker, psychologist, etc.
   C. Interview for abuser and contact tracing.
   D. Household members and others with access to the child should be screened for STD diagnosed in child.

Fig. A1.8   Management of children with suspected or confirmed history of sexual abuse. Guidelines for detection of sexually transmitted diseases.

Adapted from Davis HW: Child Abuse and Neglect, in Zitelli BJ, Davis HW (eds): Atlas of Pediatric Physical Diagnosis. New York, Gower Medical Publishing, 1987.

from sexual abuse (Fig. A1.7). Some STD infections contracted at birth may not resolve for some time. Depending on the specific agent involved, it is generally thought that the diagnosis of an STD or isolation of a sexually transmitted pathogen from a child less than 1 year of age may be due to acquisition of the disease agent during birth, whereas a similar diagnosis or isolation from older children are due to sexual transmission. Fomite transmission of sexually transmitted pathogens is not considered to be a viable explanation for STD infections in children.

N. *gonorrhoeae* infections acquired at birth include ophthalmia neonatorum and gonococcal amniotic infection syndrome, which is manifested as a nonspecific sepsis (N. *gonorrhoeae* may be isolated from the orogastric juices). These infections are symptomatic and should be treated successfully before the baby is released from the hospital. If a child less than 1 year of age is diagnosed with a gonococcal infection, a review of the patient's medical history may provide some clues as to the origin of infections.

Chlamydia infections are known to be persistent in young children. Depending on the patient population, C. *trachomatis* may be acquired frequently by babies at birth; as many as 70% of babies exposed to C. *trachomatis* organisms may acquire nasopharyngeal, vaginal, or rectal infections. These infections may persist for up to a year, but it is not known whether all such infections are resolved within this period. Anecdotal reports suggest that infections may persist for more than 2 years. Thus, when considering the significance of positive chlamydia cultures in young children it is necessary to take these facts into consideration.

Legal Requirements

Many hospitals and laboratories have standard procedures for screening victims of suspected sexual abuse. Such protocols should include a list of the sexually transmitted pathogens to be screened for and the acceptable methods for transporting specimens and isolating and identifying organisms. Specific details in the protocol will depend on specific legal requirements in each state. For example, some state laws require that specimens be transported to the laboratory by a police officer

to maintain the chain of evidence; many states do not have this requirement. States also may require isolates to be preserved when microbiological evidence pertaining to them is used as evidence. A typical set of guidelines is presented in Figure A1.8.

BIBLIOGRAPHY

Frau LM, Alexander ER: Public health implications of sexually transmitted diseases in pediatric practice. *Pediatr Infect Dis* 4:453, 1985.

Fuster CD, Neinstein LS: Vaginal *Chlamydia trachomatis* prevalence in sexually abused prepubertal girls. *Pediatrics* 79:235, 1987.

Glaser, JB, Hammerschlag MR, McCormack WM: Epidemiology of sexually transmitted diseases in rape victims. *Rev Infect Dis* 11:246, 1989.

Hamerschlag MR, Alpert S, Rosner I, Thurston P, Semine D, McComb D, McCormack WM: Microbiology of the vagina in children: Normal and potentially pathogenic organisms. *Pediatrics* 62:57, 1978.

Hamerschlag MR, Rettig PJ, Shields ME: False positive results with the use of chlamydial antigen detection tests in the evaluation of suspected sexual abuse in children. *Pediatr Infect Dis* 7:11, 1988.

Ingram DL, White ST, Occhiuti AR, Lyna PR: Childhood vaginal infections: association of *Chlamydia trachomatis* with sexual contact. *Pediatr Infect Dis* 5:226, 1986.

Khan M, Sexton M: Sexual abuse of young children. *Clin Ped* 22:369, 1983.

Neinstein LS, Goldenring J, Carpenter S: Nonsexual transmission of sexually transmitted diseases: An infrequent occurrence. *Pediatrics* 74:67, 1984.

Rettig PJ, Nelson JD: Genital tract infection with *Chlamydia trachomatis* in prepubertal children. *J Pediatr* 99:206, 1981.

White ST, Loda FA, Ingram DL, Pearson A: Sexually transmitted diseases in sexually abused children. *Pediatrics* 72:16, 1983.

Whittington WL, Rice RJ, Biddle JW, Knapp JS: Incorrect identification of *Neisseria gonorrhoeae* from infants and children. *Pediatr Infect Dis* 7:3, 1988.

Selection and Evaluation of Tests and Quality Control

J.S. LEWIS

Purpose and Selection of Diagnostic Tests

DIAGNOSIS OF DISEASE

The process of diagnosis requires two essential steps. The first is the establishment of a differential diagnosis (i.e., diagnostic hypotheses) followed by attempts to arrive at a single diagnosis by progressively ruling out specific diseases. This process requires very *sensitive* tests. Such tests, when normal, permit the physician to confidently exclude the disease. The next step is the pursuit of a strong clinical suspicion for a specific disease. This process requires a very *specific* test. Such a test, when abnormal, should essentially confirm the presence of the disease.

The use of a test to exclude or confirm a diagnosis should indicate that the physician's best estimate, after a careful evaluation of the patient's problem, is that the diagnosis in question is either unlikely or probable, respectively.

SCREENING

The primary use of screening tests in asymptomatic patients is to detect diseases whose morbidity can be reduced by early detection and treatment and to reassure patients found to be free of disease. There are several important principles in applying screening tests. First, the disease in question should be common enough to justify the effort to detect it. Next, it should be accompanied by significant morbidity if not treated, and effective therapy should exist to alter its natural history. Finally, detection and treatment of the presymptomatic state should result in benefits beyond those obtained through treatment of the early symptomatic patient. Once these criteria are met, the issue can be examined from the standpoint of laboratory tests. An acceptable test is one that will be abnormal in almost all individuals with the disease and provide the physician with confidence that the patient is free of disease when the test is normal.

PATIENT MANAGEMENT

Tests are commonly repeated for one or more of the following purposes:

1. To monitor the status of a disease process
2. To identify and reverse complications of treatment
3. To ensure therapeutic levels of one or more drugs
4. To aid in prognosis
5. To check an unexpected test result

For these purposes, the *reproducibility* of the test is the most important characteristic.

DETERMINATION OF DISEASE DISTRIBUTION

The purpose of a diagnostic test is to discriminate between patients with a particular disease and those who do not have the disease. However, most diagnostic tests measure some disease marker or surrogate (e.g., an antibody that is variably associated with the disease) rather than the presence or absence of the disease itself. The *performance level* of a diagnostic test depends on the distribution of the marker being measured in diseased and nondiseased patients and on the technical performance characteristics of the test itself (i.e., precision and reliability).

Each disease marker has a distribution in populations of diseased and nondiseased patients. Unfortunately, these distributions frequently overlap so that measurement of the marker in question does not usually permit a complete separation of the two populations (Fig. A2.1).

Evaluation of Diagnostic Tests

The first step in evaluating a diagnostic test is to determine its technical performance. Does the test measure what it claims to measure? Is the test replicable? (Replicability, or precision, reflects the variance in a test result that occurs when the test is repeated on the same specimen). A highly precise test exhibits little variance among repeated measurements; an imprecise test exhibits great variance. The greater this variation, the less faith one has in results based on a single test. However, a precise test is not necessarily a good test. A test may exhibit a high level of replicability yet be in error. Is the test reliable (i.e., unbiased)? It must exhibit agreement between the mean test result and the true value of the biologic variable being measured in the sample. Evaluations of clinical tests should consider both the replicability and the reliability of the test.

The three most commonly used measures of diagnostic test performance for STDs are sensitivity, specificity, and predictive value (Fig. A2.2). These test characteristics deal with the ability of the diagnostic test to identify correctly subjects with and without the condition of interest.

SENSITIVITY

Sensitivity, which measures the ability of a test to detect infection when it is present, is of maximum concern in patient populations having a high prevalence of disease, such as STD clinics. Sensitivity measures the proportion of patients with a positive test to all infected patients.

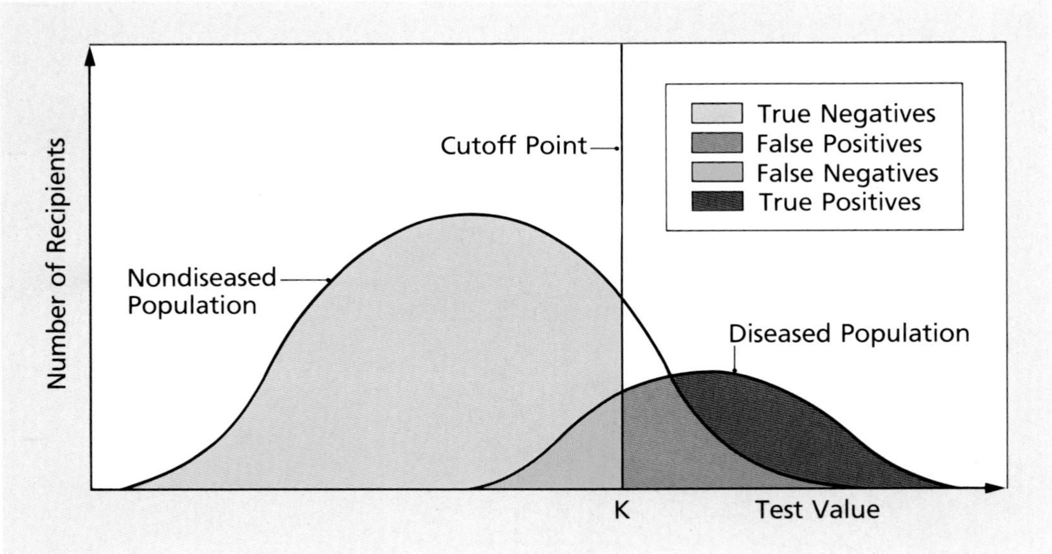

Figure A2.1 Relationship of test value to diseased and nondiseased populations for a hypothetical diagnostic test.

Legend:
- True Negatives
- False Positives
- False Negatives
- True Positives

Cutoff Point

Nondiseased Population

Diseased Population

Number of Recipients

K   Test Value

SPECIFICITY

Specificity, which measures the ability of a test to correctly exclude infection in uninfected patients, is of maximum concern when testing in patient populations having a low prevalence of disease, such as family planning clinics and most private practice settings. Specificity measures the proportion of uninfected patients with a negative test.

Sensitivity and specificity have been adopted widely because they are considered to be stable properties of diagnostic tests when properly derived from a broad spectrum of infected and uninfected patients. That is, their values are thought not to change significantly when applied in populations with different prevalences, presentations, or severity of disease. If diagnostic tests do not have a broad population base, their sensitivities and specificities change as the prevalence and severity of disease vary in the populations tested.

PREDICTIVE VALUE

When a test is to be used in a large, unselected population, it is important to know what its predictive value will be—that is, what is the likelihood that a person with a positive test result actually has the disease and, conversely, what is the likelihood that a person with a negative test result does not have the disease. This likelihood cannot be directly estimated from the test sensitivity and specificity value obtained in the preliminary evaluation since the predictive value is related to the actual prevalence of the disease in the total population.

Taken alone, test sensitivity and specificity do not reveal how likely it is that a given patient really has the condition in question if the test result is positive, or how likely it is that a given patient is not infected if the test result is negative. The fraction of those patients with a positive test result who actually are infected is called the predictive value positive (PVP) of a test. The fraction of patients with a negative test result who are actually free of the disease is called the predictive value negative (PVN).

The PVP and PVN of a diagnostic test measure, respectively, how likely it is that a positive or negative test result actually represents the presence or absence of disease in a given population of patients with a given prevalence of disease. The pos-

itive and negative predictive values of a diagnostic test, however, are not stable characteristics of that test. Rather, they depend strongly on the prevalence of the condition being examined in the population being tested. Where the disease prevalence (pretest likelihood of disease) decreases, the proportion of individuals with a positive test result who actually are infected falls and the proportion of uninfected patients falsely identified as being infected rises. Conversely, as the prevalence of disease increases, the proportion of patients with a positive test result who are in fact infected increases, while the proportion of patients with a negative test result who are not suffering from the disease falls. This fact has enormous implications for all diagnostic tests, particularly when they are used in populations with a low prevalence of disease, such as in screening for the presence of an uncommon disease.

The following example will illustrate this principle: A test for gonorrhea is evaluated in 100 individuals who are known to have gonorrhea and in 100 normal control subjects with no evidence of the disease or of any factors known to result in increased risk for the disease. It is found that 95% of the infected individuals had positive test results (sensitivity, 95%), whereas only 5% of the control group had positive test results (specificity, 95%). In comparison with other tests, this test is considered highly accurate. What is the accuracy of a positive test in predicting gonorrhea in an unselected sample of 10,000 subjects in whom the actual prevalence of gonorrhea is 2%?

By simple arithmetic, there are 200 infected individuals in a population with a 2% prevalence of gonorrhea, 190 of whom will have a positive test and 10 a negative test. There are 9,800 uninfected persons in this population, 9,310 of whom will have a negative test and 490 a positive test. Therefore, the predictive value of a positive test in detecting gonorrhea in the total population will be:

$$\frac{190}{(190 + 490)} = 27.9\%$$

The predictive value of a negative test will be:

$$\frac{9,310}{(9,310 + 10)} = 99.9\%$$

Figure A2.2 Characteristics of diagnostic tests.

CHARACTERISTICS OF DIAGNOSTIC TESTS

MEASURE OF PERFORMANCE	CHARACTERISTIC
Sensitivity =	$\dfrac{\text{True positives}}{\text{True positives + false negatives}}$
Specificity =	$\dfrac{\text{True negatives}}{\text{True negatives + false positives}}$
Predictive values positive =	$\dfrac{\text{True positives}}{\text{True positives + false positives}}$
Predictive values negative =	$\dfrac{\text{True negatives}}{\text{True negatives + false negatives}}$

Figure A2.3 shows the effect of disease prevalence on the predictive values of positive and negative test results when the sensitivity and specificity of the test are both 95%. The PVP of a test result increases with increasing disease prevalence; when the disease prevalence is 50%, PVP equals sensitivity and PVN equals specificity. Although higher disease prevalences are unlikely to occur in unselected populations, they may be obtained by preselection of the group to be tested on the basis of historical or physical data or some other test. In the example given above, the actual PVP in the positive reactor group was shown to be 27.9% under the conditions described (Fig. A2.3). The PVN of a test is not affected except at very high disease prevalences.

The value of PVP when actual disease prevalence is 2% is given for a range of sensitivities and specificities in Figure A2.4A. It is seen that the predictive value of a positive test is primarily dependent on the specificity of the test, but at this disease prevalence PVP has a maximal value of 66.9% even at very high sensitivity (99%) and specificity (99%). The values of PVN in a population with a 2% disease prevalence are shown in Figure A2.4B. Sensitivity and specificity have relatively little effect on this parameter.

One must be careful when applying results obtained during the preliminary evaluation of diagnostic tests using groups of known infected and uninfected individuals to unselected groups because of the magnification of false-positive errors by the generally low prevalences of disease in the general population. The concepts of sensitivity and specificity are not in themselves adequate to predict test reliability under these circumstances. This may be done, however, if the parameters of PVP and PVN are employed in unselected populations. These parameters take into account the known or assumed actual prevalence of disease in the general population.

Errors can be minimized by increasing the specificity of the test and by preselecting subjects at high risk of disease. This will produce a higher disease prevalence in the population to be tested. The preselection of the population by the first test will increase greatly the predictive value of the second test.

A good example is the screening use of the Rapid Plasma Reagin (RPR) or Venereal Disease Research Laboratory (VDRL) test to "enrich" the group of positives, which are then subsequently tested with the Fluorescent Treponemal Antibody Absorption (FTA-ABS) test for confirmation. A similar situation exists for the human immunodeficiency virus (HIV) enzyme-linked immunosorbent assay (ELISA) and Western blot tests. Use of the FTA-ABS or Western blot as a screening test is not indicated. These tests are no better than the screening tests for evaluation and are much more expensive and difficult to interpret.

A major problem in determining performance characteristics of many diagnostic tests is the lack of an appropriate reference standard, known as a "gold standard," against which to judge

PREDICTIVE VALUES OF POSITIVE AND NEGATIVE TEST RESULTS AT VARYING DISEASE PREVALENCES WHEN SENSITIVITY AND SPECIFICITY EACH EQUAL 95%

Figure A2.3 Predictive values of positive and negative test results at varying disease prevalences when sensitivity and specificity each equal 95%.

ACTUAL DISEASE PREVALENCE (%)	PREDICTIVE VALUES	
	POSITIVE (%)	NEGATIVE (%)
1	16.1	99.9
2	27.9	99.9
5	50.0	99.7
10	67.9	99.4
20	82.6	98.7
50	95.0	95.0
75	98.3	83.7
100	100.0	—

the test. In practice, one is often forced to accept the best available, albeit imperfect, diagnostic test as a pseudo-reference standard. Diagnostic tests should always be evaluated in terms of their use with, and contribution to, other diagnostic tests and not merely in terms of their absolute accuracy in isolating already-known clinical information.

The effectiveness of a program to control STDs depends upon its effectiveness to detect STDs. Although most laboratories will employ a number of different tests, the range that is available is rapidly increasing.

Laboratory services are an integral part of all disease control programs, and the availability of laboratory tests considerably

PREDICTIVE VALUE OF A POSITIVE TEST (PVP) OVER A RANGE OF SENSITIVITIES AND SPECIFICITIES WHEN ACTUAL DISEASE PREVALENCE IS 2%

SPECIFICITY (%)	SENSITIVITY							
	50%	60%	70%	80%	90%	95%	98%	99%
50	2.0	2.4	2.8	3.2	3.5	3.7	3.8	3.9
60	2.5	3.0	3.4	3.9	4.4	4.6	4.8	4.8
70	3.3	3.9	4.5	5.2	5.8	6.1	6.2	6.3
80	4.8	5.8	6.7	7.6	8.4	8.8	9.1	9.2
90	9.2	10.9	12.5	14.0	15.5	16.2	16.7	16.8
95	17.0	19.7	32.2	24.6	26.9	27.9	28.6	28.8
98	33.8	38.0	41.7	44.9	47.9	49.2	50.0	50.2
99	50.5	55.0	58.8	62.0	64.7	66.0	66.7	66.9

Figure A2.4 Predictive value of a positive test (PVP) (A) and a negative test (PVN) (B) over a range of sensitivities and specificities when actual disease prevalence is 2%.

A

PREDICTIVE VALUE OF A NEGATIVE TEST (PVN) OVER A RANGE OF SENSITIVITIES AND SPECIFICITIES WHEN ACTUAL DISEASE PREVALENCE IS 2%

SPECIFICITY (%)	SENSITIVITY							
	50%	60%	70%	80%	90%	95%	98%	99%
50	98.0	98.4	98.8	99.2	99.6	99.8	99.9	99.0
60	98.3	98.6	99.0	99.3	99.7	99.8	99.9	100.0
70	98.6	98.8	99.1	99.4	99.7	99.8	99.9	100.0
80	98.7	99.0	99.2	99.5	99.7	99.9	99.9	100.0
90	98.9	99.1	99.3	99.5	99.8	99.9	99.9	100.0
95	98.9	99.1	99.4	99.6	99.8	99.9	100.0	100.0
98	99.0	99.2	99.4	99.6	99.8	99.9	100.0	100.0
99	99.0	99.2	99.4	99.6	99.8	99.9	100.0	100.0

B

improves the quality of patient care. The most important characteristic and justification for the use of a laboratory test is its ability to provide information to assist patient management. The types of tests a laboratory can offer will depend on the level of its competence and its responsibilities (Fig. A2.5).

Quality Control

Quality control of diagnostic tests depends on adherence to recommendations regarding refrigeration and/or shelf life of antibiotics, culture medium, and test reagents. More important

are measures of outcome. Among these are the percentage of patients who have follow-up examinations and are found cured for each treatment regimen and, whenever possible, the level of agreement between different diagnostic tests for the same disease. For example, all intermediate and central laboratories should develop methods for comparing results of Gram-stained smears and cultures for Neisseria gonorrhoeae. This is the only practical way to continuously monitor the quality of gonorrhea diagnostic techniques that begins with medium production and ends with transmittal of results to patients.

LABORATORY TESTS COMMONLY PERFORMED IN THE DIAGNOSIS OF SEXUALLY TRANSMITTED DISEASES

DISEASE	AGENT	LABORATORY TEST	SENSITIVITY	SPECIFICITY	P	I	C
					RECOMMENDED LEVEL OF AVAILABILITY*		
Syphilis	Treponema pallidum	Dark-field microscopy	85–95	100	+/−	+	+
		VDRL (nontreponemal) test	71–100[†]	79–98[‡]	+	+	+
		RPR card (nontreponemal) test	73–100[†]	79–98[‡]	+	+	+
		FTA-ABS (treponemal) test	85–100[†]	95–100[‡]	−	+	+
		MHA-TP (treponemal) test	70–100[†]	96–100[‡]	−	+	+
		HATTS (treponemal) test	70–100[†]	96–100[‡]	−	+	+
Gonorrhea	Neisseria gonorrhoeae	Gram stain					
		Urethral, symptomatic	90–95	95–99	+	+	+
		Urethral, asymptomatic	50–70	85–87	+	+	+
		Endocervix	45–65	90–99	+	+	+
		Conjunctiva	95		+	+	+
		Vagina	Not recommended		−	−	−
		Anal canal	Not recommended		−	−	−
		Pharynx	Not recommended		−	−	−
		Culture					
		Urethral discharge	94–98	>99	+/−	+	+
		Urethral, asymptomatic	80–85		+/−	+	+
		Endocervix	85–95	>99	+/−	+	+
		Conjunctiva	95		−	+	+
		Vagina	50–85		−	+	+
		Anal canal	70–85		−	+	+
		Pharynx	50–70		−	+/−	+
		Disseminated infection					
		Gram stain					
		Blood	Not recommended		−	−	−
		Joints	5–10		+	+	+
		Lesions	5–10		+	+	+
		Culture					
		Blood	25–75		−	+/−	+
		Joint	25–75		−	+	+
		Lesions	2–5		−	+	+
		Direct antigen detection					
		Urethra	90–95	81–99	−	+/−	+
		Endocervix	60–85	76–99	−	+/−	+
		Rectum	Not recommended		−	−	−
		Pharynx	Not recommended		−	−	−
		β-lactamase tests	>99		−	+/−	+
		Direct FA	90–95	95–99	−	+/−	+
		DNA probes	95–99	99	−	+/−	+
		Confirmatory tests	95–99	>95	−	+	+
		Antimicrobic susceptibility					
		Disk diffusion			+/−	+	+
		Minimum inhibitory concentration (MIC)			−	−	+
Genital herpes	Herpes simplex virus types 1 and 2	Tzanck test	40–50	>95	−	+/−	+
		Papanicolaou smear	30–40	>95	−	+/−	+
		Direct FA	70–80	>95	−	+/−	+
		Culture	25–90[†]	>99	−	+/−	+
		Neutralizing antibody	65–70	×	−	−	+
		Direct EIA	85–90	>99	−	−	+

continued

DISEASE	AGENT	LABORATORY TEST	SENSITIVITY	SPECIFICITY	RECOMMENDED LEVEL OF AVAILABILITY* P	I	C
Trichomoniasis	*Trichomonas vaginalis*	Wet mount/saline	50–75	>99	+	+	+
		Culture	80–90	>99	−	+	+
		FA	85–90	>99	−	+/−	+
		EIA	90–95	>99	−	+/−	+
Candidiasis	*Candida albicans*	Wet mount/10% KOH	40–60	>99	+	+	+
		Culture	70–80	>99	−	+	+
		Latex agglutination	71–81	96–98	−	+	+
Chancroid	*Haemophilus ducreyi*	Gram stain	<50	50–70	+	+	+
		Culture	30–70	>98	−	+/−	+
Gardnerella vaginitis	*Gardnerella vaginalis*	Wet mount/saline	70–90	95–100	+	+	+
		Gram stain	60–80	95–100	+	+	+
		pH	75–80	60–70	+	+	+
		Culture	80–90	>99	−	+/−	+
Granuloma inguinale	*Calymmatobacterium granulomatis*	Direct stain/Wright-Giemsa	40–50	<50	+	+	+
		Culture	Not recommended		−	−	−
Chlamydia (also lympho-granuloma venereum)	*Chlamydia trachomatis*	Culture	80–90	>99	−	+/−	+
		Direct antigen-FA	80–92	95–98	−	+	+
		Direct antigen-EIA	70–90	92–97	−	+	+
		Giemsa stain	45	95	−	+	+
		Papanicolaou stain	62	96	−	+/−	+
		Conjunctiva Giemsa stain	95	90–95	−	−	+
		Conjunctiva culture	95	>99	−	−	+
		Micro-IF antibody	60–80	95	−	−	+
		Complement fixation for LGV	40–50	85	−	+/−	+
		DNA probes	90–93	96–98	−	+/−	+
Genital mycoplasma infections	*Mycoplasma hominis*	Culture	75–80	95–97	−	+/−	+
		Serology	Not recommended		−	−	−
	Ureaplasma urealyticum	Culture	90–95	90–92	−	+/−	+
		Serology	Not recommended		−	−	−
AIDS	Human immunodeficiency virus (HIV-1)	EIA	>99	>99	−	+/−	+
		Western Blot	>99	>99	−	+/−	+
Genital warts	Human papillomaviruses (HPV)	DNA probes	88–92	96–98	−	+/−	+

*Peripheral (P) = outpatient clinics or primary practitioner's laboratory (facilities limited); intermediate (I) = regional, state, hospital laboratory; central (C) = national research or reference laboratory.
†Varies with stage of disease.
‡Varies with population being tested.

Fig. A2.5   Laboratory tests commonly performed in the diagnosis of sexually transmitted diseases.

BIBLIOGRAPHY

Griner PF, Mayewski RJ, Mushlin AI, Greenland P: Selection and interpretation of diagnostic tests and procedures. *Ann Intern Med* 94:553, 1981.

Hart G: *Epidemiologic Aspects of Venereal Disease Control*. US Dept of Health and Human Services publication No. 00-3633. Atlanta, Centers for Disease Control, 1980.

Hart G: The role of treponemal tests in therapeutic decision making. *Am J Public Health* 73:739, 1983.

Holmes KK, Mårdh P-A, Sparling PF, Wiesner PJ: *Sexually Transmitted Diseases*, ed 1. New York, McGraw-Hill Book Co, 1984, pp 992–998.

Rothenberg RB, Simon R, Chipperfield E, Catterall RD: Efficacy of selected diagnostic tests for sexually transmitted diseases. *JAMA* 235:49, 1976.

Swartz JS: *Assessing Medical Technologies*. Washington, DC, National Academy Press, 1985, pp 70–175.

Vecchio TJ: Predictive value of a single diagnostic test in unselected populations. *N Engl J Med* 274:1171, 1966.

Whittington WL, Cates W Jr.: Checking out the new STD tests. *Contemp Obstet Gynecol* 23:135, 1984.

World Health Organization—VDT 85.437. Simplified approaches for sexually transmitted disease (STD) control at the primary health care (PHC) level. Report of a WHO working group. Geneva, Sept. 24–28, 1984.

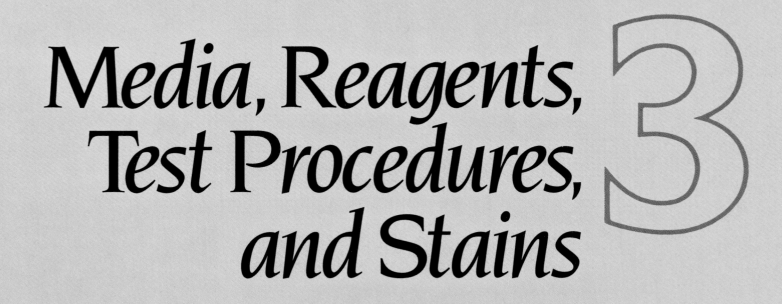

Media, Reagents, Test Procedures, and Stains

3

S.K. SARAFIAN

Transport and Culture Media

(It should be noted that inclusion or exclusion of manufacturers of media and reagents does not constitute endorsement or disapproval of any manufacturer or product.)

1. **A8 AGAR** Growth medium for *Mycoplasma hominis* and *Ureaplasma urealyticum*.

Trypticase soy broth (BBL, Cockeysville, MD)	2.4 g
$CaCl_2 \cdot 2H_2O$	0.014 g
Putrescine dihydrochloride	0.166 g
Distilled water	80 mL

Dissolve ingredients and adjust pH to 5.5 with 2N HCl. Add 1.05 g bacteriological grade agar (Gibco Laboratories, Grand Island, NY). Autoclave at 121°C for 15 minutes, and equilibrate at 56°C. The following supplements may be combined, filter sterilized, and added to the basal agar after equilibration at 56°C:

Unheated, pooled normal horse serum	20 mL
CVA enrichment (Gibco Laboratories, Grand Island, NY)	0.5 mL
Yeast extract (25% aqueous extract of pure dry yeast), pH 6.0	1.0 mL
Urea (10% solution)	1.0 mL
L-Cysteine-HCl (2% solution)	0.5 mL
GHL tripeptide (20 µg/mL solution)	0.1 mL
Penicillin G, potassium (100,000 U/mL solution)	1.0 mL

Plates are incubated at 37°C in a CO_2 gassed incubator.

2. **BIPHASIC BLOOD AGAR** Isolation medium for *Gardnerella vaginalis* composed of a basal layer of 7 mL of CNA agar base (Columbia agar, BBL, Cockeysville, MD) containing 10 µg colistin, 15 µg nalidixic acid, and 2 µg amphotericin B per mL and a 14-mL overlayer of the same medium containing 5% (v/v) human blood.

3. **BLOOD AGAR** Growth medium for *Mycoplasma* spp.

Blood agar base No. 2 (Oxoid, Columbia, MD)	40 g
Dextrose	5.0 g
Thallous acetate (or thallous sulphate)	0.125 g
Distilled water	1000 mL

Boil to dissolve and autoclave at 121°C for 15 minutes. Cool to 50°C. Add 100,000 units penicillin and 200 mL horse serum; mix and pour thick plates. Inoculate and incubate separate plates at 37°C, for up to 5 or 6 days, under aerobic and anaerobic conditions simultaneously.

4. **CHOCOLATE AGAR** A complex nonselective medium used for the growth of fastidious microorganisms such as *Neisseria gonorrhoeae*.

GC agar base (BBL, Cockeysville, MD)	7.2 g
Distilled water	100 mL

Mix and boil for 2 minutes. Autoclave at 121°C for 15 minutes. Cool to 50°C.

Hemoglobin	2.0 g
Distilled water	100 mL

Mix the hemoglobin with 2–3 mL of the distilled water to form a smooth paste. Continue mixing and gradually add all the water. Autoclave at 121°C for 15 minutes and cool to 50°C. Aseptically combine both solutions. Add 2 mL IsoVitaleX (BBL, Cockeysville, MD). Mix and pour 20–25 mL per petri dish.

5. **DULANEY SLANTS** A medium used for the growth of *Calymmatobacterium granulomatis*.

Yolks are aseptically removed from 5–8-day hen egg embryos and placed in an equal volume of sterile Locke solution containing glass beads. After vigorous mixing, the resulting homogenate is dispensed into slanted tubes and coagulated by incubating in steam at 80°C for 15 minutes.

6. **GC II AGAR BASE*** (BBL, Cockeysville, MD)[†] Basal medium used for the preparation of selective media for *N. gonorrhoeae* and *Haemophilus ducreyi*.

Pancreatic digest of casein	7.5 g
Selected meat peptone	7.5 g
Corn starch	1.0 g
Dipotassium phosphate (K_2HPO_4)	4.0 g
Monopotassium phosphate (KH_2PO_4)	1.0 g
Sodium chloride	5.0 g
Agar	10.0 g
Distilled water	1000 mL

The final pH should be 7.3 ± 0.2.

*GC medium base is supplemented with 1% (v/v) IsoVitaleX enrichment.
[†]Similar media are also manufactured by Oxoid (Columbia, MD) and Difco (Detroit, MI) Laboratories; they differ mainly in their nitrogen sources.

7. **GC-LECT** (BBL, Cockeysville, MD) A selective medium for *N. gonorrhoeae*.

This medium is prepared from a chocolate agar base supplemented with five antimicrobial agents.

8. **ISOVITALEX** (BBL, Cockeysville, MD) A supplement for media used for the isolation of *N. gonorrhoeae* and *H. ducreyi*.

Approximate formula per liter distilled water:

Vitamin B12	0.01 g
L-Glutamine	10.0 g
Adenine	1.0 g
Guanine HCl	0.03 g
p-Aminobenzoic acid	0.013 g
Diphosphopyridine nucleotide, oxidized (coenzyme 1)	0.25 g
Cocarboxylase	0.1 g
Ferric nitrate	0.02 g
Thiamine HCl	0.003 g
L-Cysteine HCl	25.9 g
L-Cystine	1.1 g
Dextrose	100.0 g

Each vial of IsoVitaleX enrichment is supplied with a vial of sterile rehydrating fluid diluent containing approximately 10% dextrose.

The composition of this enrichment is similar to that of Vitox (Oxoid, Columbia, MD) or CVA (Gibco Laboratories, Grand Island, NY).

9. **JEMBEC** This medium is used for the transport and selective growth of N. *gonorrhoeae*. The Jembec plate allows the investigator to add the CO_2 required for the growth of N. *gonorrhoeae*, after the specimen has been inoculated, by placing a CO_2-generating tablet in a well provided in the plate.

   Jembec plates are manufactured by Flow Laboratories, Inc. (McLean, VA). Plates containing either modified Thayer-Martin or Martin-Lewis medium are available; they should be used according to the manufacturers' directions.

10. **MARTIN-LEWIS MEDIUM** A selective medium for N. *gonorrhoeae* identical to modified Thayer-Martin medium except for substituting anisomycin (10 μg/mL) for nystatin.

11. **MODIFIED DIAMOND'S MEDIUM** This is a culture medium for *Trichomonas vaginalis*.

Trypticase (BBL, Cockeysville, MD)	20.0 g
Yeast extract	1.0 g
Maltose	0.5 g
L-Cystine HCl	0.5 g
L-Ascorbic acid	0.02 g
Distilled water Q.S. to	90.0 mL

    Adjust pH to 6.5 and autoclave at 121°C for 15 minutes, cool to 48°C, and add the following antibiotics: sodium penicillin G (1000 U/mL), streptomycin sulfate (1.5 mg/mL), amphotericin B (2 μg/mL). Also add 10 mL horse serum that has been heat inactivated at 56°C for 30 minutes. Dispense into 5-mL aliquots in sterile tubes and store at 4°C for up to 14 days. Warm to 35°C before inoculation. This medium, without horse serum, may be stored at −20°C.

12. **MODIFIED NYC MEDIUM** (prepared plates may be obtained from Scott Laboratories, Inc., Fiskeville, RI)

    A selective medium for N. *gonorrhoeae*.

GC agar base	36 g
Bio-enrichment	10 mL
3% lysed horse red blood cells	200 mL
Horse plasma	120 mL
Dextrose	5.0 g
Colistin	5.0 mg
Vancomycin	2.0 mg
Amphotericin B	1.2 mg
Trimethoprim lactate	3.0 mg
Distilled water	1000 mL

13. **MYCOPLASMA BROTH** This is a transport medium for *Mycoplasma* spp.

    Mix 70 mL Mycoplasma broth base with 30 mL yeast extract (1 part) and horse serum (2 parts) and add the following:

0.4% Phenol red	0.5 g
Penicillin (100,000 U/mL)	0.5 mL
Polymyxin (5000 μg/mL)	1.0 mL
Amphotericin (5000 μg/mL)	0.1 mL

    Adjust pH to 6.0 with 1N HCl and dispense into 1-mL aliquots.

14. **MYCOPLASMA BROTH BASE** A component of media used for transport and culture of *Mycoplasma* spp.

Beef heart infusion	50.0 g
Peptone	10.0 g
NaCl	5.0 g
Distilled water	1000 mL

    Autoclave at 121°C for 15 minutes and store at 4°C.

15. **NICKERSON MEDIUM** (Bacto BiGGY Agar, Difco Laboratories, Detroit, MI)

    A selective medium recommended for the detection, isolation, and differentiation of *Candida* spp.

Bacto yeast extract	1.0 g
Glycine	10.0 g
Bacto dextrose	10.0 g
Bismuth sulfite indicator	8.0 g
Bacto agar	20.0 g
Distilled water	1000.0 mL

    Final pH should be 6.8.

    Suspend 49 g Bacto BiGGY agar in 1 L distilled water. Heat to boiling to dissolve completely. Do not boil for longer than a few minutes as overheating will destroy the selective properties of the medium (do not autoclave). The medium contains a flocculent precipitate that should be evenly dispersed by swirling medium in flasks prior to dispensing in tubes or plates. Prepared medium should be stored at 4°C.

16. **SABOURAUD DEXTROSE AGAR** This is a culture medium for *Candida albicans* and other fungi.

Glucose	40.0 g
Neopeptone or polypeptone (BBL, Cockeysville, MD)	10.0 g
Agar	15–20.0 g
Demineralized water	1000.0 mL

    Final pH should be 5.6. Heat the mixture to dissolve completely. Dispense into tubes (18–25 mm in diameter) and autoclave at 121°C for 15 minutes.

17. **SP-4 MEDIUM** Growth medium for M. *hominis* and M. *genitalium*.

    Liquid medium:

Mycoplasma broth base	1.0 g
Bacto-peptone (Difco Laboratories, Detroit, MI)	1.6 g
Bacto-tryptone (Difco)	3.0 g
Distilled water	197 mL

Dissolve ingredients and adjust pH to 7.8 (0.6 mL 2N NaOH). Autoclave at 121°C for 30 minutes and cool to room temperature. Add the following sterile components:

Phenol red (0.5% solution)	1.2 mL
Penicillin G potassium (100,000 U/mL)	3.0 mL
Yeastolate (Difco) (2%)	30.0 mL
CMRL-1066 (10×) (with glutamine, without NaHCO₃) (Gibco Laboratories, Grand Island, NY)	15.0 mL
Fresh yeast extract (25%) (Flow Laboratories, McLean, VA)	10.5 mL
Fetal bovine serum (heat-treated, 56°C for 1 hour)	50.0 mL
Glucose (50% solution)	3.0 mL

Final pH should be 7.4.

Solid medium:
Add 2.4 to 6.8 g Difco Noble agar (depending on spiroplasma) to autoclavable fraction, before autoclaving and after adjusting pH. After autoclaving, cool to 56°C and allow nonautoclavable fraction to warm to 56°C. Combine both fractions aseptically before pouring plates.

18. **2SP MEDIUM** This is a transport medium for *Chlamydia trachomatis* or *Mycoplasma* spp. consisting of 0.2 M sucrose in 0.02 M phosphate buffer, pH 7.2, and the following antibiotics: gentamycin (2 μg/mL), amphotericin (0.5 μg/mL), vancomycin (10 μg/mL).

19. **SHEPARD'S 10 B BROTH** Growth medium for M. *hominis* and U. *urealyticum*.

PPLO broth (without crystal violet) (Difco Laboratories, Detroit, MI)	1.47 g
Distilled water	73 mL

Dissolve powder and adjust pH to 5.5 with 2N HCl. Autoclave at 121°C for 15 minutes. The following supplements may be combined, filter sterilized, and added to the basal broth after cooling to room temperature:

Unheated normal horse serum	20 mL
Yeast extract (25%)	10 mL
L-Cysteine HCl stock solution (2%)	0.5 mL
Urea stock solution (10%)	0.4 mL
CVA supplement	0.5 mL
Sodium phenol red solution (1%)	0.1 mL
Penicillin G potassium (100,000 U/mL)	1.0 mL

The final pH of the complete 10 B broth should be approximately 6.0. The medium is aseptically dispensed in convenient small volumes and stored at −20°C.

20. **THAYER-MARTIN AGAR** A selective medium for the isolation of N. *gonorrhoeae*.

To the complete chocolate agar (see No. 4), add 1 mL of VCN inhibitor containing (per mL):

Vancomycin	300 μg
Colistin	750 μg
Nystatin	1250 U

The modified Thayer-Martin agar also contains trimethoprim lactate at a final concentration of 5 μg/mL.

21. **TRANSGROW** This transport and selective growth medium for N. *gonorrhoeae* is similar to chocolate agar except for the addition of 2.0 g agar and 0.3 g glucose per 100 mL double-strength GC agar base before autoclaving. VCN inhibitor (1 mL) is added to cooled complete medium, as described for the Thayer-Martin agar. Dispense into sterile bottles, gas with 20% CO_2 in air, and tighten caps securely.

22. **TRANSPORT MEDIUM FOR HERPES SIMPLEX VIRUS** (Gibco Laboratories, Grand Island, NY)

Hanks balanced salt solution with 2% fetal calf serum (containing antibiotics to prevent bacterial overgrowth).

23. **TRYPTICASE SOY BROTH + 0.5% BOVINE SERUM ALBUMIN (BSA)** This is a transport medium for *Mycoplasma* spp.

Trypticase soy broth (BBL, Cockeysville, MD)	3 g
BSA	0.5 g
Distilled water	100 mL

Dissolve by mixing thoroughly and warming gently until solution is complete. Dispense and autoclave at 121°C for 15 minutes.

24. **TRYPTICASE SOY BROTH + 15% GLYCEROL** This is a freezing solution for the storage of neisseriae at −70°C.

Trypticase soy broth (BBL, Cockeysville, MD)	30 g

Dissolve in 500 mL distilled water by mixing thoroughly and warming gently until solution is complete.

Glycerol	150 mL
Distilled water Q.S. to	1000 mL

Dispense and autoclave at 121°C for 15 minutes.

25. **YEAST EXTRACT, 25%** |Difco Laboratories (Detroit, MI), Oxoid (Columbia, MD)| This is a component of medium used for the growth of *Mycoplasma* spp.

Sprinkle 250 g active baker's yeast onto the surface of 1 L distilled water in a 2-L beaker. Heat the mixture to boiling, then clarify it by centrifuging at 1000 × g for 1 hour. Adjust the pH to 8.0 with 1N NaOH and filter sterilize.

Reagents and Test Procedures

(It should be noted that inclusion or exclusion of manufacturers of reagents does not constitute endorsement or disapproval of any manufacturer or product.)

1. **ACETIC ACID** (3%) (Acetowhitening)

Glacial acetic acid	3.0 mL
Distilled water Q.S. to	100 mL

2. **ALKALINE PHOSPHATASE TEST**

p-Nitrophenyl phosphate disodium Tetrahydrate	100.0 mg
Distilled water	25.0 mL

    Dissolve the substrate and add 25 mL of a solution containing 0.1 M glycine and 0.001 M $MgCl_2$, pH 10.5.

    Filter sterilize, dispense into 0.3-mL aliquots, and store at $-20°C$. To detect alkaline phosphatase production, inoculate the substrate-containing solution with test organism and incubate at 35°C for 6 hours. Development of a yellow color is indicative of a positive test.

3. **CATALASE TEST** Add a drop of 3% H_2O_2 to a loopful of growth placed on a glass slide. A positive test is recorded when a brisk bubbling occurs upon addition of H_2O_2.

Hydrogen peroxide	3.0%

4. **CHROMOGENIC CEPHALOSPORIN** This reagent is used to detect β-lactamase.

    Cefinase is available from BBL, Cockeysville, MD.

5. **CONFIRMATORY TESTS FOR N. *gonorrhoeae***

    A. *Coagglutination Tests.* Several kits are commercially available and utilize monoclonal antibodies to epitopes on the major outer membrane protein of N. *gonorrhoeae*: Phadebact Monoclonal GC Test and Phadebact Monoclonal GC Omni Test (Pharmacia, Inc., Piscataway, NJ); Meritec-GC (Meridian Diagnostics, Inc., Cincinatti, OH); GonoGen I and GonoGen II (New Horizons Diagnostics Corp., Columbia, MD). These kits should be used for the confirmatory identification of N. *gonorrhoeae*, according to the manufacturers' directions.
    B. *Combined Tests.* These tests are based on the enzymatic hydrolysis of chromogenic substrates, the production of acid from specific sugars, and other biochemical tests. Examples of these tests and their manufacturers are: Rapid N/H System (Innovative Diagnostic Systems, Inc., Decatur, GA); Vitek *Neisseria-Haemophilus* Identification (NHI) card (Vitek Systems, Inc., Hazelwood, MO); HNID panel (American Micro Scan, Sacramento, CA).
    C. *Enzyme Substrate Tests.* These tests are based on the enzymatic hydrolysis of chromogenic substrates by N. *gonorrhoeae*. Examples of these tests and their manufacturers are: Gonochek II (E.I. du Pont de Nemours & Co., Inc., Wilmington, DE); Identicult-Neisseria (Scott Laboratories, Inc., Fiskeville, RI).
    D. *DNA Hybridization Tests.* These tests are based on the detection of gonococcal DNA using specific oligonucleotides. Examples of these tests and their manufacturers are: Orthoprobe culture confirmation test for N. *gonorrhoeae* (Ortho Diagnostic Systems, Raritan, NJ); The Gen-Probe PACE system for detection and identification of N. *gonorrhoeae* (Gen-Probe, San Diego, CA).

    E. *Rapid Carbohydrate Tests.* These tests are based on the production of acid from specific sugars.
        Examples of these tests and their manufacturers are: Minitek (BBL, Cockeysville, MD); Quadferm + (Analytab Products, Inc., Plainview, NY) (also includes β-lactamase and DNase tests); RIM-N (American Micro Scan, Campbell, CA); Neisseria-Stat (Richardson Scientific, Dallas, TX), Neisseria-Kwik (Micro Bio Logics, St. Cloud, MN).

6. **KOH (10%)**

KOH	10.0 g
Distilled water Q.S. to	100 mL

7. **KOVACS' REAGENT**

p-Dimethylaminobenzaldehyde	5.0 g
Amyl alcohol	75.0 mL

    Dissolve p-dimethylaminobenzaldehyde by warming the solution in a 56°C water bath. Slowly add 25.0 mL concentrated HCl. Dispense into a brown bottle and store at 4°C. The reagent should be a light color.

8. **LOCKE SALT SOLUTION**

Sodium chloride	0.900 g
Calcium chloride	0.024 g
Potassium chloride	0.042 g
Sodium carbonate	0.020 g
Glucose	0.250 g
Distilled water	100 mL

9. **NITRATE REDUCTASE TEST**

Heart infusion broth (Difco)	25 g
Potassium nitrate C.P.	2.0 g
Distilled water	1000 mL

    Adjust pH to 7.0. Dispense into 4.0-mL aliquots in 15 by 125-mm tubes containing inverted Durham fermentation tubes, autoclave at 121°C for 15 minutes, and store at 4°C. Inoculate the broth with the test organism, and incubate at 35°C for 48 hours. Add 5 drops of each of the reagents 1 and 2 (given below) consecutively and examine for the presence of a pink to red color. If negative, add a small amount of zinc dust and incubate at room temperature for 5 minutes to detect nitrate that has not been reduced.

    A red color at this point indicates that the nitrate has not been reduced (a negative test for nitrate reduction); if the broth remains colorless, the nitrate has been completely reduced (a positive test for nitrate reduction).

Reagent 1:	
Sulfanilic acid	2.8 g
Glacial acetic acid	100 mL
Distilled water	250 mL

Reagent 2:	
Dimethyl-α-naphthylamine	2.1 mL
Glacial acetic acid	100 mL
Distilled water	250 mL

10. OXIDASE TEST

Tetra-methyl-*p*-phenylenediamine	
Dihydrochloride	1.0 g
Distilled water	100 mL

Saturate a filter paper contained in a petri dish with the reagent. Pick a portion of the colony to be tested using a platinum wire and rub it on the filter paper. A positive reaction is indicated by a deep purple color appearing in 10 seconds.

11. PHOSPHATE BUFFER, M/15, pH 6.4

KH_2PO_4	6.63 g
Na_2HPO_4	2.56 g
Distilled water Q.S. to	1000 mL

12. PORPHYRIN TEST

Delta-aminolevulinic acid	
hydrochloride (2 mM)	0.034 g
$MgSO_4 \cdot 7H_2O$ (0.8 mM)	0.02 g
Phosphate buffer (0.1 M), pH 6.9	100 mL

Dispense filter-sterilized solution into 0.5-mL aliquots and store at −20°C.

Test procedure: Add a very heavy loopful of the test organism to the substrate solution. After incubation at 35°C for 4 hours, examine under a Woods lamp for a red fluorescence. The observation of fluorescence indicates a positive reaction. If no fluorescence is observed, incubate reaction mixture overnight and reexamine. If no fluorescence is observed after overnight incubation, add an equal volume of Kovacs' reagent (see No. 7). Shake vigorously and allow the aqueous and alcohol phases to separate. The development of a red color in the lower aqueous phase indicates a positive reaction.

13. PRODUCTION OF POLYSACCHARIDE FROM SUCROSE

Strains of some Neisseria spp. (N. *sicca*, N. *subflava* biovar *perflava*, N. *mucosa*, N. *flavescens*, N. *polysaccharea*) produce a polysaccharide from sucrose that can be detected by the addition of iodine to the colonies. Traditionally the polysaccharide test is performed by the incorporation of 5% (w/v) sucrose into a medium, such as tryptic soy agar, which does not contain starch (which will give a positive test). Strains of Neisseria spp. are inoculated by the streak-plate method or spotted onto the medium and incubated at 35°C for 5 days. It was found, however, that some strains were inhibited by 5% sucrose. The test may be performed on tryptic soy agar containing 1% (w/v) sucrose after incubation for 24 hours. A drop of Lugol's iodine (Gram's iodine diluted 1:4) is added to the growth. If polysaccharide has been produced, the colonies, and often the surrounding medium, will immediately turn a dark blue, brown, or black.

It is important that the recommended incubation time not be exceeded. Many strains that produce polysaccharide metabolize it, and if the incubation is carried out for longer than recommended, the polysaccharide may be completely consumed and thus no longer detectable. It is also possible to detect the polysaccharide in traditional sucrose-containing media in which acid production is detected. The polysaccharide may be detected as a brown-to-black precipitate when one to two drops of Lugol's iodine are added to the sucrose-containing medium. The precipitate will range from a fine brown to a coarse black flocculant precipitate. The reaction will fade if the test is allowed to sit at room temperature, but may be rejuvenated by the addition of a few drops of iodine. The test may be performed with fresh Gram's iodine that has been made according to the original formula; aged Gram's iodine and commercially prepared iodine will give negative results. The polysaccharide production test may not be performed using the rapid tests for the detection of acid production from sucrose.

14. SUPEROXOL TEST

The superoxol test is a variation of the catalase test, which is performed by adding a drop of 3% H_2O_2 to a loopful of growth placed on a glass slide. The superoxol test is performed by adding a drop of 30% H_2O_2 to a colony of the organism on a chocolate agar plate. A positive superoxol test is recorded when a brisk bubbling occurs immediately when the 30% H_2O_2 is added to the colonies. A delay of 3 seconds before a bubbling is observed is interpreted as a negative superoxol reaction. Although all human Neisseria spp. and *Branhamella catarrhalis* are catalase-positive, strains vary in their reactions in the superoxol test. Strains of N. *gonorrhoeae* are superoxol-positive whereas strains of other species vary in their reaction in this test. Strains of N. *meningitidis* serogroup A, N. *lactamica*, and B. *catarrhalis* may give positive superoxol tests. Thus the superoxol test must be used in combination with other tests to accurately identify strains of N. *gonorrhoeae*. It also must be noted that, similar to the catalase test, the superoxol test should not be performed on medium containing unheated blood, which will react with the H_2O_2.

15. TZANCK SMEARS
In the Tzanck test the cells are smeared onto a slide, fixed, and stained with Wright or Giemsa preparations.

Stains

(It should be noted that inclusion or exclusion of manufacturers of reagents does not constitute endorsement or disapproval of any manufacturer or product.)

1. **ACRIDINE ORANGE STAIN** This stain is used for the detection of bacteria in clinical specimens. At pH 4.0, bacteria stain red-orange while eucaryotic cells stain green-yellow. The specimen is spread onto a clean glass slide, air-dried, and fixed by immersion in absolute methanol for 2 minutes. It is then stained for 2 minutes by flooding the slide with a solution of 0.5% acridine orange in 0.15 M acetate buffer, pH 4.0. The slide is rinsed with water, air-dried, and examined at 400–1000× magnification under ultraviolet light.

2. **FLUORESCENT ANTIBODY STAINS FOR C. trachomatis** Fluorescent antibody staining reagents for C. *trachomatis* elementary bodies are commercially available. Reagents utilizing anti-major outer membrane protein (MOMP)

monoclonal antibodies are produced by Syva Co., Palo Alto, CA; Difco Laboratories, Detroit, MI; and Kallestad Diagnostics, Austin, TX. Reagents utilizing anti-lipopolysaccharide (LPS) monoclonal antibodies are produced by Bartels Immunodiagnostic Supplies, Inc., Bellevue, WA; Boots Celltech Diagnostics, Inc., Plainview, NY; and California Integrated Diagnostics, Inc., Berkeley, CA. In general, brighter and more consistent fluorescence is observed with those products utilizing anti-MOMP monoclonal antibodies than with those using anti-LPS antibodies. Staining with the anti-MOMP monoclonal antibodies results in the consistent appearance of elementary bodies as well-defined, rough disks of a uniform size. Anti-LPS staining results in the appearance of elementary bodies of varied shapes and sizes. More cross-reactions have been observed with the reagents utilizing anti-LPS monoclonal antibodies than with those using anti-MOMP antibodies. These products should be used according to the manufacturers' directions.

3. **FLUORESCENT ANTIBODY STAINS FOR N. *gonorrhoeae***
    Commercially available fluorescent antibody staining reagents for the confirmatory identification of N. *gonorrhoeae* include: Syva MicroTrak N. *gonorrhoeae* Culture Confirmation Reagent (Syva Co., Palo Alto, CA), which consists of a fluorescein-labeled antigonococcal monoclonal antibody (This reagent also contains Evan's blue, which decreases background staining.); Bacto FA N. *gonorrhoeae* (Difco Laboratories, Detroit, MI), a fluorescein-labeled rabbit polyvalent antigonococcal antibody reagent.

4. **GIEMSA STAIN FOR CHLAMYDIAE**

    Stock solution:

Giemsa powder	0.5 g
Glycerol	33.0 mL
Methyl alcohol, absolute, acetone-free	33.0 mL

    Dissolve the powder in the glycerol by placing the mixture in a water bath (55°C–60°C) for 90 minutes. When crystals are dissolved, add 33 mL absolute methanol. Store at room temperature.
    Working solution: Prepare fresh by diluting the stock 1:23 in phosphate buffer.

    Phosphate buffer:

    Solution 1:

Na_2HPO_4	9.47 g
Distilled water Q.S. to	1000 mL

    Solution 2:

KH_2PO_4	9.08 g
Distilled water Q.S. to	1000 mL

    Mix 72.0 mL of solution 1 with 28.0 mL of solution 2 and 900 mL distilled water.
    Staining procedure: The smear is air-dried, fixed with absolute methanol for at least 5 minutes, and again dried. It is then covered with the working Giemsa solution for 1 hour. The slide is then rinsed rapidly in 95% ethyl alcohol to remove excess dye, dried, and examined for the presence of the typical intracytoplasmic inclusion bodies. The elementary bodies stain toward purple, whereas the re-

ticulate bodies are slightly more basophilic and tend to stain toward blue. There is some variability in commercially available prepared stock Giemsa solutions; these commercial products should be screened before being accepted for routine use. Modifications of the Giemsa stain are used to stain protozoa (parasites) and *Dermatophilus* spp. and to detect intracellular Donovan bodies in tissues.

5. **GRAM STAIN**

    Crystal violet:
    Solution 1: 10% crystal violet in 95% ethyl alcohol
    Solution 2: 0.8 g ammonium oxalate dissolved in 80 mL distilled water

    Mix solutions 1 and 2 together and filter after overnight storage at room temperature.

    Gram's iodine:
    1 g iodine and 2 g potassium iodine dissolved in 300 mL distilled water

    Decolorizers:
    95% ethyl alcohol (slowest)
    95% ethyl alcohol and acetone (1:1) (intermediate)
    Acetone (fastest)

    Counterstain:
    Stock solution: 2.5% safranin O in 95% ethyl alcohol
    Working solution: 10 mL stock solution in 90 mL distilled water

6. **HEMATOXYLIN AND EOSIN STAIN** Sections are cut at 5 mm.

    A. Two changes of xylol; 2 minutes each
    B. Two changes of absolute alcohol; 1 minute each
    C. One change of 95% alcohol; 1 minute
    D. One change of 90% alcohol; 0.5 minute
    E. One change of 80% alcohol; 0.5 minute
    F. One change of 60% alcohol; 0.5 minute
    G. Two or more changes of distilled water, until slides have cleared
    H. Harris hematoxylin with glacial acetic acid (5 mL acetic acid with 100 mL hematoxylin); 1–2 minutes
    I. Rinse in distilled water
    J. Place in tap water containing 20–40 drops ammonium hydroxide; 3 seconds (section will turn blue immediately)
    K. Rinse in two changes of tap water to remove the ammonia
    L. Counterstain in picro-eosin solution; 30 seconds
    M. Two changes of 95% alcohol; 1 minute each
    N. Two changes of absolute alcohol; 1 and 2 minutes
    O. Two changes of xylol; 1 minute each
    P. Mount in neutral xylol-damar

7. **JONES' IODINE STAIN**

Potassium iodine	5.0 g
Iodine crystals	5.0 g
Absolute methanol	50.0 mL
Distilled water	50.0 mL

Combine reagents and mix until in solution. Store at room temperature in a brown bottle (to protect from direct light). Before use, filter through a #41 ashless Whatman filter paper.

8. **METHYLENE BLUE STAIN**

Methylene blue   0.3 g
Ethanol   30.0 mL

When the dye is dissolved, add 100 mL distilled water.

Staining procedure: Fix smear and flood slide with methylene blue stain for 1 minute. Wash the stain off the slide in tap water, blot dry, and examine.

9. **MODIFIED ACID-FAST STAIN FOR CRYPTOSPORIDIUM OOCYSTS IN STOOL SPECIMENS**

Basic fuchsin crystals   4.0 g
Ethanol   25 mL

After dissolving the crystals, add 12.0 mL liquefied phenol and mix well with a glass stirring rod. The following are then added:

Glycerol   25 mL
DMSO   25 mL
Distilled water 75 mL

The resulting solution is mixed well, allowed to stand for 30 minutes, and then filtered. The stain may be used immediately or kept indefinitely at room temperature in an amber glass bottle. The decolorizer–counterstain solution consists of 220 mL of a 2% aqueous solution of malachite green to which 30 mL glacial acetic acid and 50 mL glycerol are added and mixed well. Filtration is unnecessary. This solution keeps indefinitely in a closed container at room temperature.

Staining procedure: Fecal material is smeared over a 2.5 by 3.0-cm area of a clean, flamed glass slide and air-dried on a warming plate. The slide is prefixed in a Coplin jar of absolute methanol for 5–10 seconds, stained in carbol fuchsin–DMSO solution in a Coplin jar for 5 minutes, and rinsed in gently running tap water until excess solution no longer runs off. The slide is then placed in the de-colorizer–counterstain for 1 minute or until a green background appears; it is then rinsed under running tap water for 10 seconds, drained, blotted, and placed on a warming plate until thoroughly dry. Slides are examined under oil immersion ($\times 10$). This procedure yields oocysts that are brilliant pink to fuchsia against a pale green background. Organisms seen on low-power screening are checked under oil immersion ($\times 100$) for the typical *Cryptosporidium* internal vacuole and material clumped to one side of the 4- to 5-μm cyst.

10. **MODIFIED DIENES' STAIN**

Methylene blue   2.50 g
Azure II   1.25 g
Maltose   10.0 g

Na$_2$CO$_3$ 0.25 g
Distilled water   100 mL

Prepare a 3% dilution of the Dienes' stain stock solution in water and filter it through a 0.22-μ filter.

Staining procedure: Cut out a small square (1 cm^2) of agar containing suspected colonies, and place it on a microscope slide with the colonies facing up. Make a petrolatum–parafin seal around the agar section, slightly higher than the agar block. Place 1 to 4 drops of the Dienes' stain working solution on the agar surface, completely covering the agar block with stain. Place a cover slip over the stained agar block, permitting it to contact the petrolatum seal. The cover slip should be as close as possible to the agar surface without touching it. Examine under oil immersion ($\times 1000$) with a light microscope. Mycoplasma colonies stain blue, whereas most bacterial and fungal colonies appear colorless.

11. **WRIGHT'S STAIN**

Wright's stain (powder form)   3.0 g
Glycerol (C.P.)   30.0 mL
Absolute methanol (acetone-free)   970.0 mL

Place the Wright's stain in a large mortar. Add approximately 5.0 mL glycerol and 30.0 mL methanol and grind to dissolve.

Add the rest of the glycerol and methanol gradually until the dye is completely dissolved. Store in a dark, tightly stoppered bottle, and allow to mature for approximately 2 weeks. Filter before use.

Staining procedure: Cover air-dried smear with 2–3 mL Wright's stain. After staining for 2 minutes, add 2–3 mL phosphate buffer, pH 6.4, to the stain, blowing to mix stain and buffer. Rinse with buffer until all the purple stain is removed. Air dry and examine.

12. **ZIEHL-NEELSEN CARBOL-FUCHSIN STAIN**

Basic fuchsin   0.3 g
Ethanol (95%) 10 mL

Dissolve powder and add solution to 90 mL of a 5% aqueous solution of phenol. Store reagent in stoppered bottles to prevent evaporation. If crystals form during storage, the reagent should be filtered before use.

Staining procedure: Cover heat-fixed smear with absorbent paper. Add enough carbol-fuchsin (4–5 drops) to saturate paper. Gently heat the bottom of the slide until the stain begins to steam. Continue heating for 5 minutes but do not allow the stain to boil or dry. Add more carbol-fuchsin if necessary. Carefully lift paper from slide with forceps. Rinse smear with tap water and flood with acid alcohol (3 mL concentrated HCl to 97 mL of 95% ethanol) for 2 minutes. Rinse smear with tap water and flood slide with aqueous methylene blue (0.3 g methylene blue chloride in 100 mL distilled water) for 1–2 minutes. Rinse in tap water, drain, and dry.

INDEX

Note: Numbers in **bold** refer to figure numbers

A

A8 agar, A3.2
Acanthosis nigricans, 12.7, **12.23**
Acetic acid, A3.5
Acetowhite epithelium
  in carcinoma of penis, 10.7, **10.19**
  in papillomavirus infection, 10.4, 10.6-
    10.7, 10.9, **10.16-10.18, 10.23**
Acholeplasma
  laidlawii, 7.3, **7.5**
  oculi, 7.3, **7.5**
Acid-fast stain for cryptosporidium
  oocysts in stool, A3.8
Acid production tests, 5.12, 5.18, **5.23,**
  5.33, Al.4, A1.5
Acneform rashes, 12.10, **12.33**
Acridine orange stain, A3.6
Acrochordons, 12.15, **12.51**
Acyclovir in herpesvirus infection, 2.17-
  2.18, **2.42-2.43**
Adenopathy
  in AIDS, 8.34, 8.36, 8.37, **8.76-8.77,**
    8.80-8.82
  in chancroid, 3.4, 3.5, **3.12**
  in syphilis, 1.6, **1.17**
Agar
  A8, A3.2
  blood, A3.2
    biphasic, A3.2
  chocolate, A3.2
  GC II base, A3.2
  Sabouraud dextrose, A3.3
  Thayer-Martin, A3.4
AIDS, 8.2-8.40
  adrenal disorders in, 8.38
  cachexia and weight loss in, 8.25
  candidiasis in, oral, 8.24, 8.25, 8.30,
    8.49-8.50
  cardiac disorders in, 8.38
  classification system for, **8.1,** 8.2
  cotton wool spots in, ocular, 8.32,
    8.33, **8.72**
  cryptococcosis in
    bone marrow in, 8.38, **8.86**
    meningitis in, 8.25-8.26, **8.53-8.54**
    pulmonary, 8.16, 8.17, **8.31**
  cryptosporidia in, 8.21-8.22, **8.41-8.43**
  cytomegalovirus infection in
    gastrointestinal, 8.19, **8.37-8.39**
    pulmonary, 8.14, 8.15, 8.16, **8.29-**
      8.30
  dermatologic lesions in, 8.28-8.32,
    8.60-8.70
  diarrhea in, 8.18, **8.34, 8.36**
  diseases associated with, **8.2-8.3,** 8.2-
    8.3
  encephalopathy in, 8.28, **8.59**
  Entamoeba histolytica infection in,
    8.22, 8.23, **8.45-8.46**
  epidemiology of, 8.4-8.7, **8.5-8.9**
  gastrointestinal disorders in, 8.16-8.25,
    8.34-8.50

Giardia lamblia in, 8.22, 8.24, **8.47-**
  8.48
hairy leukoplakia in, oral, 8.30, **8.63**
herpesvirus infections in, 8.24, 8.31-
  8.32, **8.65-8.67**
histoplasmosis in
  blood smear in, 8.36, 8.37, **8.84**
  bone marrow aspirate smear in,
    8.38, **8.85**
  and lymphadenopathy, 8.36, 8.37,
    8.82
  pulmonary, 8.16, 8.17, **8.32**
Hodgkin's lymphoma in, 8.34, 8.35,
  8.78
ichthyosis in, 8.32, **8.69**
immune system in, 8.10-8.11, **8.16-**
  8.17
Isospora belli in, 8.22, 8.23, **8.44**
Kaposi's sarcoma in, 8.28-8.30, **8.61-**
  8.62
  in oral cavity, 8.25, 8.29, **8.61**
  pulmonary, 8.16, 8.17, **8.33**
leukoencephalopathy in, progressive
  multifocal, 8.27-8.28, **8.58**
lymphadenopathy in, 8.34, 8.36, 8.37,
  8.76-8.77, 8.80-8.82
lymphoma of CNS in, 8.27, **8.57**
molluscum contagiosum in, 8.32, **8.68**
Mycobacterium avium-intracellulare in
  and gastrointestinal symptoms, 8.20-
    8.21, **8.40**
  and lymphadenopathy, 8.36, **8.81**
myelodysplasia in, 8.36, 8.37, **8.83**
neurologic problems in, 8.25-8.28,
  8.51-8.59
ocular findings in, 8.32-8.33 **8.71-8.75**
opportunistic infections in, 8.39, **8.87**
Pityrosporum in, 8.32, **8.70**
Pneumocystis carinii pneumonia in,
  8.12-8.14, 8.15, **8.19-8.25**
in pregnancy, 8.6
proctitis in, 8.18, **8.35**
pulmonary disease in, 8.11-8.17, **8.18-**
  8.33
Reiter's syndrome in, 8.32, 8.33, **8.75**
renal lesions in, 8.38
scabies in, 11.9, **11.22**
seborrheic dermatitis in, 8.30, 8.31,
  8.64
serologic testing in, 8.8, **8.10-8.12,**
  A2.5, A2.7
syphilis with, 8.28
and toxoplasmosis of CNS, 8.26-8.27,
  8.55-8.56
transmission of, 8.6-8.7
  nonsexual, **A1.7,** A1.8
treatment of, 8.38-8.40, **8.88-8.90**
  in opportunistic infections, 8.39,
    8.87
tuberculosis in, 8.14, 8.15, **8.27-8.28**
tumors in, 8.35, **8.79**
virus in, 8.9-8.10, **8.13-8.15**
  laboratory tests for, 8.8, **8.10-8.12,**
    A2.5, A2.7
AIDS-related complex, 8.3, **8.4**

Alkaline phosphatase test, 3.11, **3.31,**
  A3.5
Alopecia in syphilis, 1.9, **1.30**
Amniotic fluid, mycoplasmas in, 7.7-7.8,
  7.15
Anaerobic chamber, 9.4, **9.7**
Anal infections, *see* Perianal or rectal
  infections
Arthritis
  diseases with, 5.8, **5.16**
  in immunocompromised hosts,
    mycoplasmas in, 7.10
  postpartum, in mycoplasmal infection,
    7.8
  in Reiter's syndrome, 6.14, 6.15, **6.36,**
    12.13
Atrophic conditions, 12.9, **12.30-12.32**
Azidothymidine in AIDS, 8.40

B

Bacteroides in vaginosis, 9.3
Balinitis
  in candidiasis, 9.14, **9.37,** 12.11, **12.36**
  circinate, in Reiter's syndrome, 6.15,
    6.37, 12.13, **12.44**
  xerotica obliterans, 12.9, **12.31**
Bartholin's gland in gonorrhea, 5.6, **5.10**
Behcet's disease, 12.18-12.19, **12.63**
Bejel, 1.2, **1.2**
Biopsy
  in granuloma inguinale, 4.8-4.9, **4.15-**
    4.16
  lymph node, in lymphogranuloma
    venereum, 6.16, 6.17, **6.41**
  punch, in scabies, 11.12-11.13
  shave
    needle technique in, 12.16, **12.54**
    in scabies, 11.10-11.12, **11.25-11.26**
Bites, human, 12.18, **12.62**
Blood agar, A3.2
  biphasic, A3.2
Boils, 12.10, 12.12, **12.33**
Bone marrow dysplasia in AIDS, 8.36,
  8.37, **8.83**
Bowen's disease of vulva, 10.10, **10.27**
Bowenoid papulosis, 10.8, **10.20-10.21**
  histopathology of, 10.12, 10.13,
    10.33-10.34
Branhamella catarrhalis
  acid production test for, **A1.4,** A1.5
  characteristics compared to related
    species, 5.12, 5.17-5.19, **5.23, 5.32,**
    5.34-5.35
  enzyme substrate test for, **A1.5,** A1.6
Buboes in chancroid, 3.4, 3.5, **3.13**
Burrow of scabies mite, 11.3, **11.4,** 11.6,
  11.11
  ink test of, 11.12, 11.13, **11.27-11.28**

C

Cachexia and weight loss in AIDS, 8.25
Calculi, urinary, *Ureaplasma urealyticum*
  in, 7.6, **7.10-7.11**
Calymmatobacterium granulomatis, 4.2;
  see also Granuloma inguinale